Virus Disease of the Eye

Contributors

W. A. BLYTH, PhD.
MRC Research Fellow, Department of Microbiology,
University of Bristol

P. G. HIGGINS
Consultant Virologist,
MRC Common Cold Unit,
Salisbury, Wilts.

SHIRLEY RICHMOND, MD
Department of Bacteriology and Virology,
Manchester University;
Honorary Consultant Virologist,
Central and North Manchester

A. B. TULLO, MD, FRCS
Senior Registrar in Ophthalmology,
Manchester Royal Eye Hospital

Virus Disease of the Eye

D. L. EASTY, MD, FRCS

Professor of Ophthalmology
University of Bristol

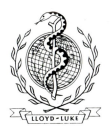

LLOYD-LUKE (Medical Books) LTD.

49 NEWMAN STREET · LONDON

1985

TYPESET, PRINTED AND BOUND IN GREAT BRITAIN BY
HAZELL WATSON AND VINEY LTD
MEMBER OF THE BPCC GROUP
AYLESBURY, BUCKS

ISBN 0 85324 157 0

Foreword

This is the third of our monographs on major problems in ophthalmology, in which we seek to cover recent advances within those areas of medicine where ophthalmology marches with a neighbouring speciality. For these are the fields where an understanding may be hard to gain either from any standard textbook or from the disparate reports in our journals.

Our output has perhaps been rather leisurely, but the rewards of instant journalism are fleeting, and after its long gestation period the elephant is renowned for its wisdom.

Professor Easty leads us reassuringly through the complexities of viral eye disease, a world of increasing importance as the bacteria, our time-honoured enemies, capitulate before successive antibiotics, and relinquish their territory to the new invaders. Many will have cause to be grateful for so succinct, so readable and so comprehensive a guide.

London, 1985   PATRICK TREVOR-ROPER

Preface

This book concerns the clinical disease which results from viruses which infect the eye, with descriptions of the microbiology and immunology. Virological eye disease causes unique symptoms and signs because of the nature of the eye as a sensory organ and its exposure to the environment. It is because of the transparency of the cornea and the ocular contents that otherwise innocuous inflammatory reactions have such deleterious effects on vision. The ophthalmologist is fortunate to be able to view ocular inflammation, be it external or internal, with ease, using sophisticated equipment for examination. In this respect perhaps he has the advantage over colleagues in other fields of medicine. However, the increased understanding of the mechanisms of inflammatory disease which should result from this have not yet emerged, which is due to a lack of close communication with workers in immunology or virology, who so often provide illumination for us in our understanding of infectious eye disease.

It is therefore the fundamentals of virology which elude ophthalmologists and, in contrast, it is the nuances of clinical disease which need clarification for microbiologists. It is the intention of this collaborative venture to present material in a way that will help microbiologists and ophthalmologists alike towards an understanding of two interrelated fields.

The first three chapters concern fundamental aspects of virology and immunology, and the inflammatory responses of the eye. In subsequent chapters, the literature is surveyed in so far as it relates to ocular disease. No apology is made for the space allocated to the Herpesviruses, which occupy so much time in the emergency room or out-patient clinics. It is to be hoped that this book will prove useful to those entering the field of ocular virus disease as clinicians, microbiologists or researchers, and that the fundamental approach will help in the prevention, diagnosis, therapy or cure of this serious group of diseases.

Bristol   D. L. Easty
January, 1985

Contents

CHAPTER ONE

Principles of Virology

S. RICHMOND

INTRODUCTION

VIRUSES differ fundamentally from all other infectious agents. Micro-organisms such as bacteria, fungi and protozoa consist of living cells which possess sufficient biochemical machinery to generate energy and to synthesise their own structural and functional macromolecules. Genetic information is stored, transmitted and modified in the form of double-stranded DNA, and reproduction occurs without the fundamental integrity of the basic cellular unit ever being lost. Viruses, on the other hand, are acellular infectious particles which are incapable of metabolic activity outside living cells. Genetic information is stored either in the form of DNA or RNA, and can only be expressed within a living cell, at the expense of that cell's own energy and metabolic machinery. A virus infection is therefore initiated when a virus particle penetrates a susceptible cell; the subsequent intracellular synthesis of viral gene products is often associated with death or damage of infected cells, which may be manifested by disease in the host.

Viruses infect virtually all living organisms. Several hundred different viruses are known which infect man, and many of these are capable of producing disease in the eye, either as part of a generalised viral illness, or as a virus infection restricted to the eye.

PROPERTIES OF VIRUSES

Size.—Size has long been used as an important criterion distinguishing viruses from other infectious agents, since viruses will pass through filters which hold back all but the smallest bacterial micro-organisms. The pox viruses, which are amongst the largest viruses known, are about 250 nm long, about the same size as mycoplasmas and the infectious forms of chlamydiae. At the other end of the scale, the parvoviruses, about 20 nm in diameter, are about the same size as large protein molecules such as haemocyanin.

Morphology.—The mature virus particle is known as the virion. In the simplest viruses this consists solely of a molecule of nucleic acid surrounded by a protein coat, the capsid, the nucleic acid and capsid together comprising the nucleocapsid. The capsid consists of morphological units, known as capsomeres, which are built up of frequently repeated polypeptide chains. The capsid protects the viral nucleic acid and confers symmetry on the virion. Two forms of symmetrical virus particles can be recognised; those with cubical symmetry in which the capsomeres surround the nucleic acid forming a regular icosahedron (for example, adenovirus and papovaviruses), and those with helical symmetry, in which the capsomeres and nucleic acid are wound together into a spiral (for example, influenza viruses and measles). All viral nucleo-capsids with helical symmetry and some viruses with icosahedral symmetry are surrounded by an envelope. This is a complex lipoprotein structure, generally derived from the cytoplasmic membrane of the host cell as the nucleocapsid is released from the cell. Virus-coded glycoprotein subunits known as peplomers are incorporated into the envelope and project from its outer surface. Both peplomers and capsid proteins are antigenic and induce specific antibody responses in the infected host.

Unlike all cellular organisms, viruses contain only one species of nucleic acid, DNA or RNA, either of which may be single- or double-stranded. RNA viruses are unique in that the genetic information is stored in the form of RNA rather than as DNA. The molecular weight of viral nucleic acid varies from 1·6 to 160 million daltons, representing from 3 to about 160 actual genes.

The ability of a virus to reproduce resides solely in its nucleic acid. When viruses are purified and analysed it can be shown that they contain 50–90 per cent protein. Since nucleic acids when in solution are susceptible to shearing and degradation it can be assumed that the protein component has a protective role. There are a limited number of ways in which the protein is arranged around the nucleic acid in order to protect it. Viruses are basically constructed from a number of subunits. Thus nucleic acid is not enveloped by a single large protein molecule but by a large number of smaller protein molecules. These subunits are not necessarily identical. Their presence endows the virus with a greater degree of genetic stability, since reduction of the size of the structural units lessens the chance of disadvantageous mutation occurring in the gene which specifies it. The subunits themselves are not symmetrical and for the maximum number of bonds to be formed they must be arranged symmetrically, and there are in fact a limited number of ways in which this can be done. One form is filamentous, as in tobacco mosaic virus. Spherical viruses occur as tetrahedrons, cubes, octahedrons, dodecahedrons (constructed from 12 regular pentagons), or icosahedrons constructed from 20 equilateral triangles. The number of subunits per face, and the number of faces, give the minimum number of subunits which can be arranged around such an object. Though electron micrographs suggest that many viruses are spherical in outline they actually have icosahedral symmetry.

A large number of animal viruses have a lipid envelope as an integral part of their structure including the herpes viruses, togaviruses, rhabdoviruses and mycoviruses. The herpes viruses replicate in the cell nucleus although the viral proteins are synthesised in the cytoplasm and transported back into the nucleus. After assembly of the nucleocapsid the virus buds off from the nuclear membrane and becomes enveloped. Prior to budding the membrane is modified by incorporation of viral specified proteins which are subsequently glycosylated. Other similar viruses acquire their envelope by budding from the cytoplasmic membrane in contrast to the herpes virus. The four events leading to maturation have now been identified: they are the formation of the nucleocapsids in the cytoplasm, the incorporation of viral glycoproteins in patches of the cellular membrane, the alignment of nucleocapsids along the inner surface of this modified membrane, and the final budding from the cell. During budding no host membranes are incorporated into the viral particles, although the bulk of the lipid in the envelope is derived from that of the host.

Many larger animal viruses are enveloped by a 65Å membrane layer. The envelope is largely derived from the host cell membrane and can be interrupted by treatment with ether or detergents which also destroys the infectivity of the virus. Examples of enveloped viruses include the influenza virus and the rhabdoviruses. The influenza and rhabdoviruses have helical nucleocapsid but other enveloped bacterial and animal viruses have an icosahedral nucleocapsid. RNA tumour viruses have even more complex arrangements where the nucleoprotein is supercoiled in the shape of a hollow sphere surrounded by an icosahedral shell which in turn is surrounded by the envelope. The envelope is derived from the cell membrane, which is modified by the insertion of virus-specific glycoprotein.

The nucleic acid of a virus contains within itself both the specific information and the operational potential such that upon entering a susceptible cell, it can subvert the biosynthetic machinery of that cell and redirect it towards the specific production of viral particles. Nucleic acids contain the nucleosides adenosine, guanosine, cytidine and either uridine or thymidine. In double-stranded molecules, base pairing occurs between guanosine and cytidine and adenosine and either uridine or thymidine. Alkali treatment or heating denatures the double-stranded arrangement which can then be separated. It is possible to separate the five possible classes of nucleic acid (double- and single-stranded DNA, double- and single-stranded RNA, and DNA-RNA hybrids) using heavy metal salts such as CsCl to generate gradients with high-speed centrifugation. Analyses such as this can also employ sucrose density gradients, or electrophoresis of nucleic acids.

There are therefore four possible kinds of nucleic acid; i.e. single- and double-stranded RNA and DNA. All these types of nucleic acid are commonly found in animal viruses. It is possible to extract the nucleic acid and determine its base composition, nuclease sensitivity, and buoyant density, etc.

Infection begins with the coming together of virus and a susceptible host cell, which is brought about by different mechanisms in plant viruses, animal viruses and bacteriophages. Animal viruses probably form a union with cells by diffusion in tissue culture. However this may not necessarily be true in the intact animal. In cultured animal cells it has been possible to measure attachments to the cell wall and to determine the effects of temperature and the ionic environment. Attachment appears to be electrostatic and is affected by the ionic environment. There is little information about specific cellular receptors for viruses except for polio and influenza viruses, where susceptible cells are known to release a virus-binding receptor substance. Non-susceptible cells lack this virus receptor so that the polio or influenza viruses cannot become attached.

Following adsorption the virus penetrates the cell wall. Living cells do not have a rigid wall, but are bounded by a plasma membrane which is mobile and active. Cells are constantly taking samples of their immediate environment by pinocytosis, or carrying out the reverse process by exporting from the cell substances such as enzymes, hormones, or neurotransmitters. Viruses therefore infect a cell, if it has an appropriate receptor molecule on its outer surface, and different receptors are probably recognised by different viruses. It is not clear how viruses enter animal cells after this attachment. It is evident that enveloped viruses can penetrate into cells by fusing with the plasma membrane, while both enveloped and non-enveloped viruses can penetrate by pinocytosis. Fusion results in the release of viral genome into the cytoplasm. After a process of pinocytosis, the virus remains contained in a vesicle of plasma membrane. Penetration followed by uncoating is not necessarily associated with the production of naked nucleic acid lying free in an infected cell. Viral internal protein may persist in association with nucleic acid which could include those enzymes necessary for further nucleic acid synthesis; the genome itself also serves as a message which associates with the ribosomes within the cell.

In the process of infection the basic mechanism whereby a DNA molecule is duplicated *in vivo* is the same regardless of whether the DNA is of cellular or viral origin. Because of the ease with which viral DNA molecules can be studied *in vitro* they have occasionally been used as the substrate preferred by biochemists in unravelling the mechanisms of DNA replication. The first DNA polymerase was isolated two decades ago, but relatively little is known about DNA replication. Theoretically a polymerase would traverse the molecule and make two daughter strands using the parental strands as templates. Theoretically also, there are several ways by which a single-stranded DNA molecule can replicate, and similarly single-stranded RNA. Whatever the mechanisms of replication are, when a virus infects a cell, not all the genes are expressed at the same time. Thus, early and late protein formation occurs, which indicates that not all protein is synthesised at the same time, nor are many proteins synthesised continuously. The regulation of gene expression by animal viruses can occur at the level of transcription, or translation, or both, and to a degree which varies not only between different viruses but during a cycle of multiplication (Figure 1.1). In an infected cell, the viral specified pure protein and nucleic acid are synthesised separately, and consequently must be brought together and assembled into mature virus particles. This may occur in two ways: either the viruses can themselves assemble in the manner akin to crystalisation whereby the various components spontaneously combine to form virus particles, or alternatively the viral genome may specify certain morpho-genetic factors which are not structurally part of the virus but whose presence is required for normal assembly. It is apparent that both forms of assembly can occur, the former being prevalent among the simpler viruses while the latter has been observed in the complex viruses such as the tailed bacteriophages. The proof that self-assembly occurs requires that purified viral nucleic acid

Figure 1.1. Schematic representation of attachment, penetration and uncoating of a virus on entering the cell. Transcription is the process of transferring the information encoded in the base sequence of one type of nucleic acid molecule to another. The enzymes involved are DNA-dependent RNA polymerase, RNA-dependent RNA polymerase and RNA-dependent DNA polymerase. Translation is the process of making a protein chain from the information in the RNA. (Taken from *Medical Virology* by Fenner and White, by permission of the authors and Academic Press.)

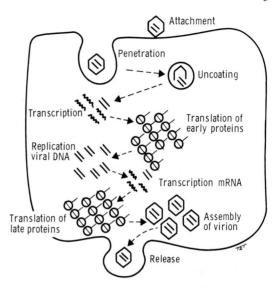

and purified structural proteins in the absence of other proteins are able to combine *in vitro* to yield particles resembling the original virus in shape, size and stability, as well as demonstrating infectivity.

CLASSIFICATION OF VIRUSES

On the basis of the above properties, it is now possible to classify animal viruses into a number of major groups or families, which are summarised in Table 1.1. The properties of the human viruses which cause infection in the eye, and which are dealt with in greater detail in later chapters, are summarised in Table 1.2.

TABLE 1.1

MAJOR GROUPS OF ANIMAL VIRUSES

	DNA viruses	*RNA viruses*
ENVELOPED VIRUSES	Herpetoviridae*	Orthomyxoviridae Paramyxoviridae* Rhabdoviridae* Retroviridae Coronaviridae Togaviridae* Bunyaviridae* Arenaviridae
NO ENVELOPE	Adenoviridae* Parvoviridae Papovaviridae* Poxviridae*	Picornaviridae* Reoviridae

*Some of the viruses belonging to these groups are dealt with subsequently in this book.

TABLE 1.2

MAJOR GROUPS OF HUMAN VIRUSES WHICH CAUSE INFECTION IN THE EYE

Family	Nucleic Acid	Shape of Virion	Symmetry	Diameter in Nanometres	Envelope	Virus Infections of the Eye
Herpetoviridae	DNA	Spherical	Icosahedral	150	YES	Herpes simplex Varicella zoster Cytomegalovirus
Adenoviridae	DNA	Spherical	Icosahedral	70–80	NO	Adenovirus serotypes 3, 4, 7, 14, 12, 21, 10, 15, 8, 19
Poxviridae	DNA	Brick-shaped	—	100×240×300	NO	Vaccinia Variola Molluscum contagiosum
Papovaviridae	DNA	Spherical	Icosahedral	45–55	NO	Wart virus
Picornaviridae	RNA	Spherical	Icosahedral	30	NO	Coxsackie A 24 Enterovirus type 70
Paramyxoviridae	RNA	Spherical	Helical	100–200	YES	Newcastle disease virus Mumps. Measles
Togaviridae	RNA	Spherical	Icosahedral	40–60	YES	Rubella. Dengue
Bunyaviridae	RNA	Spherical	Icosahedral	90–100	YES	Sandfly fever Rift valley fever
Rhabdoviridae	RNA	Bullet-shaped	—	70×180	YES	Rabies

PATHOGENESIS OF VIRUS INFECTIONS

Effect of Virus Infection at the Cellular Level

A number of sequential events occurs when a virus infects and multiplies within a living cell. The virus must first attach to the host cell surface before it can penetrate the cell either by phagocytosis, or by fusion of the viral envelope with the plasma membrane of the cell. Once within the cytoplasm, the outer protein layers of the virus are removed with consequent loss of virion integrity and of viral infectivity. Complex biochemical events within the cell then lead to replication of new viral structural proteins and nucleic acid, with eventual assembly and release of a new generation of infectious virions. These events have serious effects on the host cell which often lead to cell death. Not all viruses however have this cytocidal effect; some virus-infected cells may remain persistently infected, with continuous or intermittent shedding of virus into the extracellular environment, without destruction of the infected host cell. In other instances the viral genome persists with the cell, without production of infectious virus but with profound effects on the growth characteristics of the infected cell, which may lead to subsequent neoplasia.

These effects of virus infection at the cellular level are responsible for many of the symptoms and signs of disease in the infected host. However, although many viruses are capable of producing disease in man, infection with these viruses does not invariably produce symptoms in the host. Many infections are inapparent or subclinical, particularly in children, and different viruses vary considerably in their tendency to produce subclinical infections. Infection with measles, for example, almost always results in overt disease, whereas the majority of enterovirus infections in children are subclinical.

Entry of Virus into the Body

Before a virus infection in man can be initiated, the virus must first gain access to susceptible cells within the body. The respiratory tract, the gastro-intestinal tract and the skin provide the three main entry routes, with the mucous membranes of the eye and genital tract, and parenteral and trans-placental spread providing other important means of access (Table 1.3).

Localised Viral Infection

Viral replication occurs at first in susceptible cells at the site of entry, and many virus infections remain restricted to these areas, causing localised cellular damage. The respiratory infections caused by influenza viruses and rhinoviruses, localised skin lesions such as warts and molluscum contagiosum, and mucosal infections of the conjunctiva or genital tract are all examples of such localised virus infections.

Generalised Viral Infection

In these infections the virus, after multiplying silently at the site of entry to the body and in lymph nodes draining these sites, is then disseminated in the blood stream, lymphatics or by neuronal spread to infect and damage other susceptible cells at a distance from the original site of entry and multiplication.

TABLE 1.3

TRANSMISSION OF VIRUSES

Routes of Entry and Exit of Viruses from the Body	Viruses	Outcome of Infection
Respiratory tract (aerosol spread)	Influenza A and B Para influenza virus Respiratory virus Rhinoviruses	Respiratory tract infections (RTI)
	Adenoviruses types 3, 4, 7	RTI and/or conjunctival (Pharyngoconjunctival)
	Measles Rubella, varicella Smallpox	Systemic infections with exanthemata
Faecal-oral route	Rotaviruses Some adenoviruses	Enteric infections
	Enteroviruses Hepatitis A	Systemic infections frequently asymptomatic in children
Direct contact (a) Skin	Herpes simplex virus Papovavirus Molluscum contagiosum Vaccinia	Localised skin lesions
(b) Oral cavity	Herpes simplex EB virus	Stomatitis Infectious mononucleosis
(c) Eye	Adenovirus type 8, 10, 19 Coxsackie A24 Enterovirus type 70 Vaccinia Herpes simplex virus Newcastle disease virus	Keratoconjunctivitis Epidemic haemorrhagic conjunctivitis Vaccinia of eye Conjunctivitis
(d) Genital tract	Herpes simplex virus type 2 Papovavirus	Genital herpes Genital warts
Inoculation of (a) Saliva (b) Serum	Rabies Hepatitis B Hepatitis B Arboviruses	Systemic infections
(c) Lymphocytes	Cytomegalovirus EB virus	
Vertical transmission (a) Transplacental	Rubella Cytomegalovirus	Congenital infections
(b) Reactivation of endogenous latent infection	Herpes simplex virus Varicella-zoster	Shingles Labial herpes Dendritic ulcer Recurrent genital herpes

The exanthems of chicken pox and smallpox, the destruction of anterior-horn cells in poliomyelitis and the conjunctivitis of measles are all manifestations of such systemic viral infections. Other generalised virus infections occur in the fetus when rubella or cytomegalovirus are spread transplacentally from the infected mother. Some viruses are unable to enter the body by any of the above routes and must gain access to the blood stream in order to reach susceptible cells: arboviruses, transmitted by blood-sucking insects, and hepatitis B virus are examples of such parenterally transmitted viruses.

Virus Infection in the Eye

Eye infection may therefore result from a localised infection, when both virus replication and cellular damage are restricted either to the eye alone, or to the eye and adjacent tissues; in such infections the virus usually gains entry to the eye via the conjunctiva and damage is restricted to the external eye. Alternatively eye infection may be part of a generalised infection in which the eye is only one of several organs in which the virus is replicating. In these infections the deeper structures of the eye may also be involved as in congenital infections with rubella or cytomegalovirus.

In certain instances a virus may gain access to the body through the eye whilst not causing specific eye disease; splashing of blood products which contain hepatitis B virus into the conjunctiva, and accidental transmission of viruses in corneal transplants are rare examples of such infections (Duffy *et al.*, 1974).

Consequences of Virus Infection

There are various possible outcomes to a virus infection.

Elimination of virus and subsequent immunity of host: in many instances the host's immune defences are effectively mobilised in response to the invading agent (see Chapter 2), the virus is eliminated from the body and the host is immune to subsequent infection by the same virus. The consequences of such an infection then depend on the capacity of the cells damaged by the infection to regenerate normally. Respiratory mucosal cells damaged by respiratory viruses are replaced quickly, so there are generally no long-term sequelae to these infections. Anterior horn cells on the other hand have little regenerative capacity, so paralytic poliomyelitis frequently causes permanent damage. Similarly in the eye, conjunctival and corneal epithelial cells usually regenerate after a virus infection so that complete healing occurs, whereas if the corneal stroma is involved, subsequent recovery is often associated with vascularisation and the development of opacities, with consequent impairment of vision due to reduction in the transparency.

Latency

In some virus infections, in particular those caused by herpes viruses, the virus is not eliminated from the body but may persist as a subclinical or inapparent infection within certain cells of the body, where they are inaccessible to circulatory antiviral antibodies. Such infections are liable to reactivate, often many years after the primary exogenous infection, and these reactivated endogenous infections often have severe consequences in the eye.

Oncogenicity

Though of little relevance to virus infection of the eye, an oncogenic potential of certain viruses depends on the ability of some viruses to alter the growth characteristics of the infected host cell. Some viruses, particularly RNA viruses of the family Retroviridae, which commonly infect birds and rodents, induce cancers in their host under natural conditions. These viruses have not yet been implicated in any human cancers. Certain viruses of the herpes group are also oncogenic in animals under natural conditions, and in man there are associations between herpes viruses and malignancy, both between EB virus and Burkitt's lymphoma or nasopharyngeal carcinoma, and between herpes simplex virus type 2 and carcinoma of the cervix. However, a definite causal relationship between herpes viruses and human cancers has not yet been proven. Other viruses, such as certain human adenovirus serotypes, induce tumours when injected into baby rodents, although there is no evidence that they cause malignancy in their natural host.

EPIDEMIOLOGY

Since viruses may reach the eye not only by direct contamination of the conjunctival mucous membrane but also by blood-borne spread of a general-ised infection, the general principles underlying the maintenance and trans-mission of viruses in the community are relevant when considering virus diseases of the eye and their control.

Source of Virus

Most viruses are host specific, so the majority of human virus infections are acquired from previously infected humans, man himself forming the reservoir of infection. Certain viruses, however, may be acquired from animals, man in this instance forming an 'accidental' susceptible host. These infections, whilst they may have serious consequences for the infected individual, are irrelevant to the long-term survival of the virus. Many arborvirus infections, rabies and Newcastle disease conjunctivitis all fall into this category in which man is an 'accidental' host.

Entry and Exit of Viruses from the Body

Viruses usually enter and leave the body via either the respiratory tract, the alimentary tract or the skin. The mucous membranes of the eye and genital tract are also important sites for virus entry and shedding, whereas other viruses require injection into the body in order to reach susceptible cells. In addition, vertical transmission of virus, that is infection of a new generation by an individual or a previous generation, may occur either by transplacental spread of virus to a fetus *in utero*, or by infection of the young susceptible population by reactivation of an endogenous infection in an older person. Thus transmission of the varicella-zoster virus from an elderly person with shingles causes chickenpox in young, exposed susceptibles. The major ways in which viruses are transmitted between humans are summarised in Table 1.3 (p. 8).

In transmission by the respiratory route, virus particles are released in aerosols in the expired air of infected persons and inhaled, causing fresh infection in susceptible subjects. The conjunctiva is also exposed to such virus aerosols, so provided the conjunctival cells are susceptible to infection with the virus, conjunctival as well as respiratory tract infection and shedding may occur. This mode of transmission is probably important in the spread of certain adenovirus serotypes which infect both the eye and respiratory tract (Chapter 10). Both localised and generalised virus infections are commonly transmitted in the form of aerosols. In general the incubation period is short (2–5 days) in infections which are localised to the respiratory tract (as for example rhinoviruses and influenza viruses) but it is longer (10–21 days) in generalised infections (e.g. rubella, measles, mumps). In both instances virus is shed from the mucous surfaces towards the end of the incubation period and for a few days after onset of clinical illness.

The faecal-oral route, though an important mode for spread of viruses in general, is of little importance in viral infections of the eye, though it is possible that adenoviruses shed in the faeces may cause conjunctivitis if transferred to the eye.

Viruses which are spread by the faecal-oral route must be able to survive passage through the gastro-intestinal tract, and they may be shed in the stools for long periods after the acute stage of the clinical illness, or in the absence of a clinical illness.

Minor trauma, which allows virus particles already in contact with the skin to penetrate susceptible cells below the stratified squamous layers of epithelium must usually precede infection of the skin by viruses such as herpes simplex and vaccinia.

Direct spread from eye to eye, which occurs in certain adenovirus infections (serotypes 8, 10 and 19, Chapter 10) and in haemorrhagic conjunctivitis due to enterovirus type 70 and a new antigenic variant of Coxsackie A.24 (Chapter 11), is particularly common in underdeveloped countries with overcrowded living conditions and poor standards of hygiene. In developed countries transmission of virus in this way may occur in inadequately chlorinated swimming-pools and in eye hospitals and clinics where either unsterile instruments or contaminated fingers of the staff themselves may inadvertently transmit the infection.

Persistence of Virus in the Community

The spread of a virus in the community is considerably influenced by the degree of immunity to the virus in the population as a whole. Primary infection with viruses such as measles, which exist as a single antigenic type, confers long-lasting immunity on the individual. Such viruses therefore spread predominantly in children, who represent the susceptible section of the community. In isolated societies with insufficient numbers of fresh susceptible subjects to maintain the chain of infection, such viruses disappear and the herd immunity is lost. Re-introduction of virus then leads to devastating spread through the whole population. Influenza viruses, unlike measles, are not antigenically stable, and frequent changes in the surface antigens of these viruses (antigenic shift and drift) lead to frequent world-wide epidemics, since previous infection does not confer immunity to newly evolved strains. Similar pandemic spread of virus was recently seen in Africa and the Middle and Far East, when two apparently new strains of enterovirus emerged which infected the conjunctiva and transmitted from eye to eye. These viruses spread rapidly in the absence of any herd immunity, causing large epidemics of haemorrhagic conjunctivitis during the early 1970s (Chapter 11).

Viruses which form endogenous latent infections capable of reactivation and spread to fresh hosts (e.g. herpes viruses) do not require a chain of susceptibles for their maintenance in the community. These viruses survive in small populations, since reactivation of infection in an adult allows transmission to young, susceptible individuals in the community who then in turn become persistently infected.

CONTROL OF VIRUS INFECTIONS

Prevention of virus infection, either by public health measures or by specific immunisation programmes designed both to protect the individual and to increase herd immunity, has been highly successful in controlling some serious virus infections over the last 30 years. In contrast, the development of effective antiviral agents for the treatment of established virus infections has proved exceedingly difficult to achieve, and although this approach is now yielding some therapeutic advantages in a few selected clinical situations, notably in the treatment of herpes simplex virus infections of the eye, up to the present it has had little impact either on treatment or on overall control of virus infections in the community.

Public Health Measures

These are of particular value in controlling virus spread by the faecal-oral route (e.g. hepatitis A) and by eye-to-eye transmission. However, the improvement in living conditions required in order to limit such spread is still difficult to achieve in many areas of the world, and even in developed countries virus transmission by these routes is still common in certain sections of the community, in particular in institutions for the mentally subnormal, where an improvement in the standard of hygiene is difficult to maintain. Hepatitis A and adenovirus type 8, for example, once introduced, spread rapidly in these communities.

Recent improvements in living standards in developed countries has reduced the transmission of viruses which require close contact for spread (e.g. herpes viruses). However, the effect of this has been rather to postpone the age of primary infection from early childhood to young adult life, rather than to prevent infection altogether. Effective control of aerosol-spread viruses is very difficult, and modern urban life, which concentrates large numbers of people in relatively small areas, in general encourages the spread of viruses by the respiratory route. Control of parenteral spread of viruses is sometimes possible; for example, eradication of insect vectors, if feasible, will prevent certain arbovirus infections (e.g. urban yellow fever) and careful screening measures will reduce the risk of viruses transmitted by accidental inoculation of blood and blood products (e.g. hepatitis B). In addition, strict quarantine regulations for imported birds and animals may be used to prevent the introduction of viruses such as rabies and Newcastle disease virus into countries free of infection.

Immunisation

Immunisation against viruses can be achieved either by injection of specific protective antibodies (passive immunity), or by stimulating the host's own immune defences by administration of vaccines (active immunisation). These vaccines consist either of live attenuated virus strains, or of killed viruses, or purified viral antigens. Passive immunity is short-lasting, since donor antibodies usually only survive a few weeks in serum, and this form of immunisation is used either for protection of individuals against specific viruses to which they have been or may be exposed, or to attenuate established infection in patients at special risk. Active immunisation in contrast confers long-lasting immunity, and is used both to protect the individual and to increase herd immunity and thus reduce transmission of virus in the community as a whole.

Passive Immunity

Immunoglobulin preparations from normal pooled human sera contain sufficient neutralising antibodies to common virus infections such as hepatitis A and measles to protect against these infections. Immunoglobulins with high antibody titres against specific viruses, which are prepared from convalescent sera obtained from infected patients, are also available to prevent or attenuate with varicella-zoster, hepatitis B, vaccinia and mumps. These antibodies all act by neutralising virus particles, which then cannot attach to, and hence penetrate and replicate within, susceptible cells; immunoglobulins are therefore of limited value once substantial virus replication and cell damage has already occurred.

Active Immunisation

Active immunisation against antigenically stable viruses such as polio, measles and variola major and minor (all viruses which require a chain of susceptible hosts to maintain transmission) has proved highly successful. During the past 20 years a WHO programme which involved an intensive search to identify new cases of smallpox combined with vaccination of all smallpox contacts has led to global eradication of variola viruses. Vaccination against smallpox, which itself has serious complications, including accidental vaccination of the eye, is therefore now no longer justified. Active immunisation against polio and measles has been successful in controlling these infections in developed countries with resources for delivering immunisation to the young, susceptible section of the community. In underdeveloped countries however, both infections remain important causes of childhood mortality and morbidity, with blindness one of the serious sequelae of measles infection (see Chapter 13). Active immunisation programmes against rubella are being carried out at present to prevent congenital rubella infections, the aim being to ensure that all women are immune by the time they become pregnant. Safe and effective vaccination against rabies is now available both after possible exposure to the virus, and prophylactically for those at risk.

Immunisation is less effective against antigenically unstable viruses such as influenza A and B. To be effective, the vaccine must contain the antigens of currently circulating influenza strains, and since these change every few years continual modification of the vaccine and re-immunisation is necessary. Repeated immunisations with different vaccines are, however, of doubtful value since they tend to boost antibodies against similar antigens encountered in earlier vaccines ('original antigenic sin') rather than inducing antibodies to the new antigens incorporated in the latest vaccine. Herpes viruses, because of their tendency to form latent infections which may subsequently reactivate, are particularly difficult to control, and effective vaccines against these viruses are not at present available. With these viruses, there is the additional risk that immunisation with attenuated strains might promote persistent infections or increase viral oncogenicity.

Antiviral Agents

The development of effective agents for the treatment of established virus infections is fraught with difficulties. Since the host cell's biochemical apparatus is used to generate viral gene products it is difficult to devise agents which act selectively against the virus without also producing severe toxic reactions in the host. Secondly, the manifestations of virus disease do not occur until considerable viral replication and therefore host-cell damage has already occurred. Thirdly, accurate diagnosis in the early stages of infection is difficult, since many virus infections present with similar non-specific symptoms, and a rapid definitive laboratory diagnosis is not usually possible. In addition, effective therapy for viral infections, even if feasible, would do little to control virus transmission, because of the large number of mild or asymptomatic infections in which virus shedding occurs.

Three types of antiviral agent are currently under investigation: synthetic compounds which interfere selectively with viral replication within host cells, substances which stimulate the host's own immune response to viral infection, and interferon, which acts by rendering cells resistant to virus infection.

Synthetic Antiviral Agents

Viruses of the herpes group, particularly herpes simplex virus, have proved the most amenable to treatment by this means up to the present. Nucleoside analogues such as the thymidine analogue 5-iodo-2-deoxyuridine (idoxuridine, IDU), the cytidine analogue cytoside arabinoside (cytarabine, Alexan, Cytosar) and the purine analogue adenine arabinoside (vidarabine, Vira-A) are effective against herpes simplex and varicella-zoster both *in vitro* and in certain clinical situations. These compounds interfere with normal host cell and viral DNA replication, as they are incorporated into DNA in place of the normal nucleosides. IDU is too toxic to be used systemically, but it has proved valuable when used topically for herpetic infections of the skin (e.g. zoster and herpetic whitlow) and in the treatment of herpes simplex infection of the eye. In these situations the turnover of viral DNA is greater than that of the host cells, so a selective antiviral action is obtained. Vidarabine and cytarabine are less toxic than IDU and have been used systematically in the treatment of severe infections such as herpes simplex encephalitis and generalised zoster in immunosuppressed patients.

These analogues are likely to be superseded in the future by acycloguanosine (acyclovir or Zovirax), the most promising antiviral agent produced to date, which has specific activity against herpes viruses without significant toxic side-effects in the host. It acts by entering virus-infected cells preferentially where it is converted by a virus-coded enzyme into an active form which inhibits viral but not cellular DNA synthesis. Acyclovir has been shown to be effective in the treatment of dendritic ulcers, and trials are currently in progress to assess its efficiency in the treatment of severe systemic herpetic infections.

Other drugs such as amantadine (Symmetrel) and methisazone (Marboran), which are active against influenza A and smallpox viruses, respectively, have proved effective in clinical trials only if given prophylactically, and are generally of little clinical value.

Interferon

Theoretically, human interferon should be the ideal antiviral agent; it is a natural product of human cells, is therefore not toxic, and it has a broad spectrum of activity against many different viruses, so that accurate diagnosis of the virus infection is not necessary before it can be given. In practice, however, clinical trials have not been encouraging and interferon has had little impact so far on antiviral therapy. Work has also been hampered by the technical difficulty of producing large quantities of interferon. In attempts to overcome this problem synthetic polynucleotides which, like viruses, induce interferon production, have been used to stimulate interferon output in the virus-infected host. Although successful in inducing raised levels of interferon in serum, these compounds appear to have little effect on the course of virus infections in humans; moreover the interferon inducers themselves have undesirable side-effects.

Immune Response Stimulators

The effectiveness of drugs which enhance the host's CMI responses is currently under investigation for the treatment of viral infections, but these compounds are not used in routine clinical practice at present.

LABORATORY DIAGNOSIS OF VIRUS INFECTIONS

Diagnosis of a virus infection may be made either by isolating the infectious agent, by demonstrating the virus or viral antigens directly in material obtained from the patient, or by detecting antibodies formed by the host in response to the invading virus. These methods are summarised in Table 1.4.

Isolation Methods

Since all viruses are obligate intracellular parasites they can only be propagated within living cells. Laboratory animals and embryonated eggs have been widely used for this purpose in the past, but these methods have now been largely superseded by *in vitro* cell culture techniques. Virus growth in cultured cells is recognised either by the production of a cytopathic effect

TABLE 1.4

SUMMARY OF METHODS USED FOR LABORATORY DIAGNOSIS OF VIRUS INFECTION

A *Isolation of infectious agent*	1 Embryonated eggs ⎫ Largely superseded by 3 2 Laboratory animals ⎭ 3 Cell culture (virus recognised by CPE or haemadsorption)
B *Demonstration of infectious agent*	1 Direct visualisation (electron microscope) 2 Recognition of viral antigens with specific antisera (Fluorescent antibody tests, RIA, ELISA)
C *Serological diagnosis*	1 Appearance of antibodies to invading virus Complement fixation and FAB tests recognise group-specific antibodies Neutralisation and HAI tests recognise type-specific antibodies 2 Virus-specific IgM (Primary and congenital infections)

(CPE) or by adsorption of certain species of red blood cell to the surface of the infected cell (haemadsorption). The latter effect is due to modification of the surface of the infected cell by virus-specific proteins. Both CPE and haemadsorption may be inhibited by antisera which neutralise viral infectivity. Such neutralising antisera are virus-specific, so that neutralisation or haemadsorption inhibition tests may be used to identify virus isolates.

Alternatively, more recently developed immunofluorescent techniques with specific antisera may be used for identification (see below). Since it usually takes several days, and sometimes several weeks, for the effects of virus growth to appear in culture cells, diagnosis by isolation of the virus is seldom quick.

Direct Demonstration of Virus on Viral Antigens

In general these techniques allow the diagnosis to be made more rapidly than by isolation methods, but not all virus infections are yet amenable to diagnosis by these rapid methods.

Direct Visualisation of Virus Particles

Virus particles can be seen directly in the electron microscope with the use of negative-staining techniques, if they are present in sufficient quantity. Specimens of vesicle fluid or crusts from virus-infected skin lesions, for example, generally contain sufficiently large numbers of virus particles to allow quick and easy identification by this method. This technique allows differentiation between viruses of different families, but it does not distinguish viruses within the same group. Pox viruses such as vaccinia can be distinguished from herpes viruses, for instance, but herpes simplex virus cannot be differentiated from varicella-zoster viruses by electron microscopy alone.

Immunological Methods

Fluorescent antibody staining methods, in which specific antisera tagged with fluorescent dyes are used to visualise antibody-antigen reactions by fluorescence miscroscopy are now frequently used in diagnostic virology. In this way specific viral antigens within infected cells may be demonstrated. These techniques have proved particularly successful in identifying respiratory viral antigens in exfoliated cells from the nasopharynx. Antigens within corneal or conjunctival cells have been demonstrated by the same technique. Rabies antigens, for instance, can be demonstrated in impression smears of corneal epithelium obtained from infected patients, and this has been used as a diagnostic test for rabies.

Other recently developed, sensitive immunological methods of detecting viral antigens, such as radioimmune assays (RIA) and enzyme-linked immuno-sorbent assay (ELISA) are likely to be used increasingly in diagnostic virology laboratories in the future.

Serological Diagnosis

This is useful in primary viral infections, and diagnosis usually depends on the demonstration of a rising titre of antibodies to a particular virus in paired serum specimens collected from the patient during the acute and convalescent stages of an illness. Since detectable antibodies produced by the host in response to an invading virus often do not appear until one week or more after onset of symptoms, such a diagnosis can usually only be made retrospectively. Information obtained from a single serum specimen is often difficult to interpret since the presence of antibodies to a particular virus may be due either to concurrent or to past infection.

A number of different serological techniques are available for measuring viral antibodies, of which the complement-fixation test is most widely used in diagnostic laboratories (Figure 1.2). The viral antigens which can be detected in this way are generally specific to a particular virus group, so complement-fixing antibodies to these antigens do not distinguish between different virus serotypes within the same group. For instance, complement-fixing antibodies resulting from infection with adenovirus type 8 are induced by an antigen common to all adenoviruses. A rising titre is therefore evidence of a recent adenovirus infection, but it does not indicate which adenovirus serotype caused the infection. Proteins on the surface of the virion induce antibodies which neutralise infectivity or which inhibit the ability of certain viruses to haemagglutinate red blood cells (Figure 1.3). In contrast to complement-fixing antibodies, these neutralising and haemagglutination-inhibiting (HAI) anti-bodies are specific to a particular virus serotype, so detection of these antibodies allows identification of the particular virus. For instance, HAI antibodies induced by adenovirus type 8 do not cross-react with the haem-agglutinins of other adenovirus serotypes, so the appearance of such antibodies indicates infection with adenovirus type 8.

In general, neutralising and HAI antibodies persist in serum for many years after infection, and account for the lifelong immunity to re-infection which occurs after primary infection with many viruses. Complement-fixing anti-bodies, on the other hand, last for a shorter time, so absence of complement-fixing antibodies to a particular virus indicates lack of recent infection with the virus rather than no previous infection.

Demonstration of the class of immunoglobulin involved in antibody reac-

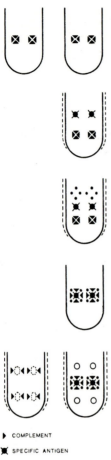

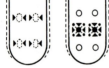

Figure 1.2. The complement-fixation test. Complement is added, followed by specific antigen. Serum is then added to be tested for the presence of complement-fixing antibodies. The tubes are incubated and antigen-complement-antibody complexes are formed. Sensitised sheep red blood cells are then added; in the absence of complement-fixing antibodies, complement causes lysis of sensitised red blood cells. (Courtesy, Dr. Elizabeth H. Boxall and Geigy Pharmaceuticals.)

▶ COMPLEMENT

✖ SPECIFIC ANTIGEN

• COMPLEMENT-FIXING ANTIBODY

○ SENSITISED SHEEP RED
   BLOOD CELLS

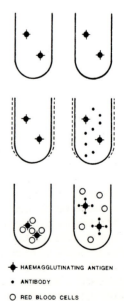

Figure 1.3. The haemagglutination inhibition test. Haemagglutinating antigen is added, followed by serum, the two reagents being incubated to form antigen-antibody complexes. Red blood cells are added; in the absence of anti-haemagglutinin antibody, red blood cells are agglutinated. (Courtesy, Dr. Elizabeth H. Boxall and Geigy Pharmaceuticals.)

◆ HAEMAGGLUTINATING ANTIGEN

• ANTIBODY

○ RED BLOOD CELLS

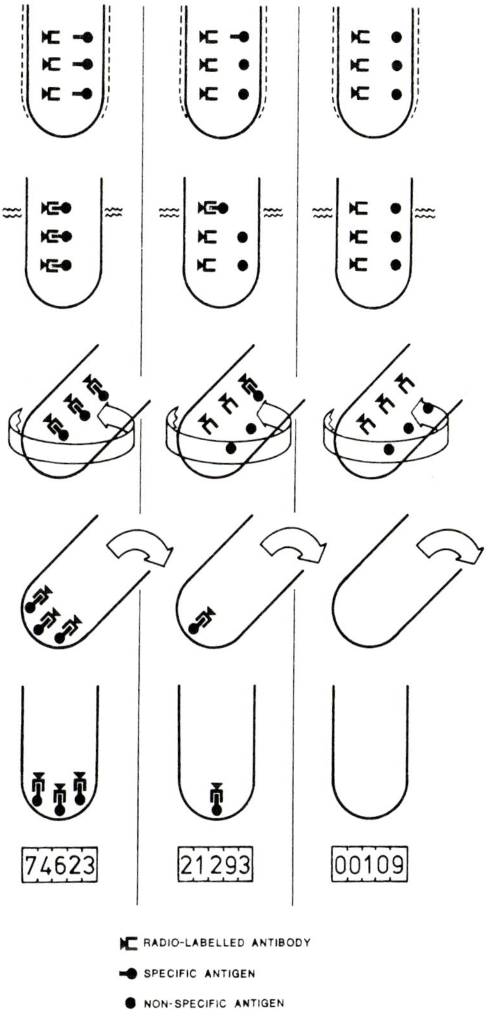

Figure 1.4. Radioimmune assay. Serum plus excess labelled antibody is added, and incubated to form antigen-antibody complexes. Following centrifugation to deposit the complexes, excess liquid is decanted and the deposit is washed. Radioactive material is counted. (Courtesy, Dr. Elizabeth H. Boxall and Geigy Pharmaceuticals.)

tions is sometimes of help in diagnosis, particularly in babies suspected of having a congenital rubella infection. Whereas most sera from neonates contains rubella-specific IgG which is maternally acquired, congenitally infected babies produce appreciable levels of rubella-specific IgM. Fractionation of the serum on a sucrose density gradient and demonstration of rubella-specific HAI or fluorescent antibodies in the IgM fraction is therefore diagnostic of a congenital rubella infection (Chapter 12).

As in the identification of viral antigens (see above) new immunological techniques such as fluorescent antibody methods, radioimmune assays (Figure 1.4) and ELISA techniques are now being developed for the detection of viral antibodies, and are likely to be of increasing importance in serodiagnosis in the future.

SUGGESTED READING

DUFFY, P., WOLF, J., COLLINS, G., DE VOE, A. G. *et al.* (1974). Possible person to person transmission of Creutzfeld-Jakob disease. *New Engl. J. Med.*, **290**, 692.

EVANS, A. S. (1978). *Viral Infections of Humans*. Chichester: John Wiley & Sons.

FENNER, F. J. and WHITE, D. O. (1976). *Medical Virology*. New York: Academic Press.

PRIMROSE, S. B. and DIMMOCK, H. J. (1980). *Introduction to Modern Virology*. London: Blackwell Scientific Publications.

ROWSON, K. E. K., REES, T. A. L. and MAHY, B. W. J. (1981). *A Dictionary of Virology*. London: Blackwell Scientific Publications.

CHAPTER TWO

Essential Concepts in Immunology

VERTEBRATES possess a surveillance mechanism called the immune system that protects them from disease-causing (pathogenic) micro-organisms, such as viruses and bacteria, and from cancer cells. This system specifically recognises and selectively eliminates foreign invaders. The immune system is complex and not yet understood completely. Further information is being gathered constantly, and this chapter presents concepts much of which are based on experiments on laboratory animals or on artificial *in vitro* systems which may not necessarily prove applicable to man.

Adaptive and Non-adaptive Immune Responses

Immunity to infection may be based on *non-specific factors* which can act independently of the immune system, and *specifically acquired immunity* which frequently operates in concert with non-specific factors, thereby increasing its effectiveness. The non-specific physical factors which help to protect the eye will be described (Chapter 3). It is also known that mucous secretion can inhibit the penetration of cells by viruses through competition with cell-surface receptors for the viral neuraminidase. The bactericidal enzyme lysozyme is present in many secretions including tears and saliva, and is also found in the granules of polymorphs and macrophages and in body fluids. Bacteria can be removed by phagocytosis. They become adherent to polymorphs and macrophages by some primitive recognition mechanism on the part of the phagocytic cell. The microbes are then engulfed into a phagosome by arms of cytoplasm which wrap around them. Phagosomes fuse with a lysosomal granule to form a phagolysosome in which the bacterium is killed by many factors such as low pH, a variety or proteolytic enzymes, lysozyme, peroxidase and a number of bactericidal basic polypeptides. The importance of polymorphs in combating infectious disease is shown by the seriousness of chronic granulomatous disease, and the Chediak-Higashi syndrome in children where there are deficits in neutrophil leucocytes which are able to ingest, but not to finally kill, bacteria. These infants suffer persistent infections by many common bacterial agents.

The acute inflammatory response to foreign organisms and to products of tissue injury caused by them has a beneficial role. Increased capillary permeability leads to rapid entry of polymorphs, and later monocytes, into the site of infection from the blood stream, where they may combat the microbes by phagocytosis. Massive transudation of serum bactericidal factors also occurs which include C-reactive protein properdin, with the constituents of the complement system, which together can kill a variety of micro-organisms in the presence of magnesium ions through activation of the alternative pathway. Non-specific antiviral agents include interferon, which inhibits intracellular viral replication and is synthesised by cells in response to viral infection.

Where an infection is a primary one, adaptive responses occur which are highly specific for the invading organism. This process involves the sensitisation of lymphocytes and plasma cells to produce cell-mediated immune responses and immunoglobulin respectively. Where a re-infection occurs, then the degree of specific protection afforded against the invading organisms is often such that it is unable to gain a foothold in a target tissue and it may be said that the host is immune. Because viruses are often intracellular organisms, cell-mediated immunity is usually involved in this protection; however, where there is a phase of extracellular existence by the virus, then specific antibody is important in the prevention of invasion and in the inhibition of spread.

The Lymphocytic Response

Two systems of immunity protect vertebrates, both of which may respond specifically against foreign antigens, although one response is generally favoured (Figure 2.1). The cellular immune response is particularly effective against fungi, parasites, intracellular viral infections, cancer cells and foreign tissue. The humoral immune response defends primarily against the extracellular phases of bacterial and viral infections. Cellular immunity resides in the cells of the lymphoid system, while the humoral immunity ultimately exists in the serum. This dual system results from two essentially different populations of lymphocytes. Each lymphocyte in the two populations is potentially able to recognise and respond to one of a few closely related antigens. One class, the T-cells, mediate the cellular immune response, so that when a foreign substance is recognised these cells are activated, initiating reactions which include binding and eliminating the substance. The second class of lymphocytes, the B-cells, initiate the humoral immune response. These cells are stimulated by the presence of foreign invaders to form plasma cells which secrete antibodies which bind specifically to the foreign substance and initiate a variety of elimination processes.

The cell surfaces of lymphocytes carry membrane-bound antibodies or antibody-like molecules that function as antigen receptors; those on B-cells are known to be antibodies, while those on T-cells have similar binding properties but their molecular nature is not known. Since each lymphocyte

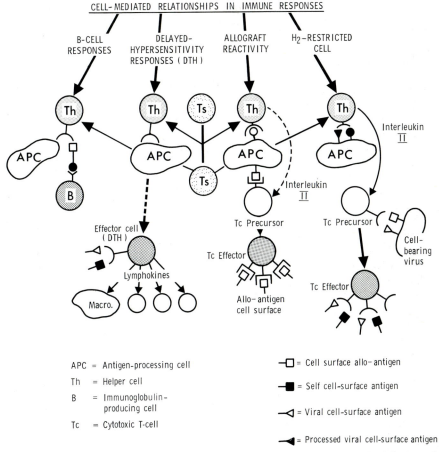

CELL-MEDIATED RELATIONSHIPS IN IMMUNE RESPONSES

Figure 2.1. Cell interactions in immune responses. A balance exists between the influence of helper and suppressor T-cells. The immune responses denoted are the production of antibody by B-cells, the induction of delayed-hypersensitivity T-cells, and the production of effector T-cells against homologous tissue or altered cells in the host induced by viruses. (From *Immunology Today*, December 1981; Courtesy, Elizabeth Simpson and Philip Chandler, and the publishers, Elsevier Biomedical Press.)

carries one kind of specific receptor which responds to only a few closely related antigenic determinants, it might be considered that the number of antigens to which a vertebrate might respond would be limited. However, a mammal contains 10^8 to 10^{12} lymphocytes which effectively possess the capacity to respond to an enormous number and variety of antigens. The lymphocyte population is thought to consist of 10^5 to 10^8 clones of cells with different receptor specifications, and the sizes of these clones are estimated to range from about 1 to about 10^7 cells. However, it must be remembered that antigens present many determinants, and at the same time a given determinant may be recognised by more than one receptor.

Lymphocytes which bind antigen may be triggered to proliferate and differentiate to form clones of progeny cells which possess surface receptors of the same idiotype as the parent cell. Certain of the progeny differentiate into effector cells which are the functional end-products of the immune response. The B-lymphocyte effector cells are known as plasma cells which secrete humoral antibodies of the same idiotype and antigen-recognition specificity as their cell-surface receptors. Successive stages in the development of mature plasma cells after antigen challenge takes about five days and eight cell generations. The mature plasma cell has an extensive endoplasmic reticulum whose internal cavities are filled with antibody molecules.

T-cells give rise to several types of effector cells with different functions, such as the cytotoxic or killer T-cell which eliminates foreign cells directly. Other types of effector T-cells are responsible for delayed hypersensitivity, for helping B-cell differentiation and proliferation, for amplifying killer T-cell differentiation and proliferation, and for suppressing immune responses (suppressor T-cells) (Figure 2.1). The progeny of lymphocytes contain not only effector cells, but also expanded clones of memory cells, which retain the capacity to produce further progeny cells of both effector and memory types upon subsequent stimulation by an original antigen. Memory cells may exist for decades in contrast to effector cells, the life of which are measured in days.

Lymphocytes compose 20–45 per cent of the nucleated cells in the blood, and over 99 per cent of the nucleated cells in the lymph. However, these cells contact and respond to immunising antigens in specialised lymphoid organs that provide accessory cells and tissue architecture appropriate for antigen processing and presentation. This system has three functions: to concentrate antigens, to circulate the lymphocyte population through these organs so that every antigen is exposed to the organism's repertoire of antigen-specific lymphocytes in a short period of time, and to carry the product of the immune response, i.e. specific T-cells and humoral antibodies, to the blood stream and tissues.

Antigens are collected and processed by different lymphoid organs depending upon the route of entry into the body. In the eye, the conjunctiva acts as a layer which is capable of responding to antigens by the accumulation of large numbers of lymphocytes which may line the tarsal plates and on occasions may form themselves into clear-cut follicles. In inflammatory disease, large numbers of lymphatic cells collect at the corneal limbus and in the ciliary body. In external eye disease the local lymphatic node subserving the conjunctiva may become clinically apparent in the pre-auricular region. Processing of an antigen in a lymphatic node involves macrophages, which take up antigens from circulating fluid for presentation of lymphocytes.

The typical lymph node contains a cortex and medulla throughout which a reticular network supports macrophages. The reticulum and its adherent cells trap antigens. Lymphocytes circulate through the blood stream and lymphatic channels to reach a lymphatic node where they contact processed antigen. In a resting lymph node the cortex is divided into discrete B-cell domains known as primary follicles and adjacent T-cell domains which compose the diffuse cortex. T- and B-cells adhere to the large endothelial cells of venule walls which they traverse to enter the node. B-cells then migrate to the follicles, and

T-cells to the cortex. After entering their specific cortical domains, recirculating lymphocytes enter the medullary sinusoids, whence they are transported via the main lymphatic ducts into the blood stream. There are specialised lymphatic organs attached to the respiratory system and gastro-intestinal tracts in mammals, including the adenoids, tonsils, Peyer's patches and appendix, which have postcapillary venules serving as lymphocyte entry sites into specific B-cell and T-cell domains. Most lymphocytes enter and leave the spleen via the blood stream. Once again, the spleen contains primary follicles which are B-cell domains, while T-cells are located in the sheath which surrounds the area between the central arteriole and the marginal sinus.

The products of the immune response in any lymphoid organ are effector T-cells and humoral antibodies produced by plasma cells. These products, which must reach the tissues to play a defensive role, are distributed by the blood stream, having entered it via efferent lymphatic vessels and lymphatic ducts. Of the five classes of humoral antibodies, IgG can traverse blood-vessel walls and enter the interstitial spaces of tissues most efficiently. About 50 per cent of an organism's IgG antibodies are found in the interstitial fluid and 50 per cent in the blood stream. The remaining classes of circulating antibodies, IgA, IgD, IgE and IgM, are confined primarily to the blood stream or to specific location sites. T-cells in the blood stream collect on blood-vessel walls near a site where antigens have invaded the tissues. These cells then migrate through the vessel walls into the tissues, where they initiate inflammatory responses to the invading agent.

Antigen which enters a lymph node via afferent lymphatics is taken up by macrophages in the afferent sinusoids, the diffuse cortex and the medulla within minutes of infection. Much of the antigen is incorporated in the cytoplasm of the macrophage in phagosomes, which then diffuse to form lysosomes. These contain hydrolytic enzymes known as phagolysosomes. The enzymes degrade the antigenic components so that they are no longer antigenic, following which the macrophage surface receives a certain amount of highly immunogenic material for presentation to antigen-specific lymphocytes. Antigen which is not associated with macrophages begins to collect within primary follicles about 24–48 hours after injection in the laboratory animal. The antigen is retained in dendritic reticular cell processes which lie in close proximity to many B-cells within the follicle.

The B- and T-cells entering a lymph node are small cells, with dense nuclei surrounded by a thin layer of cytoplasm that contains few mitochondria, no polysomes and little endoplasmic reticulum. Binding of an antigen to the surface of either type of lymphocyte triggers activation, with enlargement of the cell, swelling of the nucleolus, formation of microtubules and increased rate of macromolecular synthesis. This *blast transformation* is accompanied by concomitant changes in the morphology of the lymph node. The wave of T-cell divisions in the diffuse cortex following their encounter with processed antigen is following by transformation of small B-cells to large B-cells in the follicle. These cells give rise to memory and effector cells of the B lineage. Some of the T-cells migrate towards the primary follicle, where a focus of dividing T- and B-cells as well as active macrophages build up to form a germinal centre which compresses the follicle into a crescent around it; the follicle now becomes a secondary follicle. Plasma cells begin to settle in the medulla to form cords. Other lymph nodes are then populated by B-cell progeny together with activated T-cells which also enter the blood stream. Most B effector cells remain in the lymph nodes, but T and B memory cells and T effector cells re-enter the general circulation following antigenic challenge. The combination of specific cellular proliferation, increased fluid in the tissues, increased numbers of non-lymphoid cells and retention of normally recirculating lymphocytes causes the node to enlarge, producing the typical swollen gland associated with infection.

It is clearly important that the body distinguishes accurately between what are constituents of its own normal tissues (self) and what are not (non-self). Foreign substances are reacted against in order to maintain the integrity of the body. At a molecular level, the greater the disparity between foreign substances and self, the more violent will be the immune response. The general function whereby the body is policed is known as surveillance. The most obvious example is surveillance against the presence of invading organisms, but other essential aspects include surveillance against the emergence of lymphocytes capable of reacting against self, against the development of mutant or neoplastic cells, and against transplanted or transfused foreign tissue cells. The distinction between self and non-self is the task of the small lymphocyte. These cells comprise about 90 per cent of both central and peripheral lymphoid tissue and continually recirculate between the central lymphoid tissue and the blood stream via the lymphatics. They are active and mobile so that they continually gain access to other organs by passing through the walls of the capillary blood vessels. They are therefore suitable for policing the body for any macromolecules carrying foreign molecular determinants.

Immunoglobulins

An individual B-cell activated by an antigen proliferates and differentiates to form plasma cells that begin to synthesise identical antibodies with a single specificity at the rate of 3,000 to 30,000 molecules per cell per second. However, the response is heterogeneous with respect to antibody specificity because most antigens have multiple antigenic determinants that trigger the activation of different B-cells, and even a single antigenic determinant generally activates several different B-cells that display receptor immunoglobulins with similar but not identical specificity. Thus the serum of any vertebrate contains an extremely heterogeneous collection of immunoglobulin molecules whose specificities reflect the organism's past antigenic history. A schematic representation of the human immunoglobulin molecule is shown in Figure 2.2.

The B-cell response may therefore produce, as a result of a challenge by a single antigen, antibody molecules of all five classes of immunoglobulin, IgA, IgD, IgE, IgG and IgM. IgM is the first antibody produced in response to an immunogen, and is the pentamer of the basic antibody structural unit (Figure 2.3). IgM is principally an antibody of the blood because its large size prevents its entry into the interstitial fluid. It fails to cross the placenta from the maternal to the fetal circulation. It may be displayed as a monomer on the surface of B-cells where it acts as a receptor immunoglobulin.

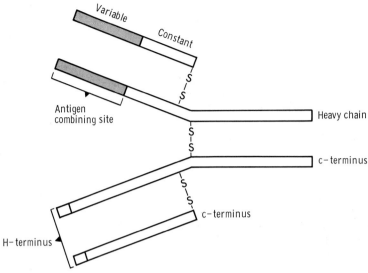

Figure 2.2. A schematic representation of a human immunoglobulin molecule showing some of the principal structural features. The antigen-combining site is to a variable region of the light chains which can exhibit a broad range of specificities. The constant domains carry out various effector functions which include the stimulation of B-cells to proliferate and differentiate, activation of the complement system, opsonisation, and transfer of immunoglobulin in milk, sweat, tears, saliva and the gastro-intestinal secretions. The C-terminus may attach to cell receptors on the macrophage monocyte series.

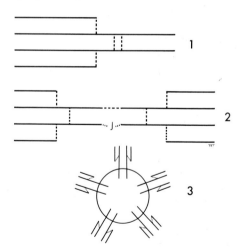

Figure 2.3. Simplified representation of the structure of the common immunoglobulin classes.
1. IgG
2. Secretory IgA; the J chain or secretory piece joins two molecules to form the secretory molecule
3. IgM; five subunits are joined by a J chain

IgG is a monomeric antibody, produced later in the immune response than IgM. Higher doses of antigen are required to stimulate IgG than IgM. IgG is the most prevalent antibody in the blood and in the tissue spaces. It is one of the major triggers of complement fixation, although on a molar basis it is less effective than IgM at exciting this process. IgG also initiates macrophage ingestion of antigenic particles by coating with antibody. It is the only antibody which is able to pass across the placenta to provide a measure of humoral protection for a developing fetus.

IgA is produced later in the immune response than IgM, and can exist as a monomer, dimer, or trimer of the basic structural unit (Figure 2.3). IgA is thought to act as a protective barrier directed against micro-organisms at potential points of entry through mucous membranes. The epithelial cells produce a polypeptide called *secretor component* which complexes with the Fc region of the IgA antibody and specifically mediates their transport from interstitial spaces on to the epithelial surface. IgA is a major component in milk and colostrum, where it may function to protect the gastro-intestinal tracts of newborn infants. IgA is found in saliva, tears and sweat.

IgD is a monomer which is found in small quantities in serum and for which there is no known function at the present time. It is found on the surface of the majority of B-cells in the blood.

IgE is found in the blood in small quantities in normal circumstances and is a monomer which may bind tightly to mast cells in connective tissues, and to basophils in the blood via their Fc regions. IgE bound to mast cells may react with external antigens and trigger the mast cell to degranulate, allowing the release of its intracellular contents in the form of heparin, histamine and other substances.

Humoral antibodies initiate several effector mechanisms for elimination of foreign cells and macromolecules by neutralisation, coating with antibody (which aids phagocytosis by polymorphonuclear leucocytes and macrophages), and contact lysis by killer cells. In addition, IgM and most subclasses of IgG activate the complement system when they bind foreign antigens.

Mechanisms of Tissue Injury

The eye, with its optical system, is particularly sensitive to the transient or permanent effects of damage to its transparent tissues which can be initiated by invading viruses. In contrast to the tissues of the eye, disease processes in other tissues reach advanced stages of tissue injury before either the patient or the clinician becomes aware of it. The eye is thus a microcosm where disease processes are recognized at an early stage in their development.

In this section tissue damage is described in clinicopathological terms in relation to the biology of vascular, cellular and matrix components. The extent and manner in which viruses induce such changes in the eye will be examined in the specific chapters devoted to them. To understand how immune mechanisms may lead to such changes, the processes which can be observed in affected tissues are first described.

Damage to blood vessels may lead to transient and reversible dilatation and increased capillary permeability, allowing escape of plasma proteins and blood cells as in acute inflammation with all its clinical signs. Vasculitis, which is a morphological alteration in the structure of blood vessels, may vary in severity and type, and affects different sizes of arteries and veins as well as capillaries. Changes resulting from vasculitis include deposition of macromolecular space-occupying immune complexes, infiltration of the vessel wall with polymorphs and mononuclear cells, fibrinoid necrosis, deposition of fibrin, degeneration of collagen and elastin, fibrogenesis, intimal hyperplasia, vascular thrombotic occlusion, vascular rupture, and avascular necrosis of tissues.

Cells may undergo necrosis or suffer damage owing to interruption of their blood supply, but may also suffer ill-effects from cytotoxic immune reactions which have been classified by Coombs and Gell (1975). Immediate hypersensitivity reactions (Type 1 reactions) are those in which an antigen reacts with sensitised mast cells and basophils passively coated with cytophilic antibody, usually of IgE type, which triggers the release of stored vasoactive amines such as histamine and slow reactive substance from these cells. Although these mechanisms are known to be important in allergic disease of the respiratory tract and conjunctival sac, together with the skin in anaphylaxis, they are also thought to increase vascular permeability, leading to deposition of immune complexes in the tissues. Although there is no absolute proof, it has been suggested that such mechanisms could be of importance in the pathogenesis of diseases in which immune complexes are thought to play a role, where the complexes are deposited in the vessel walls, e.g. serum sickness, nephritis, vasculitis and arthritis following meningococcal and gonococcal infections, and autoimmune diseases such as systemic lupus erythematosus.

In Type II reactions, antibody is cytotoxic to the cell or its membrane-bearing specific antigen. In these reactions, complement may be required for the completion of the tissue-damaging process on the surface cell membranes. *In vitro* tests indicate a possible mechanism involving mononuclear cells which bear immunoglobulin heavy-chain receptors on their surfaces which collaborate in attacking target cells coated with antibody. The so-called K-cell activity may be demonstrated by typical phagocytic macrophages, but even when these cells are removed from a white cell suspension prepared from blood, lymphoid tissue or bone-marrow, considerable K-cell activity remains. It has been established that these non-phagocytic K-cells are either T- or Ig-bearing B-lymphocytes.

Isoimmune reactions occur in transfusion of mismatched blood or in a mother with an Rh-negative blood group carrying a baby with Rh antigens, and also in organ transplantation. A long-standing homograft which has withstood the first onslaught of the cell-mediated reaction can evoke humoral antibodies in the host directed against surface transplantation antigens on the graft. These may be directly cytotoxic, or cause adherence of phagocytic cells or non-specific attack by K-cells.

In autoimmune reactions, antibody is produced against the patient's cells, such as in the case of haemolytic anaemia. In Hashimoto's thyroiditis, antibodies are found which in the presence of complement are directly cytotoxic for isolated human thyroid cells in culture. In Goodpasture's syndrome, antibodies to kidney glomerular basement membrane are present. Biopsies demonstrate complement components as well as antibody bound to the basement membrane, where serious damage may occur as a result. Type II reactions are probably operative in certain diseases of the eye, particularly in the case of ocular inflammation induced by release of sequestered lens and retinal antigens (see Chapter 3).

Type III or immune-complex-mediated reactions result from the union of antibodies and antigen which may give rise to an inflammatory reaction in a number of ways. If complement is fixed (see next section) anaphylatoxins will be released as split products of C3 and C5, and these will release histamine and cause vascular permeability changes. The simultaneous production of chemotactic factors leads to the influx of polymorphonuclear leucocytes which begin the phagocytosis of the complexes. The polymorph granules release proteolytic enzymes including collagenase, kinin-forming enzymes and polycationic proteins, which further increase vascular permeability. Cellular damage may also occur through reactive lysis in which activated C5,6,7 becomes attached to the cell surfaces and binds C8,9. Under certain conditions platelets may be aggregated to provide either a further source of vasoactive amines, or they may form micro-thrombi which lead to local ischaemia. The outcome of the formation of immune complexes depends upon both the absolute and relative amounts. In gross antibody excess the complexes are rapidly precipitated and tend to be localised to the site of the introduction of antigen. In contrast, when there is antigen excess, soluble complexes are formed which may cause systemic reactions and be widely deposited in kidneys, joints and skin.

Where there is antibody in excess a localised lesion may occur following the introduction of antigen, similar to the reaction described by Arthus, who induced a hyperaemic oedematous skin reaction in hyperimmunised rabbits. The reaction is characterised by intense infiltration of polymorphonuclear leucocytes. The antigen is precipitated with antibody often within the venule and the complex binds complement. Anaphylatoxin may be generated and cause histamine release. Chemotactic factors may be formed, leading to the influx of polymorphonuclear leucocytes. Where relatively large amounts of foreign serum are injected (e.g. horse serum as in the use of antidiphtheria serum) serum sickness can occur, when there is a rise of temperature, swollen lymphatic glands, a generalised urticarial rash, joint swelling and pain. These symptoms and signs result from the deposition of soluble antigen-antibody complexes which are formed in the presence of antigen excess. Larger complexes may induce some of the features of anaphylaxis, possibly through the release of vasoactive amine. These complexes induce increased vascular permeability and allow smaller complexes to be deposited in differing parts of the vascular bed, particularly in the capillaries of the kidney where they may be seen to build up as lumpy granules containing antigen, immunoglobulin and C3, on staining with immunofluorescence.

When sera taken from patients with immune complex disease is stored at 4°C a precipitate may sometimes form containing IgM and IgG. The IgM is an antibody to IgG which is thought to bind it, thus acting as an effective antigen-antibody complex. Synovial fluid taken from patients with rheumatoid arthritis may form immune complexes which produce cryoprecipitates of aggregates of IgG with antiglobulin factors.

In vivo recognition of immune complex formation can be performed on sera or biopsy material. In sera, abnormal peaks may form following ultracentrifugation, IgG may be found in high-molecular-weight fraction on Sephadex gel filtration, precipitation may occur with Clq or rheumatoid factors, cryoprecipitation may occur, and inhibition of K-cell activity may be seen *in vitro*. Evidence may be obtained from biopsy using immunofluorescence.

Erythema multiforme, whether induced by drug allergy or by the immuno-logical reaction with an infective organism such as mycoplasma, is consistent with being caused by circulating immune complexes. Ocular inflammatory disease involving the conjunctiva can be severe and can induce lasting sequelae with keratinisation of the tarsal plates, and the aberrant ingrowth of lashes.

Cell-mediated hypersensitivity (Type IV) is encountered in allergic reactions to bacteria, fungi and viruses, the rejection following organ transplantation, and following sensitisation to certain chemical and pharmacological agents. Histologically, there is perivascular cuffing at an early stage with mononuclear cells, followed by an extensive exudation of mononuclear and polymorpho-nuclear cells, the latter migrating towards the lesion, leaving behind the mononuclears together with cells of the monocyte or macrophage group. The predominant feature of cell-mediated hypersensitivity reaction is that it can be transferred from sensitised to non-sensitised animals by cells of the small lymphocyte series, rather than by serum antibody. Studies in children with thymic insufficiency show that they lack cell-mediated hypersensitivity reac-tions, these reactions being unimpaired in children with primary immunoglobu-lin deficiency, indicating that the thymus-dependent T-cells are critically important in these reactions. It is likely that the hypersensitivity process is initiated by the processing of the antigen by macrophage, and then combining with receptors on the surface of the lymphocyte present as memory cells following an earlier sensitisation process. This activates the cell membrane, following which the interior of the cell responds with the formation of a large blast cell which eventually undergoes mitosis. During the period of blast-cell transformation, mediators are produced which participate in the ensuing hypersensitivity process. These mediators were designated lymphokines by Dumonde *et al.* in 1969 to cover all biologically active factors other than antibodies which can be detected in cell-free supernatants of stimulated lymphocytes. Most circulating lymphocytes are inactive cells, which can be activated if they are suitably stimulated by antigen or by non-specific mitogens. Antigens require pre-treatment by macrophages before being able to activate lymphocytes, although phytohaemagglutinin can do so without the help of macrophages (Figure 2.4).

The important feature which distinguishes cell-mediated reactions from those mediated by antibody are the delayed and localised nature of the former. The sequence of reactions can theoretically be divided into three major components which may be responsible for delay, in contrast to humoral reactions where the responses are brought about by preformed molecules meeting with the antigen. In CMI antigenic material initially activates a small number of lymphocytes which are specifically reactive. This activation leads to the production of a chemotactic factor which attracts other lymphocytes to the site. Thereupon unsensitised lymphocytes are activated by mitogenic factors and thereby start to amplify the reaction further by releasing active mediators which recruit and stimulate more lymphocytes. Blood monocytes are also attracted and are then transformed into activated macrophages by lymphokines. The macrophages then demonstrate enhanced phagocytic action, microbiocidal activity, and increased lysosomal enzyme activity. At this stage the CMI reaction has reached a level of expression, which may take the form

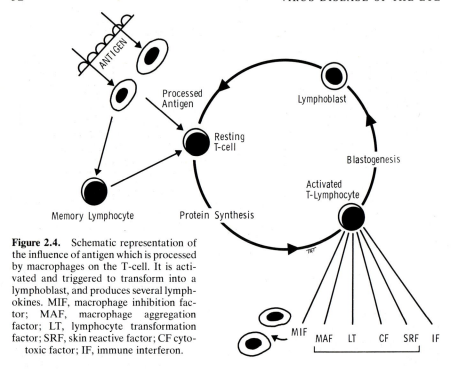

Figure 2.4. Schematic representation of the influence of antigen which is processed by macrophages on the T-cell. It is activated and triggered to transform into a lymphoblast, and produces several lymphokines. MIF, macrophage inhibition factor; MAF, macrophage aggregation factor; LT, lymphocyte transformation factor; SRF, skin reactive factor; CF cytotoxic factor; IF, immune interferon.

of a delayed hypersensitivity reaction, or increased efficiency in killing and digesting pathogens. The co-operative cytotoxic effect of K-lymphocytes and macrophages causes the death of a virus-infected cell with specific antigenic determinants on its surface.

The Complement System

The WHO definition of the complement system is 'a system of factors occurring in normal serum activated characteristically by antibody-antigen interactions and which subsequently mediate a number of biologically significant consequences.' Complement belongs to a series of plasma systems termed 'triggered enzyme cascades' by McFarlane in 1969. It is an effector mechanism which can produce a rapid and amplified response to a stimulus. The response may have beneficial or adverse effects, depending upon the circumstances. The system is complex in its reaction pathway and in the homeostatic mechanism which has evolved to control it. The complement system may be thought of as occurring in three stages (Figure 2.5); the generation of C3 splitting enzymes, the activation of C3 and the activation of the terminal components. C3 activation is probably the most significant part of the sequence. C3 may be split by non-immunological enzymes such as trypsin, thrombin, plasmin and leucocyte cathepsins. The two immunological C3 converting enzymes are the end-products of the classical and alternative pathways of complement activation. The classical pathway is triggered by the presence of an antigen-antibody

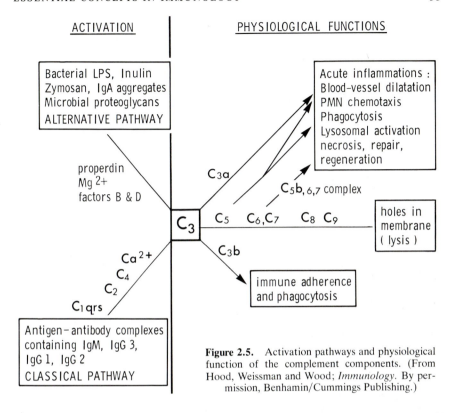

ACTIVATION | PHYSIOLOGICAL FUNCTIONS

Bacterial LPS, Inulin
Zymosan, IgA aggregates
Microbial proteoglycans
ALTERNATIVE PATHWAY

Acute inflammations :
Blood-vessel dilatation
PMN chemotaxis
Phagocytosis
Lysosomal activation
necrosis, repair,
regeneration

properdin
Mg $^{2+}$
factors B & D

C_{3a}

$C_{5b,6,7}$ complex

C_3 C_5 C_6,C_7 C_8 C_9

holes in
membrane
(lysis)

Ca^{2+}
C_4
C_2
C_1qrs

C_{3b}

immune adherence
and phagocytosis

Antigen–antibody complexes
containing IgM, IgG 3,
IgG 1, IgG 2
CLASSICAL PATHWAY

Figure 2.5. Activation pathways and physiological function of the complement components. (From Hood, Weissman and Wood; *Immunology*. By permission, Benhamin/Cummings Publishing.)

complex. The alternative pathway is triggered by certain substances which fix large amounts of the late components C3–9, but very little of C1, C4 or C2. The best known of these is Gram-negative endotoxin and a factor from cobra venom, in addition to which there are various immunoglobulin aggregates and antigen-antibody complexes which behave similarly, such as aggregates of human IgA. The latter part of the complement activation system consists in the formation of a multi-molecular complex.

Complement fixation is initiated by the binding of one IgM or several IgG molecules to an antigen on a foreign cell surface. This binding exposes a complement-binding site of the Fc region of the antibody molecule. Complement component C1 binds to the antigen-antibody complex and the activation of the classical pathway is achieved. C3 is cleaved; C3a causes local blood-vessel dilatation and also may attract polymorphonuclear leucocytes. C3b attaches over the entire cell membrane, promotes opsonisation and combines with the C4-2 complex to initiate cleavage of C5. Subsequently a trimolecular complex, C5,6,7, which in turn can bind C8 and 9, leads to the formation of fenestrations in the cell wall, with subsequent influx of ions and eventual cell lysis.

Mechanisms of Ocular Protection

The remarkable fact that the cornea does not often become infected is due not only to the evolution of physical mechanisms but also to immunological protective mechanisms. The palpebral conjunctiva has been compared to a lymph node, and indeed histological examination of this conjunctiva shows it to be crowded with a wide range of inflammatory cells together with lymphocytes and plasma cells, many of which are actively producing immunoglobulins. Although the cornea has been regarded as privileged with respect to the immune system, it nevertheless continues to enjoy the special protective mechanisms against invasion by infective agents. The intra-ocular structures however are sequestered from the immune system by an adaptation in the walls of the capillaries of the retina and iris; these possess tight junctions between their endothelial cells which prevent the egress of immunoglobulin or immunocompetent cells of the lymphatic system in the absence of specific inflammatory stimuli, although when the latter enter the internal eye, inflammatory responses may quickly occur, as is seen by the immediate onset of acute endophthalmitis due to infection which can follow intra-ocular surgery. There is nevertheless likely to be a relative delay in the inflammatory responses which allows microbial proliferation to occur with greater intensity than in other tissues. The contents of the eye are therefore at risk when invaded by micro-organisms because of the sequestral nature of this internal environment.

The factors which operate to protect the surface of the eye are also of importance in the control of established disease. Where immunological mechanisms of protection are at fault, then microbes have an increased chance to gain entry into the cells of the surface epithelium and thereby cause clinical disease. Once an organism has entered the deeper structures such as the corneal stroma, then, although immunological processes act to control the further spread of the virus, they may also lead on to tissue damage. One of the most important defence mechanisms of the mucous membranes of the body is the local production of specific immunoglobulin as secretory IgA.

The Secretory Immunological System

The interface between the body and its environment is divided into two very different areas, the skin and the mucosae. The former is nearly impermeable to potential invaders from the outer world, in contrast to the latter which lacks the protection of a keratin sheath and may be composed of a single layer of epithelium, although in the cornea the epithelium is multi-layered. Nature has reinforced this flimsy protection by adding, beneath the epithelium, a lymphoid tissue that reacts to antigen applied to the mucosa and excretes the corresponding antibody into the appropriate external secretion, such as the tears in the case of the eye, providing what Burnet called an 'antiseptic paint' for the mucosa. The cornea is a continuation of the mucosal interface of the conjunctival sac and does not have the advantage of a subepithelial depot of immunocompetent lymphocytes.

A considerable amount of scientific investigation has been carried out on the immunological defences in the mucosae of the gut. One of the major stimuli to immunoglobulin production arises from intestinal colonisation by viruses, bacteria and parasites, and from the ingestion of dietary antigens. The recognition that the gut is a major contributor to the development of local immune mechanisms has followed the realisation of the importance of the lymphatic organs in the mucosae.

The two arms of the lymphoid system have already been discussed. Central primary lymphoid organs provide foci where stem cells develop into small lymphocytes, while the peripheral lymphoid organs harbour mature, immunologically competent cells. In the central organs lymphocyte proliferation is independent of antigenic stimulation, whereas in the peripheral organs, antigenic stimulation results in the proliferation of immunologically competent cells which subserve cell-mediated immunity or antibody formation.

It has been found that in birds, stem cells develop in two discrete areas, T-cells developing in the thymus and B-cells in the bursa of Fabricius. The B-cells in the bursa modulate antibody formation, bursectomy resulting in hypogammaglobulinaemia. It is interesting that the avian bursa of Fabricius is anatomically connected with the gut, being situated close to the cloaca, a fact which prompted a search for the mammalian equivalent in the gastro-intestinal tract. It is now considered that the lymphoid tissue of the gut is part of the peripheral lymphoid system but that it has a more complex role and structure than lymph nodes.

Though there are substantial differences between the mucosa of the gut and the epithelium of the conjunctival sac, it seems likely that there is a linkage between humoral mechanisms for the protection of these membranes. The precise mechanisms in the production of local immunoglobulin in the form of IgA are complex, but in the case of the gastro-intestinal tract it seems likely that antigen gains access to Peyer's patches through a specialised microfold epithelial cell (M cell). In Peyer's patches, antigen interacts with T and B small lymphocytes, some of which are IgA precursor cells. These cells migrate to the mesenteric lymph nodes and undergo a process of differentiation during which some of them develop the capacity to produce IgA locally. They thereafter enter the thoracic duct and, via the blood circulation, home selectively to the gut mucosa, where over 90 per cent of the lymphoid cells in the lamina propria are IgA-secreting plasma cells. Whether production of local antibody in the gastro-intestinal tract can be associated with production of specific IgA-producing cells at other mucous membrane sites such as the conjunctiva is not yet clear.

The majority of cells in human lacrimal gland and rabbit conjunctival and lacrimal glands contain immunoglobulin A. Since the epithelial cells adjacent to these IgA plasma cells contain secretory component, these two tissues may constitute part of the secretory immune system (Franklin et al. 1973; Tomasi and Bienenstock, 1968). The B-cells thought to be committed to IgA production may arise in the gut-associated lymphoid tissue and possibly other tissues as well. The circulating B-cells are then preferentially laid down along mucosal surfaces and differentiate into IgA-producing cells. The mechanism responsible for this preferential lodging is unknown, but a role for antigen has been suggested. Using ocular models to study antigen-independent localisation of secretory IgA-producing plasma cells, Franklin et al. (1978) concluded that there was evidence that in the absence of antigenic stimulus, factors produced by activated mammary gland implanted experimentally in rabbit anterior chambers induced localisation of IgA-committed lymphoid cells which differentiated to plasma cells. Such a response occurred after hormonal activation and was not induced by non-lactating mammary gland. Activated mammary tissue probably liberates a lymphokine-like substance which non-specifically arrests or induces to differentiate certain B-lymphocytes during their passage through tissue. The evidence for such an equivalent occurrence in lacrimal gland or conjunctival tissue remains unclear and there is a possibility that other mechanisms exist which operate to direct the localisation of IgA-producing cells in these tissues. Notwithstanding these findings, antigen is regarded as being responsible for the homing of IgA-committed lymphocytes to mucous membranes where they proceed to produce IgA as plasma cells.

In the rabbit, palpebral conjunctival aggregates of lymphoid tissue in the form of multiple nodules exist on the conjunctival surface. The conjunctiva-associated lymphoid tissue is morphologically similar to gut-associated lymphoid tissue and bronchus-associated tissue. Axelrod and Chandler (1978) have suggested that the conjunctiva-associated tissue may play a role in the secretory immune system similar to that proposed for gut- and bronchus-associated lymphoid tissue.

The capacity of the external eye to react against non-evasive antigens has recently been demonstrated by Hall and Pribnow (1981). New Zealand white rabbits were immunised by dropping ovalbumin into the conjunctival sac four times daily for three weeks. Many rabbits developed detectable haemagglutinating antibody by day 7, and all had antibody by day 14. The serum antibody persisted for at least six months after the beginning of immunisation. Plaque-forming cells were found in the lymph nodes, spleens, conjunctiva and limbal tissue. Fc receptor cells were found in all of the tissues examined but the number of Fc receptor cells did not seem to have any relationship to the numbers of plaque-forming cells in the same tissues. Such evidence points towards the possibility of future preventative measures against widespread ocular pathogens.

Protection against Virus Diseases

Protection against re-infection was one of the first mechanisms which linked virology and immunology with the observation that persons recovering from smallpox or measles would not get a second attack, i.e. they were immune. Variolation was the deliberate inoculation of virulent smallpox virus; this was protective on occasions, but in some cases caused death or permanent disfigurement. People living in the countryside had long known that those tending cows suffering from cowpox did not catch smallpox from them but merely got blisters on their hands. Also, they did not catch smallpox when it was prevalent in the rest of the community. Jenner investigated this systematically and his work culminated in the experiment on James Phipps and his writings on the subject published in 1798.

Pasteur, although trained as a chemist, turned his interest to infectious diseases in man, and made important contributions to immunology (Parish, 1965), including the development of live attenuated vaccine in 1880 with a bacterium, the chicken cholera bacillus, and in 1885 with the virus of rabies.

Pasteur coined the term vaccination in recognition of the similarity of his observations to the work of Jenner. In 1888 Roux and Yersin discovered diphtheria toxin and it was readily shown that immunity could be developed against such a toxin; the important observation was made in 1890 by Behring and Kitasato that this immunity could be transferred passively by inoculating serum from an immunised animal into an untreated one, i.e. that there was a specific antibody in the serum. The eventual elucidation of the chemical structure of the five immunoglobulins which act as antibodies is now part of the history of immunology.

The Role of Humoral Immunity

In primates natural passive transfer of antibody occurs from mother to newborn across the placenta and via milk and colostrum, the latter antibodies possibly being active in the gut lumen, although they may not enter the circulation. In mammals the placenta is permeable to IgG but not IgM or IgA, a fact which can be exploited in the diagnosis of congenital rubella where IgM in the cord blood represents the fetal synthesis of antibody, whereas IgG is maternal antibody secreted across the placenta.

The antibody response in laboratory animals is a dynamic one in the first instance, which in the case of viruses resembles the response to other antigens. There is a short inductive phase with an initial appearance of IgM antibodies followed by IgG which is persistent. In viral infections the initial antigenic dose is minute, but subsequently there is a dynamic relationship between the multiplying virus and its components, and the developing immune response which is of considerable significance in the immunopathogenesis.

Serum antibodies attracted considerable attention for many years and immunologists were mainly preoccupied with the 'spillover' concept of mucosal protection. However, the demonstration that IgA, a minor immunoglobulin in serum, was the predominant immunoglobulin class on mucosal surfaces such as those of the respiratory and gastro-intestinal tracts, led to the acceptance of its major role in the protection against respiratory and enteric infections.

Although the development of serum antibody responses constitutes a characteristic of most viral infections, its protective role varies from virus to virus. With most enteroviruses, myxo- and paramycoviruses, and arthropod-borne viruses, the circulating antibody, by its ability to limit viraemia and spread of virus to susceptible target organs, appears to be the major source of protective immunity. Mucosal antibody responses when stimulated locally are probably independent of the systemic response. However, mucosal antibody may also be generated following infection or immunisation with replicating or non-replicating viral agents, regardless of the route of administration, provided adequate amounts of viral antigen becomes available to the mucosal immuno-competent tissues. It is probable that many immunoglobulins must attach to a virus surface to render it non-infectious. From currently available data, there are three mechanisms for virus neutralisation: coating of the virus surface, aggregation of particles, and virolysis. Antibody alone may coat or aggregate, but complement may cause all three of these mechanisms of neutralisation to take place. Which one of these mechanisms takes place *in vivo* depends upon the relative quantity of virus, antibody and complement, as well as the type of virus and antibody involved (Daniels, 1975).

Though *in vitro* studies have demonstrated that antiviral antibodies and complement can interact with antigens at the surface of virus-infected cells and cause cell lysis, the role of this mechanism *in vivo* is not known. The nature of immunological injury to cells may be influenced by a number of factors, such as the nature of the expression of viral antigens on the cell surface. Where there are few antigenic sites, the cell surface might escape injury because it is necessary for the sites to be close enough to each other to allow IgG doublet formation, which is a requirement for complement activation. Such a concept might explain the persistence of virus-infected cells in the presence of antibody. There is indeed a parallel between the amount of surface antigen as determined by immunofluorescence and the sensitivity of antibody-induced cytotoxicity which has been demonstrated for measles. The effects of antibodies on cells could also be influenced by fluctuations in the amount of virus antigen on the surface; thus measles virus carrier cultures have been shown to undergo cycles of disappearance and reappearance of antigens, while intracellular antigens did not differ appreciably. It is not known whether fluctuations in surface antigen correlates with the variations in sensitivity to cytotoxic antibodies which have been noted in measles-infected cells.

Where antibody becomes attached to virus-infected cells there may be variable effects on the immunopathology of the infection. In one instance, normal leucocytes might attach to antibodies bound to target cells and initiate a cell-mediated cytolytic effect. This has been shown to occur with cells infected with herpes simplex virus *in vitro*. In other cases antibody may not have a cytolytic effect against target cells and can actually protect the cells against cell-mediated immune cytolysis by blocking the specific antigenic sites on the cell surface (Cole *et al.*, 1973); although this effect has been demonstrated *in vitro* no such effects have yet been demonstrated *in vivo*. Such a mechanism might go some way to explain persistent infections. There is data to suggest that binding of antibody to surface-associated viral antigens may indirectly influence intracellular viral DNA and antigen synthesis. Antibody-induced virus suppression has been postulated to be important in maintaining latent herpes infections in ganglion cells (Stevens and Cook, 1974).

Cell-mediated Immunity

The primary role of antibody is in protecting against infection and restricting the spread of extracellular virus, while that of the cell-mediated response is to promote recovery from infection by eliminating or restricting virus-infected cells. There is good evidence that effective cell-mediated reactions are crucial in recovery from certain virus infections. Analysis of patients with the immunodeficiency diseases has indicated that patients with hypogammaglobulinaemia recover normally from virus infections such as measles and varicella, and from vaccination. In contrast, patients with defects in cell-mediated immunity suffer from a variety of recurring and often fatal viral infections such as vaccinia, measles, varicella zoster, cytomegalovirus and herpes simplex virus. In animal systems it has been possible to demonstrate that thymic impairment, either by neonatal thymectomy or treatment with anti-thymus globulin can increase susceptibility to such viruses as herpes simplex virus. It has also been possible in some instances to restore immune competence and promote recovery from infection by transfer of immune T-cells, as in the case of studies carried out in lymphocytic choriomeningitis by Gilden *et al.* (1972).

The greatest progress in the understanding of cell-mediated immune reactions has come from the study of simplified *in vitro* systems. These models are of interest because they permit dissection and elucidation of the basic mechanisms underlying the response *in vivo*, and they also offer a potential for useful diagnostic tests. The mechanisms which are derived from these *in vitro* studies offer insight into the possible mechanisms which might occur *in vivo*. Interferon, which is one of the lymphokines, is produced by activated lymphocytes *in vitro* and *in vivo*. Other lymphokines are macrophage chemotactic factor and migration inhibition factor which are probably involved in attracting mononuclear phagocytes to the focus of infection, thus helping to limit its spread. A second general mechanism involves cell-mediated destruction of infected cells which display viral-induced antigens on their membranes. It is in this situation that the infected cells are recognised as foreign and presumably rejected. Assuming that the antigens are expressed prior to the time of full maturation, the cells will be destroyed by cellular immune lysis and virus replication will be aborted. On the other hand, in the absence of antibody excess and interferon, lysis of infected cells containing large amounts of already intact infectious virion could in fact serve to spread the infection. In the case of acute viral infections, the principal effect of cell-mediated cytotoxy is likely to assist recovery. In contrast it has also been shown that cell-mediated cytotoxicity of infected cells with LCM may be a major cause of the pathological process in the disease in question.

The Macrophage

Mononuclear phagocytes are effector cells in cell-mediated immune reactions which are influenced by activated T-cells. They may also act when they are specifically armed by antibody. Macrophage ingestion of viruses has been shown by immunofluorescence. Viruses can also be inactivated in Kupffer cells in the liver and in the macrophages lining the spleen. Macrophages may also act as non-permissive hosts for a variety of viruses such as the herpes simplex virus, vaccinia, and Coxsackie. It is of interest that viruses capable of producing cytopathological effects in various organs, if they also replicate in macrophages, usually produce lethal infections in adult animals. On the other hand, viruses which are not cytopathic but are nevertheless capable of replicating in macrophages may result in persistent infections. In studies using colloidal silica the vital role of mononuclear phagocytes is shown; after phagocytosis they cause intracellular breakdown of lysosomes leading to death of the macrophage. Using these techniques it can be demonstrated that adult mice normally resistant to intraperitoneal challenge with HSV, following pretreatment with silica, succumb to lethal hepatitis. This indicates that macrophages within the liver of an experimental animal play a crucial role as effector cells in the restriction of infection by the herpes simplex virus. Macrophages may act specifically by virtue or their Fc-C receptor which allows them to have ready access to complexes of all sorts. They are able to endocytose and inactivate antibody-virus complexes for which they are non-permissive.

Interferon

Interferon (IF) production is a fundamental cellular response to the presence of foreign nucleic acid in the form of double-stranded RNA. It is a low-molecular-weight protein (about 30 000) coded for by the cell in which it is produced. Possibly all cells, including epithelial cells, are capable of producing interferon when stimulated. Viruses are the most potent inducers of interferon, the foreign double-stranded RNA being formed in the course of their replication within the cell. The infected cell liberates interferon for a few hours, and acts on uninfected cells causing them to synthesise another protein that remains in the cell which protects against all viruses by inhibiting the action of viral messenger RNA. Interferon has no direct action on virus itself and does not interfere with entry of the virus into the cell itself. It has never been conclusively shown that IF is a vitally important part of the defence mechanism against viruses. The introduction of IF passively into experimental animals or its induction by the administration of a synthetic double-stranded RNA preparation (Poly I; poly C) has allowed demonstrable antiviral activity in experimental infection. It has been particularly evident in infections of epithelial surfaces such as the conjunctiva or respiratory tract when treatment is begun before rather than after the initiation of infection. IF would therefore seem to be an ideal antiviral chemotherapeutic agent for use in man, being non-toxic, non-allergenic, and active against a broad spectrum of viruses. However, systemic investigations in human patients have not produced dramatic results.

The inflammatory responses to virus infections therefore consist of many elements, including T-cells which are capable of killing infected target cells, macrophages which are able to inactivate and limit the spread of viruses, and antibody which can neutralise virus, but which possibly blocks T-cell killing. Antibody may also function as a cytophyllic antibody to help macrophage clearance of virus. Antigen-antibody complexes on cell surfaces have also been shown to permit target-cell killing by non-sensitised lymphocytes but the *in vivo* importance of this mechanism is not clear.

The effect of the inflammatory reaction probably depends largely on the nature and virulence of a virus and on the timing of the response. It is therefore not surprising that generalisations concerning the role of the inflammatory response in viral infections are difficult to make. In practical terms, enhancement or suppression of humoral or cell-mediated responses may have very different beneficial or adverse effects in different viral infections, and indeed different effects at varied times within the same infectious process.

SUGGESTED READING

BELLANTI, J. A. (1978). *Immunology II*. London: W. B. Saunders Co.
GELL, P. G. H., COOMBES, R. R. A. and LACHMAN, P. (1975). *Clinical Aspects of Immunology*, 3rd edit. Oxford: Blackwell.

Mims, C. A. (1977). *The Pathogenesis of Infectious Disease.* London: Academic Press.
Roitt, J. (1974). *Essential Immunology.* London: Blackwell Scientific Publications.

REFERENCES

Axelrod, A. J. and Chandler, J. W. (1978). Morphologic characteristics of conjunctival lymphoid tissue in the rabbit. In: *Immunology and Immunopathology of the Eye*, p. 292. Ed. A. M. Silverstein and R. O'Connor. New York: Masson.

Cole, G. A., Prendergast, R. A. and Henney, C. S. (1973). In: *Lymphocytic Choriomeningitis Virus and Other Arenaviruses*, p. 61. Ed. F. Lehman-Grube. Berlin: Springer Verlag.

Coombes, R. R. A. and Gell, P. G. H. (1975). In: *Clinical Aspects of Immunology*, 7th edit., p. 761. Ed. P. G. H. Gell, R. R. A. Coombes and P. J. Lachman. Oxford: Blackwell Scientific Publications.

Daniels, C. A. (1975). Mechanisms of viral neutralisation. In: *Viral Immunology and Immunopathology*. Ed. A. L. Notkins. London: Academic Press.

Dumonde, D. C., Wolstencroft, R. A., Panayi, G. S., Mathew, M., Morley, J. and Howsom, W. T. (1969). "Lymphokines", non-antibody mediators of cellular immunity generated by lymphocyte activation. *Nature (Lond.)*, **224**, 38.

Franklin, R. M., Kenyon, K. R. and Tomasi, T. B. (1973). Immunohistological studies of human lacrimal gland: Localisation of immunoglobulins secretory component and lactoferritin. *J. Immunol.*, **110**, 984.

Franklin, R. M., Prendergast, R. A. and Silverstein, A. M. (1978). Antigen-independent localisation of secretory IgA-producing plasma cells. In: *Immunology and Immunopathology of the Eye*, p. 302. Ed. A. M. Silverstein and R. O'Connor. New York: Masson.

Gilden, D. H., Cole, G. A. and Nathanson, N. (1972). Immunopathogenesis of acute central nervous system disease produced by lymphocytic choriomeningitis virus. II. Adoptive immunisation of virus carriers. *J. Exp. Med.*, **135**, 874–889.

Hall, J. M. and Pribnow, J. F. (1981). Topical ocular immunisation of rabbits. *Invest. Ophthal. & Vis. Sci.*, **21**, 753.

McFarlane, R. G. (1969). A discussion on triggered enzyme systems in blood plasma. *Proc. Roy. Soc. B.*, **173**, 259.

Parish, H. J. (1965). *A History of Immunisation.* Edinburgh: Livingstone.

Stevens, J. G. and Cook, M. L. (1974). Maintenance of latent herpetic infection: apparent role of antiviral IgG. *J. Immunol.*, **113**, 1685–1693.

Tomasi, T. B. and Bienenstock, J. (1968). Secretory immunoglobulins. *Adv. Immunol.*, **9**, 1.

CHAPTER THREE

The Eye and its Inflammatory Responses

The human eye is composed of an optical system which focuses light onto the retina whence the inverted image is conducted via the optic nerve to the cerebral cortex. These images are then processed and are eventually perceived and recognised according to previous experience.

The essential anatomy of the eye is based on an outer coat composed of the scleral/corneal capsule, on the inner side of the posterior two-thirds of which is found a highly vascular layer known as the uvea (Figure 3.1). The anterior portion of the uvea is separated from the cornea to form the anterior chamber, the uvea persisting as a diaphragm which is the iris, in the centre of which is the pupil. Immediately posterior to the iris is the ciliary body, which is a vascular layer responsible for the production of aqueous humour, and for the control of the variable power of the crystalline lens. The uvea continues as the choroid which underlies the retina and is responsible for supplying the outer layers of the retina which are avascular and which contain the rods and cones.

The transparent optic media consist of the cornea, aqueous humour, crystalline lens and vitreous humour; the lens plays a role in accommodation for near vision, while it is at the air-cornea interface that most of the refraction of light entering the eye takes place. The cornea has a number of functions in addition to its transparency, the fact that it is part of the outer coat of the eye indicating that it also has a protective role. The air-corneal interface is maintained as an optically perfect convex surface by the presence of a layer of tears. The tears are produced from glands in the bulbar conjunctiva which maintain the tear film in normal conditions. Where the eye become irritated by a foreign body, trauma, or inflammation, excessive watering of the eye may occur, due to the action of the lacrimal gland. In normal circumstances, evaporation of the tear film is prevented by an overlying oily lipid layer on the surface of the film.

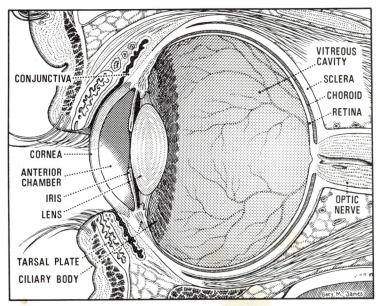

Figure 3.1. Coronal section of the human eye situated within the orbit. The uvea is composed of the iris, ciliary body and choroid. Most virus diseases involve the external eye, which is defined as the tissues of the lids, the conjunctivae both tarsal and bulbar, together with the conjunctival fornices, and the corneal layers. The sclera may be involved in some diseases. (Courtesy, M.T.P. Press Ltd.)

The external eye is composed of the lids, the lacrimal apparatus (which both produces tears and conducts them away via the nasolacrimal ducts) and the conjunctiva. The eyelids are thin curtains of skin, muscle, fibrous tissue and mucous membrane that protect the eye from external irritation, limit the amount of light entering the eye, and distribute moisture over the surface of the eye. Located in the free margin of the lids are the openings of the lacrimal canaliculi (the puncta lacrimalia), the eyelashes and the opening of glands. The intramarginal sulcus, or grey line, divides the eyelashes anteriorly from the orifices of the tarsal glands posterior to it. Opening into the follicle of each lash are the ducts of sebaceous glands and large sweat glands. The sebaceous secretion from the tarsal (Meibomian) glands prevents the overflow of tears, produces an airtight closure of the lid, and covers the eyeball with a layer of oily fluid which prevents the evaporation of tears.

The conjunctiva is a thin, transparent mucous membrane lining the inner portion of the lids, from where it is reflected onto the sclera. Between the scleral and tarsal portions is a cul-de-sac or fornix which forms a considerable extension to the conjunctival sac. The conjunctiva lining the lid is composed of marginal, tarsal and orbital portions. The portion on the lid margin forms a mucocutaneous junction at the grey line. The tarsal portion is closely adherent to the fibrous tissue of the tarsal plate and the orbital portion is thrown into folds. The bulbar portion is closely adherent to the sclera. At the medial angle of the eye are two specialised structures known as the caruncle and the semilunar fold. The conjunctiva consists of stratified epithelial cells and a well vascularised loose connective tissue. It is divided into the following subdivisions: marginal, tarsal, orbital, fornical, limbal and bulbar. These subdivisions possess distinct ultrastructural characteristics which reflect their different functions. The bulbar conjunctival epithelium consists of polygonal cells which are piled up in an irregular fashion, in contrast to the more orderly arrangement in the corneal epithelium. The surface epithelial cells contain plicae which are similar to those observed in the cornea. It is thought that the plicae are coated with mucopolysaccharides. The basal lamina is not complete, which enables wandering cells to migrate from the stroma to the epithelial cell layer. There are Langerhans cells (corneal histiocytes) in the suprabasal portion of the conjunctival epithelium.

The stroma resembles other connective-tissue networks and is composed of collagen fibres, fibroblasts, and a vascular system. Macrophages, polymorphs, lymphocytes, plasma cells, and eosinophils as well as mast cells may be present. The capillaries within the conjunctival stroma contain fenestrated and non-fenestrated endothelial cells.

The tear film has considerable importance and has several functions. It acts as a lubrication for corneal and conjunctival surfaces, and provides the first important optical surface for incoming light waves. Evaporation from the surface may account for corneal deturgescence to some extent. The film contains lysozyme and immunoglobulins, which are important in antibacterial protection. The tear film contains three layers: a superficial layer made of lipids produced and secreted by the glands of Zeis and Moll as well as the Meibomian glands. This prevents or retards the evaporation of tears, and also prevents spillage of tears from the lid margins. The middle layer is watery and is a lacrimal-gland secretion. The posterior layer of the tear film is in contact with the microvilli of the anterior surface of the corneal epithelium, and is mucoid. It is elaborated by the goblet cells of the conjunctiva.

The cornea in adults is oval with a horizontal diameter of 12 mm and a vertical diameter of 11 mm. The centre of the cornea is 0·5 mm in thickness. The anterior corneal epithelium is made up of 5 or 6 layers of squamous epithelium. The posterior layer is the basal layer which has its own basement membrane and rests on the anterior surface of Bowman's membrane. The basal cells are anchored in place to these structures by hemidesmosomes. The base of the basal cell is flat, whereas the anterior surface is dome-shaped. When the basal cells mitose, daughter cells are pushed anteriorly, where they are called wing cells. They are attached to neighbouring cells by desmosomes (Zinn, 1973). Superficial to the wing cell layer is a layer of flattened desquamated epithelium. On the anterior surface of the epithelium are villous projections which are thought to be important in tear-film stabilisation. In contrast to the basal cells, the superficial cells possess few intracellular organelles. Epithelium has high metabolic activity and is also a source of collagenase which may play a role in stromal melting problems. Bowman's membrane is an acellular zone of collagen fibrils 10–16 μm in thickness. The stroma comprises 90 per cent of the total thickness of the cornea. The cells are made up of keratocytes which are believed to be a form of fibrocyte. Under certain conditions, fibrocytes can be converted to fibroblasts, which can manufacture new collagen fibrils as well as mucopolysaccharides. The keratocyte is shaped like an amoeba with pseudopodal extensions or cell processes. The extracellular space consists of layers containing collagen fibrils and acid mucopolysaccharides. The collagen fibrils have a periodicity or 640 Å and a diameter ranging from 240 to 280 Å. They run parallel to each other in their own particular lamella, this ordered arrangement accounting in part for corneal transparency. Descemet's membrane has a smooth appearance and stains with PAS. It is a thick basement membrane which is secreted by the endothelium and composed of collagen and polysaccharides. The endothelium is a single cell layer which lines the posterior surface of the cornea. The cells are attached to each other by terminal bars. They have mitochondria and are rich in endoplasmic reticulum, which is an indicator of their high metabolic activity.

Because of the nature of the eye as a sensory organ, and its influence on survival, it seems that specific physical mechanisms have evolved to ensure its protection from damage (Figure 3.2). The blink reflex itself is one of the most rapidly occurring reflexes in the body, and is of the greatest significance in protection of the ocular surface. A reflex increase in flow of tears occurs following any ocular insult, such as the introduction of a foreign body onto the cornea, or beneath the tarsal plate. The corneal epithelial cells show a rapid turnover, and where they are disrupted following trauma they rapidly regenerate to cover the recently denuded surface. The epithelial cells characteristically possess tight junctions between them, which create a barrier to the entry

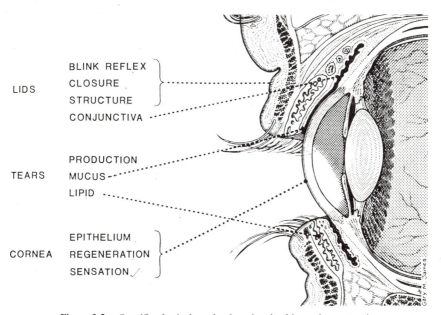

PHYSICAL FACTORS IN OCULAR SURFACE PROTECTION

LIDS

BLINK REFLEX
CLOSURE
STRUCTURE
CONJUNCTIVA

TEARS

PRODUCTION
MUCUS
LIPID

CORNEA

EPITHELIUM
REGENERATION
SENSATION

Figure 3.2.   Specific physical mechanisms involved in ocular protection.

of micro-organisms. The surface of the eye is exquisitely sensitive and foreign materials are rapidly dispelled from the surface by a copious flow of tears (Table 3.1).

A disease process affecting the conjunctiva presents some risk to the cornea, and it is because of this that infective conjunctival disease should be regarded as serious until it has been overcome. Severe infective corneal disease is not encountered very often, which is surprising in view of the many objects, such as contact lenses or cosmetics, introduced into the eye or onto the lid margins, which is an index that a high level of corneal protection has evolved. Because of the avascular nature of the cornea it has in the past been considered to be a privileged tissue, but it seems clear that specific protective mechanisms have developed which appear to be extremely efficient, although this is not so evident in less developed regions of the world. Where faults occur in the physical mechanisms of protection, there is increased risk of ocular infection (Table 3.2) (Easty, 1980).

On the other hand the ocular contents are privileged in an immunological sense by the presence of a blood-vitreous and blood-aqueous barrier. The optic media, composed of the crystalline lens, the aqueous humour and the vitreous humour, are separated from the vascular system by the presence of tight junctions in the vascular endothelium of the retinal vessels, the vessels of the ciliary body, and those of the iris. The inner layers of the pigmentary epithelium of the retina, ciliary body and iris also possess tight junctions between each cell, and are therefore part of the blood-aqueous and blood-vitreoretinal barrier. The contents of the eye are therefore free of the immunoglobulins and immunocompetent cells which might be present in other tissues of the body. Because of the isolation of the ocular cavity it has traditionally been thought to be at risk of severe microbial infection because of the ease with which such agents proliferate in this environment, which seemingly responds with a delayed inflammatory reaction that may eventually result in the loss of useful vision.

It is clear from this brief account of the anatomical structure of the eye and its sensory nature, with its transparent optical media, that it presents special immunological problems when it becomes infected. Viruses may enter via the external surface, where they may proliferate in the conjunctival sac or the corneal epithelium. Special protective mechanisms have evolved on the surface of the eye which appear to be extremely efficient. However, once a micro-organism penetrates to the subepithelial tissues, those immunological mechanisms which are stimulated in the epithelial phase of the disease continue to operate against invading organisms in the stroma. These reactions may combat spread, but at the same time may be responsible for causing persistent tissue damage, and hence produce lasting visual loss. Because of the presence of a blood-aqueous and blood-retinal and vitreal barrier, it is rare for blood-borne viruses to enter these tissues. The inflammatory responses of the conjunctival sac and the cornea show characteristic changes that can often be seen to bear a relationship to the original viral agent. Therefore the clinical examination of the conjunctival sac can help in making the preliminary diagnosis. Precise documentation of the clinical appearance of the disease is necessary so that the response to treatment may be accurately evaluated.

TABLE 3.1

MECHANISMS OF CORNEAL PROTECTION

Anatomical/physiological
  Full lid closure
  Good resting blink reflex
  Normal Bell's phenomenon
  Normal corneal sensation
  Good tear flow
  Maintenance of the epithelial barrier

Immunological
  Lactoferrin ⎫
  Mucus   ⎬ in tears
  IgA   ⎪
  IgG   ⎭
  Immunocompetent cells in limbus, conjunctiva and ciliary body (T- and B-cells)
  Presence of specific immunoglobulin in corneal stroma
  Systemic humoral and cell-mediated immune responses induced by microbial invasion of eye
  Production of neutrophil chemotactic factor by epithelial cell damage

TABLE 3.2

RISK FACTORS IN OCULAR INFECTIONS

External eye
  Disruption of epithelium (by abrasion or foreign body)
  Chronic infections of lids or lacrimal sac
  Poor lid closure
  Nocturnal corneal exposure
  Corneal anaesthesia
  Other ocular disease, for example allergic eye disease, peripheral corneal melting syndrome,
    cicatricial mucous membrane pemphigoid, tear-film anomalies, sicca syndrome, etc.
  Systemic immunosuppression
  Immunodeficiency syndromes
  Topical therapy to the eye
    corticosteroid
    prolonged use of antibiotics
  Genetic susceptibility to recurrent disease
  Contact-lens wear

Internal eye
  Penetrating injuries
  Intraocular surgery in the presence of extraocular infection
  Contamination of instruments and irrigating solutions
  Non-sterile technique
  Maternal infection during the first trimester (rubella, toxoplasma)

Immunological Protection of the External Eye

Immunological mechanisms may operate to protect against invasive micro-organisms prior to their entry into tissues, or against organisms which have already penetrated the tissues. The eye is protected by adaptive mechanisms, and the response to invasive organisms is modified by the presence or absence of these adaptive responses.

Tears contain lysozyme, a cationic low-molecular-weight enzyme which reduces the local concentration of susceptible bacteria by attacking the mucopeptides on their walls. Many Gram-positive bacteria are affected by lysozyme but *Staphylococcus aureus* is not, and it is this organism which is responsible for the chronic inflammatory external eye disease which accounts for many ophthalmic problems. Lysozyme is produced by the lacrimal gland in high concentration, and is elevated during the morning and reduced during sleep. Another tear protein, lactoferrin, has bacteriostatic properties, possibly due to the fact that it makes certain metals unavailable to micro-organisms (Broekhuyse, 1974). Complement is detectable in human tears, and C3 and C4 have been quantitated. The relationship of complement to protection or disease is at present unclear.

Langerhans' or dendritic cells have been identified in the corneal and conjunctival epithelium (Figure 3.3). The distribution in human epithelial sheets was demonstrated by histochemical, immunofluorescent, and electron-microscopic methods. Langerhans' cells stained positive with ATPase and with antibodies to HL-A Dr antigen. Human conjunctiva showed 250 to 300 Langerhans' cells per mm^2 compared to 15–20 per mm^2 in the peripheral third of the corneal epithelium. The position of these cells in the epithelial cells of the periphery of the cornea and in the conjunctiva possibly supports the concept of immune surveillance of chemical, microbial, or viral intrusions (Rodrigues *et al.*, 1981).

The *non-specific immune responses* (non-adaptive) (Figure 3.4) may be activated by physical mechanisms; trauma to the cornea resulting in an epithelial abrasion is accompanied by severe pain, photophobia, and vaso-dilatation of the microvasculature in the bulbar and tarsal conjunctiva. At the same time there is rapid entry of PMN cells into the tears and stroma, which find their way by chemotactic mechanisms to the injured area.

Normal conjunctiva forms a barrier to invasion by exogenous substances. There are large numbers of inflammatory cells present in the subepithelial layers, including lymphocytes, plasma cells and neutrophils. There are also fixed tissue mast cells. The epithelial cells of the conjunctiva may participate in phagocytosis. They may also bear surface receptors for invasive organisms as shown by conjunctival infection with Listeria and Chlamydia.

Invasion of the surface of the conjunctiva or cornea results in *adaptive humoral or cell-mediated immune responses*, both dependent upon the organism concerned (Figure 3.5). Infections with adenoviruses, *Chlamydia trachomatis* or herpes simplex virus may result in specific responses in local tissues, the draining lymph nodes, or the systemic circulation. The responses help to curtail infective disease and prevent entry of micro-organisms to deeper tissues.

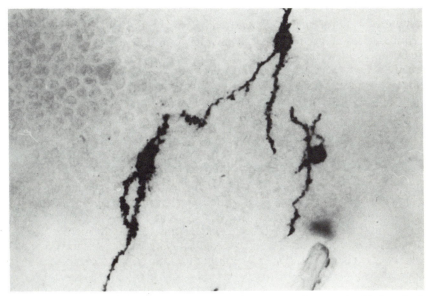

Figure 3.3. Langerhans' cells with 'streamer' dendritic processes in corneal epithelium in the guinea-pig. These cells may be capable of capturing and distributing antigen. (Courtesy, Mitchell H. Friedländer.)

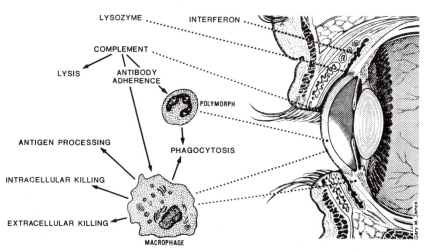

Figure 3.4. Natural non-specific immune responses in ocular-surface infective disease.

ADAPTIVE SPECIFIC RESPONSE

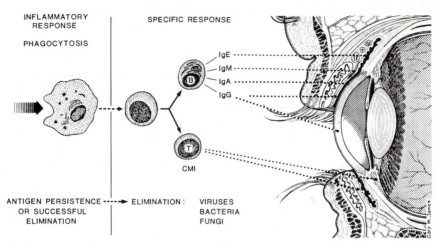

Figure 3.5. Adaptive immune responses occur following primary disease. In secondary infection they already exist.

Corneal stroma contains IgG, which probably acts against microbial agents (Allansmith *et al.*, 1973). The inflammatory reaction seen in the corneal stroma is determined by many factors, but the relative quantities of antigen and antibody probably decide whether antigen-antibody complexes are precipitated in the transparent tissue, or whether they remain in solution and escape towards the limbal vasculature and lymphatics.

Specific (adaptive) immune responses may exist prior to tissue invasion as secretory IgA in tears (Bluestone *et al.*, 1975), as with other external secretions. The presence of specific IgA would act to neutralise susceptible organisms prior to secondary invasion; for example, in the case of herpes simplex virus, which can be cultured from the conjunctival sac in the absence of clinically apparent disease, it is probable that IgA often neutralises and prevents attack of corneal epithelial cells by virus.

Once micro-organisms gain entry into the conjunctival or corneal epithelial layers, the mechanisms which prevent the spread of the virus are thought to include activation of the complement system, and the attraction of poly-morphonuclear leucocytes. When adaptive responses have already occurred in the host, modulation of infective disease occurs, with quick resolution. In primary infections the non-specific responses would operate to contain infection, but in many situations, resolution occurs only after the adaptive responses are stimulated.

Immunological Eye Diseases

There are a number of targets in or around the eye which are involved in immunological disease. The external eye may be subject to damage due to mechanisms which are aimed at combating infection by micro-organisms, or it may respond adversely as a hypersensitivity to external allergens. The cornea and the conjunctiva are affected, together with other mucous membranes and the skin, in autoimmune disease such as cicatricial mucous membrane pemphigoid. The cornea and sclera may demonstrate inflammatory responses associated with generalised immune complex or autoimmune diseases. The privileged nature of the contents of the eye allows corneal grafting to be carried out, although rejection can occur and is a well-recognised cause of failure.

The metastatic penetration of micro-organisms into the internal eye rarely occurs in systemic infections, but occurs in the newborn following maternal infections when the barrier between the systemic circulation and the ocular contents is not complete. Maternal toxoplasma infection is a well-recognised cause of retinochoroiditis, with its typical appearance; recurrences of inflammation can occur at the edge of a lesion later in life.

Entry of micro-organisms can occur following ocular surgery, when they produce sight-threatening infections. There may be delay in entry of antibody phagocytes and immune-competent cells, because of the avascularity of the ocular contents and the presence of the blood-aqueous and blood-vitreous barriers.

In contrast, because the uveal tract is in intimate contact with the intravascular compartment of the body, inflammatory disease is sometimes associated with systemic disease which has an immunological basis, for example ankylosing spondylitis.

The eye may be of help in the diagnosis of *immunodeficiency disease*, or may itself become infected as a result of deficits in immunological protection (Easty, 1977). The Chediak-Higashi syndrome is an autosomal recessive disorder characterised by recurrent and severe pyogenic infections, partial oculocutaneous albinism, and giant cytoplasmic granules in many cells, particularly the peripheral blood leucocytes. The phagocytic action of the leucocytes is defective against bacteria.

Ataxia telangiectasia is associated with immunodeficiency and is characterised by conjunctival telangiectasia, strabismus, and disconjugate gaze movement. There is also progressive ataxia and a variable immunodeficiency involving humoral or cellular immune responses. There is susceptibility to infection by bacterial and viral agents. Eye disease occurs in mucocutaneous candidiasis, which is characterised by persistent infection with *Candida albicans* involving mucous membranes associated with an endocrinopathy. The upper half of the cornea may demonstrate superficial stromal opacification and vascularisation (pannus). A punctate epithelial keratitis with the formation of micro-erosions produces a disturbing degree of photophobia. Selective IgA deficiency may be associated with allergic eye disease in the form of vernal catarrh, or with keratoconus. Severe generalised virus infections may cause immunodeficiency against other organisms, so that other secondary invaders may cause corneal infection.

Systemic therapy with immunosuppressive drugs may be associated with ocular infection usually by one of the herpes viruses. Herpes simplex keratitis can occur with considerable severity in renal-transplant patients, and cytomegalic inclusion disease of the retina may also be found. Topical corticosteroid medication induces local immunosuppression, which may allow uninhibited proliferation of the herpes simplex virus if prescribed erroneously, producing the amoeboid ulcer which may have serious consequences for vision.

The conjunctiva can act as a target and be sensitised by external airborne allergens which settle on the cornea, whence they are cleared by the flow of tears so that they eventually come into contact with the conjunctiva lining the tarsal plates.

Allergic conjunctivitis occurs in children and young adults. It may be mild and seasonal, or it can be persistent and severe. There may be mild itching, soreness and hyperaemia, with limited change in the tarsal plates (Figure 3.6). Where there is established disease, fine papillae form excrescences which disguise the normal vertical blood vessels of the tarsal plate. In the severe form of the disease there are large, persistent cobblestone papillae (Figure 3.7). During active disease the papillae become hyperaemic and engorged, and there is a profuse discharge. Patients with vernal disease of this type are generally atopic with strongly positive skin tests to a wide range of external allergens, elevation of serum IgE, and positive RAST. Specific antibodies can be found in the tears. Where the disease is persistent and severe, keratitis occurs and a corneal ulcer may be formed which may represent a threat to vision. The chronic ulcer is due to the deposition of layers of thick mucus which inhibit regeneration of the corneal epithelium so that the ulcer becomes chronic. There is clinical evidence that patients with atopic disease, or allergic conjunctivitis, may occasionally suffer from quite severe infection with the herpes simplex virus.

Autoimmunity causes disease of the eye according to a number of clinically recognisable syndromes. The criteria which are used to define the autoimmune diseases however have not been fully met in ocular disease, in contrast with other classical examples such as autoimmune thyroiditis, or experimental allergic encephalitis. Cicatricial mucous membrane pemphigoid involves the conjunctiva and is frequently a troublesome disorder. Shrinkage of the conjunctival sac occurs, and subepithelial bullae form which, on rupturing, induce a fibrotic reaction at the base of the lesion. Areas of denuded epithelium produce adhesions known by ophthalmologists as symblepharon. During this process, mucous glands in the conjunctiva are destroyed. Ultimately a reduced tear production occurs. Scarring of the tarsal plates induces inturned lashes which cause corneal epithelial abrasions. The immunopathology observed in the conjunctival epithelium resembles that seen in bullous pemphigoid lesions affecting the skin. Pemphigus vulgaris occasionally produces lesions affecting the conjunctiva but, unlike pemphigoid, is associated with circulating antibodies to an intracellular substance in the deeper layers of the conjunctival epithelium. There is evidence for complement binding at the site of antibody-antigen reaction in diseased tissues.

The periphery of the cornea is especially at risk of developing autoimmune-like changes because of the proximity of the tissue to a rich vascularised area at the limbus. In Mooren's ulcer, chronic ulceration begins at the periphery with a steep undermined and sometimes infiltrated border. The ulcer may spread around the corneal edge and then may extend towards the central area leaving a thinned, scarred and vascularised cornea. Ulcers may spread

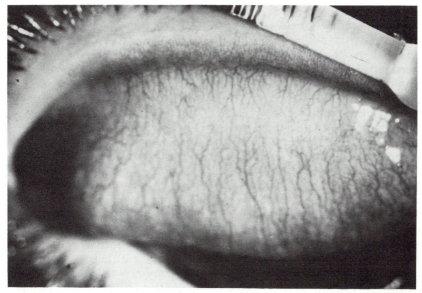

Figure 3.6. Mild inflammatory response in the everted upper tarsal plate in a patient with hay-fever conjunctivitis. The vascular system of the tarsal plate is normal and clearly seen.

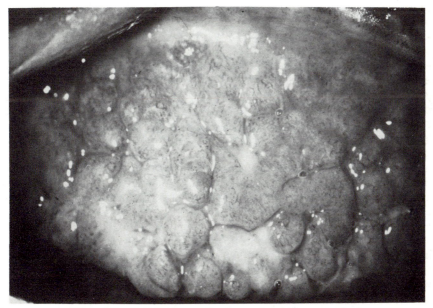

Figure 3.7. Cobblestone papillae in a patient with vernal catarrh.

remorselessly or may be self-limiting. In patients with severe disease an elevated island of cornea remains which eventually sloughs away. Occasionally, particularly when the condition is unassociated with other systemic disease, the prognosis for vision is poor. There are many associated conditions such as rheumatoid arthritis, Wegener's granulomatosis, and polyarteritis nodosa. The peripheral corneal melting syndromes as they are also called may follow peripheral infiltrates which are typical of those associated with staphylococcal disease of the lids, and also may follow herpes zoster ophthalmicus. In spite of the suspected autoimmune mechanisms, the evidence for such is not very convincing at the moment. Circulating antibody to corneal epithelium has occasionally been found, and immunoglobulins and complement have been noted to become bound to the conjunctival epithelium in the neighbourhood of the peripheral cornea. The melting process has been found to be associated with excessive production of collagenase from the conjunctiva, and attempts have been made to inhibit the enzyme degradation with anti-collagenases such as l-cysteine introduced topically. It seems likely that the peripheral corneal melting syndrome is the end-process caused by a number of systemic or local immunological mechanisms.

Sjögren's syndrome. Keratoconjunctivitis sicca, xerostomia, and rheumatoid arthritis or other connective-tissue disease coexist to form a disease pattern known as Sjögren's syndrome. Ninety per cent of patients are female; the disease presents in middle age, with dryness of the mouth due to reduced salivary-gland secretion, and difficulty with swallowing. There may be parotid-gland enlargement and dryness of the nasal mucosa. The eyes become gritty and sore with a reduced tear flow. Keratitis develops when micro-erosions occur, associated with mucus production, which may become attached to the corneal surface to form filaments in the upper part of the cornea. Tear lysozyme levels are reduced. Patients develop lymphoid infiltration of the salivary glands with eventual tissue destruction, scarring and fibrosis. Anti-nuclear factor may be found in 70 per cent of sera, and rheumatoid factor in 48 per cent. Lymphocytes show impaired transformation responses to mitogen and contact allergens. Management consists of control of the associated connective-tissue disorder with appropriate systemic therapy. Oral manifestations require dental examination, and careful hygiene. The dry eye can be treated with artificial tears, and occlusion of the tear-drainage system into the nasal cavity.

Uveitis may occur in isolation or in association with systemic infective or immunological disease. The term refers to inflammation of the uveal tract and may involve primarily the iris (iritis), the ciliary body (cyclitis), or choroid (choroiditis). The blood vessels of the iris and ciliary body become permeable to plasma protein, which escapes into the intra-ocular fluid together with inflammatory cells which can be seen in the anterior chamber with a slit-lamp microscope. Cells may form coin-like deposits on the corneal endothelium, when they are known as keratic precipitates, and may be either plasma cells or lymphocytes. The inflamed pupil margin may become adherent to the lens, producing adhesions leading to cataract.

The pathogenesis of uveitis has been investigated in animal models and it has been found that there are multiple auto-antigens associated with retinal receptors and the pigment epithelium, and these antigens have therefore been implicated in the pathogenesis of experimental allergic uveitis, and their role in patients with undiagnosed uveitis has been assessed. It has been shown that a soluble ('S') antigen exists surrounding the photoreceptor cells (Wacker *et al.*, 1977), together with a particulate ('P') antigen which is found in the rod outer segments. An insoluble ('U') antigen has also been located at the base of the pigment epithelium towards the choroidal surface. The S antigen has been identified in animal models as acting as a primary agent in uveitic inflammatory disease. Both humoral and cell-mediated immune responses appear to play a role in the disease produced by the S antigen. S antigen was able to induce a transformation of lymphocytes taken from patients with ocular inflammatory disease. This was particularly true where there was retinal involvement as a component of their disease. It is therefore apparent that certain cases of uveitis where the aetiology is unknown may represent an autoimmune response in the choroid directed against certain of the retinal antigens which may reach it via the pigment epithelial layer. It remains a possibility that the antigens may become significant in uveitis which is initiated by viral infection.

Retinal Vasculitis

Vasculitis predominantly involves the venous system in the retina, although it may occasionally affect the arterial system. Because the vessels of the retina are similar to those of the brain and the anterior uvea in that the endothelial cells have tight intercellular junctions, the escape of fluid from the intravascular compartment is minimal. In inflammatory disease this blood-retinal barrier is broken down, producing oedema together with retinal haemorrhages and exudates. The changes in vascular permeability are best demonstrated by fluorescein angiography of the retina. A peripheral type of disease which was originally described by Eales is found particularly in young adults, and is associated with intra-ocular haemorrhages, sometimes into the vitreous. The occasional association of retinal vasculitis with systemic inflammatory disease has suggested that it may be due to deposition of circulating immune complexes, and there is evidence of this at laboratory level.

Corneal Graft Rejection

The success of corneal transplants was for long thought to be due to the lack of antigenicity of the corneal elements, and the death of donor cell layers and their replacement by the host cells, before an immune response could be mounted. This adaptation was thought to render the tissue less susceptible to specific rejection even when the host became sensitised, in addition to which it was thought that the privileged nature of the cornea would sequester it from antibody and lymphocytes. It was subsequently shown experimentally that corneal graft rejection could occur, and that the layer involved was the endothelium. This layer is vital to corneal transparency because it is a fluid pump so that damage to it results in corneal swelling and graft failure. It is considered that the endothelium possesses little power to regenerate, so that once the rejection episode has taken place it means that a further transplant must be carried out. It has been shown that lymphocytes can react against the endothelium, which they reach via the scar of the interface or from the uveal tissue of the anterior segment. A lymphocyte line forms at a leash of vessels which may have reached the interface, which then progresses across the endothelium leaving a layer of dead cells in its wake (Figure 3.8). This process can be inhibited with the use of topical corticosteroid. There is a certain amount of evidence which suggests that sharing of two or more HL-A antigens between the donor and the recipient will reduce the incidence and severity of rejection, particularly in high-risk patients with active inflammatory disease of the anterior segment or with new vessels in the cornea.

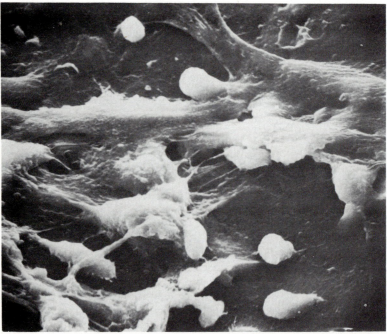

Figure 3.8.   Cytotoxic lymphocytes involved in active endothelial rejection (SEM×18 700). (Courtesy, Dr. Frank Pollock and MTP Press Ltd.)

There are therefore certain features of the eye which make it unique for the clinical and experimental immunologist. Its transparency makes it possible to observe inflammatory reactions in the cornea, retina and uvea with precision. Allergic reactions of the external eye can be equally well seen. The contents of the eye are privileged because of the special adaptation of the blood vessels of the retinal and anterior uvea. When the barrier between the blood and the aqueous and vitreous is broken down, there is a risk that the host may become sensitised to lens or retinal antigen.

Infective disease of the external eye is a common cause of visual disturbance. The spread of micro-organisms from the corneal epithelium into the stroma can be witnessed, although the mechanisms of tissue injury are as yet not understood (Easty, 1980). Nevertheless it is clear that the processes involve protective mechanisms directed against invading micro-organisms, or a sensitivity reaction to microbial antigen which is persistent in this tissue.

The Clinical Response in Microbial Disease

Although there are a number of viral agents which may invade the eye or its adnexa, it is those involving the external eye which are the more common in Western communities. The slit-lamp microscope allows detailed examination of the conjunctiva, of the tarsal plates and bulbar region, and the fornices of the lower lids. Examination of the upper fornices requires the aid of a lid retractor which enables the observer to 'double evert' the upper lid. Bacterial, mycotic and viral infections may produce characteristic changes in the conjunctiva and cornea which help the observer to diagnose (Table 3.3). The response of the conjunctiva to external allergens and to contact-lens wear may also produce changes which may confuse the unwary, and so care should be taken in documenting a precise history and description of the clinical findings.

The Chlamydiae are a cause of follicular conjunctivitis. These organisms are closely related to bacteria because they possess both DNA and RNA, and are sensitive to antibiotics. They cause inclusion conjunctivitis in adults and the newborn, and in endemic areas, trachoma. Chlamydia are obligate intracellular parasites which divert the synthetic capabilities of the cell towards their own metabolic requirements and towards the production of more organisms. Antibodies to Chlamydia of the IgG or IgA class can be found in tears of patients with trachoma or inclusion conjunctivitis. Antibodies can also be found in the serum by complement fixation tests. Since many people in Western communities are seropositive for chlamydial disease, it is important to establish an increasing antibody titre as an aid to diagnosis. Inclusion conjunctivitis in adults is comparatively rare, and is generally associated with a high antibody level.

Inclusion conjunctivitis may occur in the newborn as a result of infection via the birth canal. The lids become swollen and a papillary conjunctivitis may be present with a purulent discharge. In adults follicular conjunctivitis with palpable pre-auricular nodes may develop. The lower tarsal plate and upper fornix demonstrate large follicles (Figures 3.9 and 3.10). A superficial keratitis in the form of minute epithelial opacities may also be noted. Endemic trachoma is associated with corneal scarring and visual loss.

History and Examination

The patient's preliminary complaints help in diagnosis. Acute conjunctivitis due to bacterial causes may be present with a purulent or mucopurulent discharge, with stickiness of the lids on waking. There is a complaint of grittiness, or sand in the eyes, and some irritation. The patient may also complain of lid swelling and redness of the eyes, which may feel sore and uncomfortable. There may be tenderness in the region of the pre-auricular gland.

Patients with chronic involvement of the lid margins due to staphylococcal infections producing chronic blepharitis, with histories of recurrent styes or

TABLE 3.3

THE CLINICAL SIGNS OF CONJUNCTIVITIS AND THEIR CAUSES

	Bacteria	Staph. blepharitis	Chlamydiae	Primary HSV infection	Adenovirus	Haemorrhagic conjunctivitis	Type 1 HS	Foreign material e.g. CL prosthesis	Molluscum contagiosum	Warts	Thygeson's keratitis
Lid margins											
swelling	++	+	−	+	++	+	+	−	+	−	−
hyperaemia	++	++	−	+	+	+	+	−	+	−	−
meibomitis	+	++	−	−	−	−	−	−	−	−	−
notching	−	+	−	−	−	−	−	−	−	−	−
vesicles	−	−	−	+++	−	−	−	−	−	−	−
masses	−	Staph. chalazia	−	−	−	−	−	−	+	+	−
Palpable pre-auricular gland	+	+	+	+	+	+	?+	−	−	−	
Tarsal plates											
fine papillae	−	+	+	+	++	+	++	+	−	+	−
giant papillae	−	−	−	−	−	−	++	++	−	−	−
follicles	+ (moraxella)	+	+++	++	++	++	−	−	++	−	−
papillae and follicles	+	++	+	−	++		−	−	+	−	−
non-specific hyperaemia	++	+	−	−	−	−	+	+	+	+	−
haemorrhage	−	−	−	−	+	++	−	−	−	−−	−
inflammatory membrane	++ Haemolytic strep	−	−	−	+ (rare)	−	−	−	−	−	−
Cornea											
punctate epithelial keratitis	+	+	+	++	+	−	+	−	+	+	+
superficial stromal keratitis	−	−	+	+	+	−	+	−	−	−	−
diffuse stromal keratitis	−	rarely	+	+	rarely	−	−	−	−	−	−
Limbal reaction	+	+	+	+	+	+	+	+	+	−	−
Pannus		++	++	−	+		+	+	+	−	−

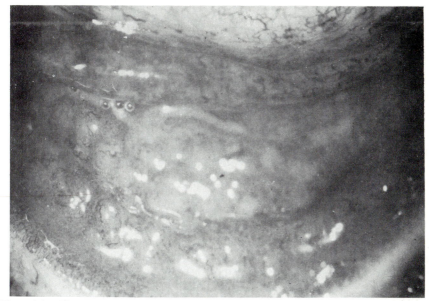

Figure 3.9. The lower fornix and tarsal plate in a patient with inclusion conjunctivitis. Many follicles are present.

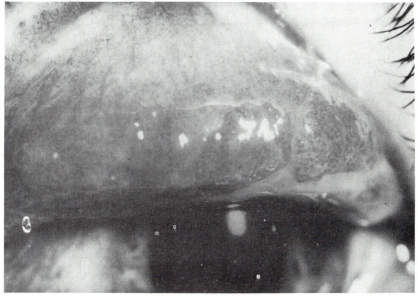

Figure 3.10. The everted upper tarsal plate with exposure of the fornix in a patient with inclusion conjunctivitis. Large follicles are apparent at the upper margin (i.e. the lower part of the tarsal plate as illustrated in the everted position).

chalazions, complain of redness of the lid margins, grittiness, photophobia and soreness and redness. Allergic conjunctivitis involving immediate type 1 hypersensitivity reactions causes similar symptoms, added to which itching can be pronounced. Generally such symptoms are transient and relate to an increase in one of the common environmental allergens such as tree or grass pollen, although in perennial disease an episodic history is no longer helpful in reaching a diagnosis.

Recognition of inflammatory disease of the tarsal plates requires experience. The reactions may often tell the observer a great deal about the cause of the conjunctivitis (Table 3.3). Experience is first gained from examination of the normal conjunctivae, so that subtle abnormality may be easily discerned.

In order to examine the tarsal conjunctiva it must be exposed; in the case of the lower lid this requires slight downwards and backwards pressure on the tissues immediately inferior to the lid which exposes the tarsal plate and the lower fornix for observation. To examine the upper lid, the lashes of the upper lid are taken between the finger and thumb of the left hand and counter-pressure is exerted at the upper margin of the tarsal plate on the external surface of the lid using a glass rod or an orange stick. The procedure should be carried out with care as it can cause discomfort for the patient in inflammatory disease. Once the upper lid has been everted it may be examined with the binocular microscrope without any further discomfort to the patient.

The inflammatory reactions occurring in the upper and lower lids are designated papillary or follicular according to their appearance and pathology. In the normal tarsal plates the conjunctiva is thin and transparent with a smooth surface. There is no sign of an inflammatory reaction and the vessels possess a regular appearance and anatomical arrangement. The vascular arcades of the upper tarsal plates can be seen and there is no vascular dilatation or new vessel formation. The lower tarsal plate shows a similar appearance and the fornix presents a series of folds without follicles.

Papillae change the anatomy of the tarsal conjunctiva, and present as an outgrowth from the conjunctival surface, with a central vascular core and an increase in the layers of the stratified epithelium. This is associated with increased cellular infiltration which may include polymorphs, plasma cells, lymphocytes, macrophages, mast cells and eosinophils. The reaction is generally seen as a response to external allergens (Figure 3.11), but also may accompany many other infective external diseases including adenoviral infections (Figure 3.12) (Easty, 1978). Papillary reactions can be quantified at a clinical level according to a simple scoring system which is helpful in the documentation of active disease, and in the performance of clinical trials where an insight into the influence of topical drug therapy may be required over a period of time.

Follicles may present in a number of diseases of the external eye where the infective agent is usually intracellular. Follicles have smooth, rounded surfaces and may be up to 0·25 mm in diameter. They are easily detected in the lower fornix but their differentiation from papillae is more difficult in the upper tarsal plate. Double eversion of the tarsal plate may be required to demonstrate them in the upper fornix (Figure 3.13), while in the tarsal plate they can be disguised by the presence of fine papillae, the follicles presenting as elevations

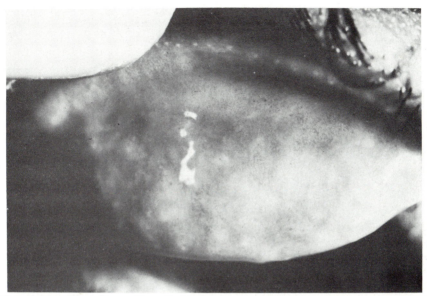

Figure 3.11. Diffuse fine papillae with infiltration and scarring in an adult atopic patient with persistent allergic conjunctivitis.

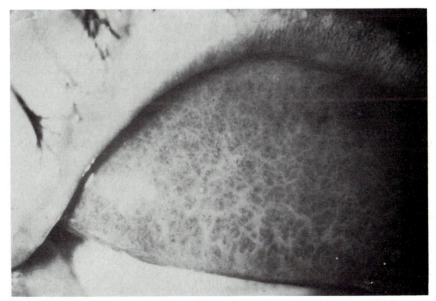

Figure 3.12. A marked papillary reaction in the tarsal plate as a result of adenoviral infection. There is no sign of the vertical vascular arcades that are seen in the normal tarsal plate.

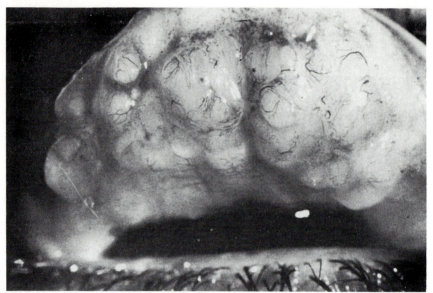

Figure 3.13. Massive chronic follicles seen in the doubly everted upper lid, in a patient with endemic trachoma. (Courtesy, Dr. Sorab Darougar and MTP Press Ltd.)

of the mucous membrane due to cell collections in the deeper tissues (Figure 3.14). They are seen more easily at the upper margin of the tarsal plate.

Active inflammation is accompanied by vascular hyperaemia of varying grades of severity, and by neovascularisation, which may present as central vessels in the papillae (Figure 3.15), or on the outer surface of the follicles (Figure 3.16). In addition neovascularisation occurs in chronic inflammatory conditions where there is a loss of the regular architecture which is seen with papillae or follicles, and the appearance of the vessels is haphazard.

Inflammatory cell infiltration is a feature of all reactions in the tarsal plates, be they due to external allergens or microbial agents, but the nature of these infiltrations can only be surmised from the examination. There is little known about the correlation between the clinical appearance and histopathology changes, neither is the effect of topical therapy on these inflammatory responses understood. Epithelial hyperplasia is frequently seen associated with chronic inflammation, particularly in the case of type 1 hypersensitivity responses (Easty, 1981). There may also be oedema of the surface epithelium, with separation of cells and escape of inflammatory cells into the tear film through these interruptions (Easty *et al.*, 1980). As a result of the various changes which can occur in the tarsal plates following inflammatory disease the normal vertical vascular arcades may be masked. The typical lid changes in a number of external ocular diseases due to various causes are demonstrated in Table 3.3. Occasionally, scarring of the tarsal plates or fornices may result (Figure 3.17) particularly following endemic trachoma.

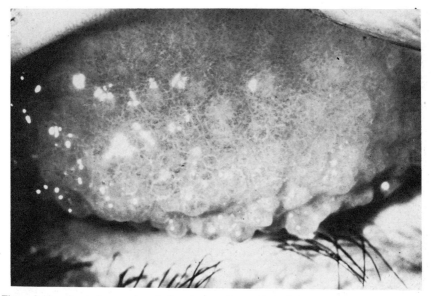

Figure 3.14. Everted upper tarsal plate in a patient with inclusion conjunctivitis; there is a papillary reaction in association with deeper follicles. There are also follicles at the upper border of the everted tarsal plate.

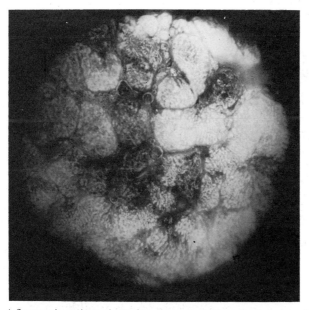

Figure 3.15. A fluorescein angiography study to demonstrate the vascular nature of conglomerate papillae in vernal disease. There are many micro-vessels which form a vascular core to each papilla.

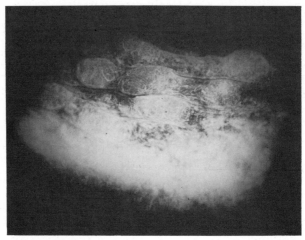

Figure 3.16.   Fluorescein angiography to demonstrate mainly surface vessels around follicles situated in the lower fornix in a patient with inclusion conjunctivitis.

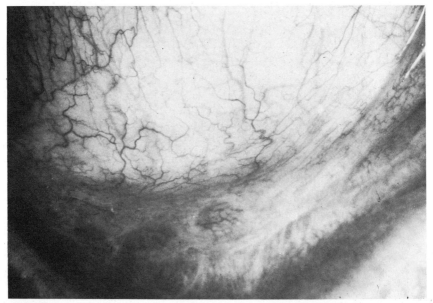

Figure 3.17.   Scar-tissue formation in the lower tarsal plate following membranous conjunctivitis due to adenovirus infection.

The bulbar conjunctiva becomes injected in association with infective disease, and at the limbus demonstrates formation of collections of inflammatory cells which produce a subtle nodular appearance or a diffuse swelling with vascular hyperaemia. A number of external ocular diseases induce ingrowth of conjunctival vessels in to the cornea at the cornea-scleral junction, in its upper half (pannus). It requires some experience to be sure that early pannus formation is present. An irregular pannus is seen following inclusion conjunctivitis, and is helpful in reaching a diagnosis (Figure 3.18). In contrast, pannus is rarely present in adenoviral conjunctivitis, and when there is any vascular ingrowth, it has a regular profile (Figure 3.19).

The cornea, because of its avascularity, is at risk of infective disease and is dependent on physical and immunological mechanisms for protection. Infective and allergic disease may affect the corneal epithelium in a number of ways. Spread of the disease into the stroma may have more lasting sequelae because of the disorganisation of the collagen fibrils and scar-tissue formation. It is these permanent changes in the stroma which lead to visual deterioration or blindness.

Documentation of Corneal Disease

Changes in the stroma should be documented in a simple and standard way so that other observers can comprehend the state of corneal disease; this helps in assessing the response to treatment when multiple observers are involved.

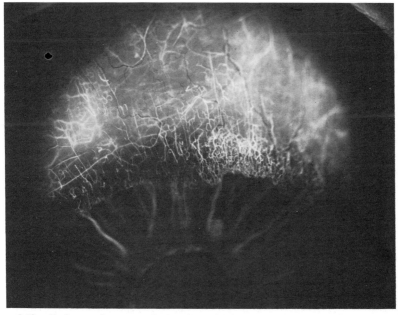

Figure 3.18. Early vascular pannus in a patient with inclusion conjunctivitis demonstrated by fluorescein angiography. The edge of the pannus is irregular.

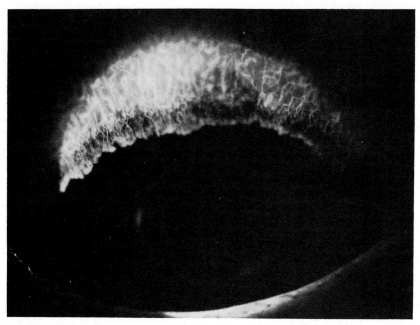

Figure 3.19. The limbal vascular reaction in a patient with adenovirus infection. Although there is a tendency for fluorescein leakage to occur at the apices of the vascular network, there is little sign of ingrowth.

Bron (1973) attempted to formalise the recording of clinical observations and has identified the problems which can be encountered in translating observations into documentary terms. It is difficult to identify exactly what composes a lesion which may be visualised in the cornea, and to understand how this relates to histological and immunological processes. However, careful attention must be aimed at precise documentation of corneal disease (Figure 3.20). Thus, corneal oedema can be represented by pencil shading, corneal scarring or opacity by vertical hatching, infiltrate by oblique single hatching, and a corneal abscess by oblique double hatching; oedema, scarring or opacity, infiltration and abscess formation can be coded with symbols O, S, I and A respectively. The corneal thickness must be assessed and identified by an estimate of the degree of swelling in comparison with the normal thickness, which can be expressed as a fraction. Corneal vessels are easily shown using a colour code, which can be red for deep vessels and blue for superficial vessels. However, vascular beds in opaque corneas may be very complicated and defy easy documentation (Figure 3.21). Staining reactions are also well shown using simple colour codes. Keratic precipitates can be represented as small round circles and annotated. Anterior synechiae can be demonstrated as a series of small crosses. Whatever the method of corneal documentation chosen it remains important that the method is comprehensible to other observers, so that either improvement or deterioration may be recognised when set against the record of previous corneal disease.

O = shading
S = vertical IIII
I = oblique single hatch
A = oblique double hatch

THE EYE AND ITS INFLAMMATORY RESPONSES   67

A surprising number of external diseases of the eye may be accompanied by punctate keratitis which may effect the epithelium, superficial stroma, or both. Table 3.3 indicates some of the causes of punctate keratitis. It may be difficult to recognise the aetiology without taking a full history and, on occasions, completing a series of investigations. For example, the herpes simplex virus can cause superficial stroma opacities which may be punctate in nature (Figure 3.22a, b). Chlamydial infection causes inclusion conjunctivitis with a superficial punctate keratitis at an early stage, and later stromal opacities (Figure 3.23). There is a rare punctate keratitis where opacities remain predominantly in the epithelium as minute conglomerations of white spots described by Thygeson. There is an absence of signs in the lids and tarsal plates, and the cause is not yet known (Figure 3.24). Because it is commonly misdiagnosed, patients may receive incorrect treatment. The lesions generally disappear with small quantities of topical corticosteroid, although they have a tendency to recur.

Corneal inflammatory diseases may be associated with involvement of the anterior uvea, and the reaction in the anterior chamber can be noted by observing the degree of proteinaceous exudate, which produces a flare, together with the appearance of inflammatory cells, both of which can be immediately scored by experienced observers. Inflammation in the uvea can produce adhesion of the pupil margin to the surface of the lens, so that the reaction of the pupil to light is disturbed; this may become apparent on dilatation of the pupil so that it has an irregular appearance.

Observation should be extended to the crystalline lens because both inflammatory disease in the anterior segment involving the uvea, the formation of posterior adhesions between the pupil margin and the lens surface (synechiae), and the tendency of prolonged corticosteroid medication to induce opacities in the posterior subcapsular region of the lens, all may contribute to the formation of permanent opacities which can affect vision.

In conclusion, it can be seen that the eye is subject to many diseases which affect the surface, some of which have a predominantly immune basis, while others, where external infection occurs, excite immune responses which may in themselves cause permanent effects on the eye as a visual organ. There are a large number of viruses which may cause eye disease, more commonly of the external eye (Table 3.4). Where viral disease is suspected, liaison should be made with microbiological teams so that a diagnosis may be made within the shortest possible time. Viral swabs should be taken; the technique should be meticulous, the swab being introduced into the fornices of the conjunctival sac to ensure a good yield of virus. Wet swabs dipped in transport medium probably give the most rewarding results. Where a particular virus is suspected, serum antibody should be requested on at least two occasions in order to identify a rising titre against a specific virus. The use of tear samples taken by capillary tubes and examined with electron microscopy following centrifugation is a method with potential, although its true status as a diagnostic aid has not yet been fully assessed. It has the important benefit of providing a dependable diagnosis at an early stage of the disease, which in the case of adenoviral conjunctivitis can be valuable. In the next chapters some of the work which has been carried out in virus disease of the eye is set against a background of

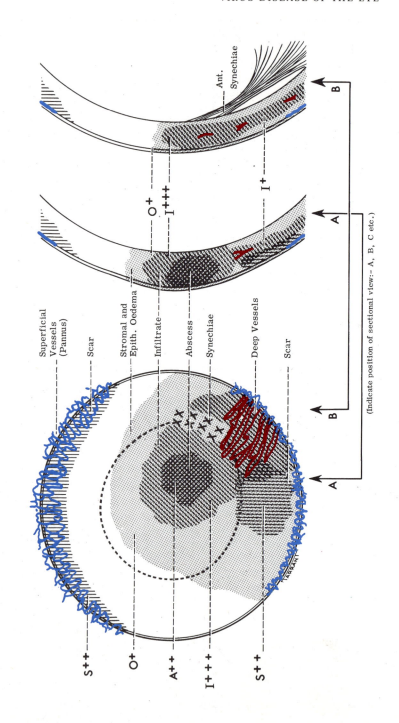

CHARTING CORNEAL DISEASE

Superficial
Vessels
(Pannus)

Scar

Stromal and
Epith. Oedema

Infiltrate

Abscess

Synechiae

Deep Vessels

Scar

Ant.
Synechiae

(Indicate position of sectional view:- A, B, C etc.)

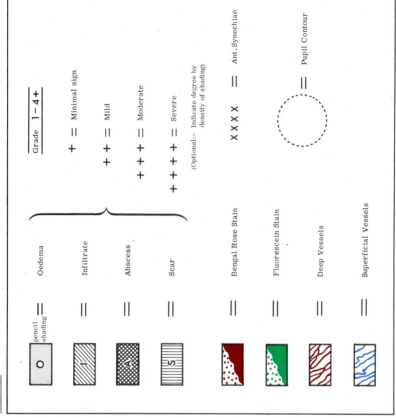

Department of Clinical Ophthalmology

Figure 3.20. A scheme suggested by Bron for accurate documentation of corneal inflammatory disease. (Courtesy Mr A. J. Bron, and the Editor of the *British Journal of Ophthalmology*.)

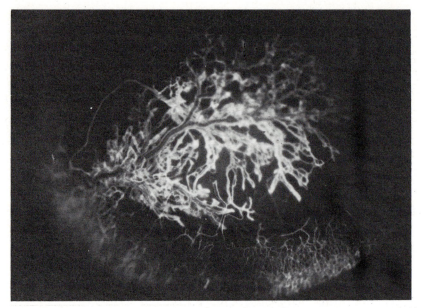

Figure 3.21.   Complicated vascular plexus in a patient with a dense corneal scar demonstrated by fluorescein angiography.

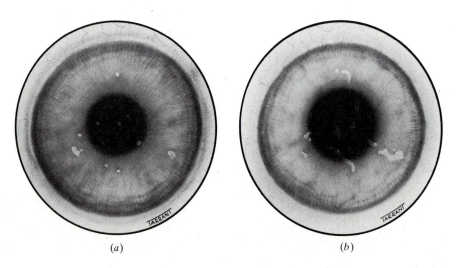

(a)   (b)

Figure 3.22.   (a) and (b) Bilateral superficial stromal punctate keratitis due to herpes simplex virus.

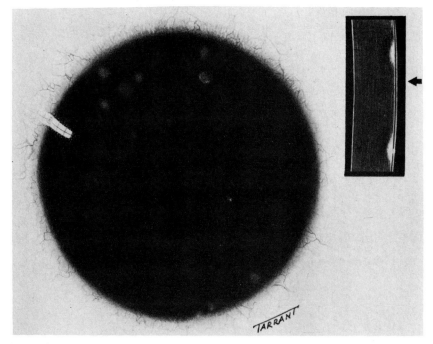

Figure 3.23. Superficial stromal punctate keratitis following inclusion conjunctivitis in a young adult.

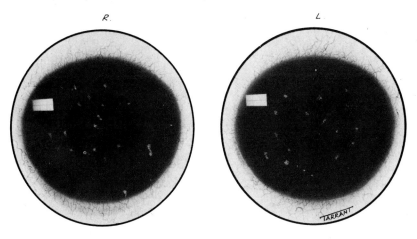

Figure 3.24. Thygeson's punctate epithelial keratitis.

TABLE 3.4
VIRUSES CAUSING EYE DISEASE

	Discharge: (W=watery, P=purulent)	PAG*	Lid margins: (H=hyperaemia, S=swelling)	Tarsal plates: (F=follicle, P=papillae, H=hyperaemia)	Bulbar conjunctiva: H=hyperaemia	Cornea*	Inner eye
Herpetoviridae							
HSV (primary)	W++ P++	+	vesicles H++ S++	F+++	H++	PEE dendrite	uveitis
Varicella	P++	++	vesicles H++ S+	F+	H+ limbal phyctenae	PEE, PEK DK	uveitis
Zoster	P++		H+ S++ vesicles++	F+ haemorrhage	H++	PEE dendrite DK	uveitis scleritis
CMV	–	–	–	–	–	–	uveitis retinitis congenital abnormality
EBV	++	+	S+ F+	F+ haems membrane	H++	DK	
Adenoviridae	W++	+	H+ S++	H++ F++ P++	H++	PEK SSPK	
Poxviridae							
Variola	P++	++	S++ H++	F++	H++ pustules	ulcers	uveitis
Vaccinia	P++	++	S++ H++	F++ P++	H++	PEE DK	uveitis
Molluscum contagiosum	W++	–	molluscum body	F++	H++	PEE, SSPK pannus	
Papovaviridae							
Wart virus	W++	–	warts	F+ multiple papillomata	H+	PEE	

	Discharge: (W=watery P=purulent)	PAG*	Lid margins: (H=hyperaemia S=swelling)	Tarsal plates: (F=follicle P=papillae H=hyperaemia)	Bulbar conjunctiva: H=hyperaemia	Cornea*	Inner eye
Picornaviridae							
Coxsackie A	P++	+	S+ H+	membrane	H++ phyctenae	pannus	uveitis
Enterovirus 70	P++	+	S+ H+	F+ P+	haems	–	–
Paramyxoviridae							
Newcastle disease	P+	++	S+ H+	P+ F+ haems		PEE	
Mumps	–	–	H+ oedema	–		PEE DK	–
Measles	++	+	S+ plica & caruncle	?membrane ?Koplick's spots		PEK PEE 2° infection	–
Togaviridae							
Rubella	–	–	–	?2F+	–	–	Congenital rubella syndrome
Bunyaviridae							
Sandfly fever	+	+		H++			
Rift-valley fever	+	+		H+			Retinal disease

* DK = disciform or diffuse keratitis; PAG = pre-auricular gland; PEE = punctuate epithelial erosions; PEK = punctate epithelial keratitis; SSPK = superficial stromal punctate keratitis.

immunological mechanisms, epidemiology and basic virology. Since herpes simplex keratitis provides severe problems in management, considerable efforts have been made by research teams in many parts of the world to learn more about the manner in which it causes eye disease. The balance of interest has therefore been directed at the pathological and immunological processes which follow and govern infection with this virus. The rapid expansion in synthetic antiviral therapy, which would be expected to continue in the future, has been largely directed against the herpes viruses. No apology is made, therefore, that much of the information in the following chapters is directed at this common and important infective agent.

RECOMMENDED READING

FRIEDLÄNDER, M. H. (1979). *Allergy and Immunology of the Eye*. London: Harper and Row.

REFERENCES

ALLANSMITH, M. R., WHITNEY, C. R., McCLELLAN, B. H. and NEWMAN, L. P. (1973). Immunoglobulins in the human eye. *Arch. Ophthal.*, **89**, 36.

BLUESTONE, R., EASTY, D. L. and GOLBERG, L. S. (1975). Lacrimal immunoglobulins and complement quantified by counterimmuno-electrophoresis. *Brit. J. Ophthal.*, **59**, 279.

BROEKHUYSE, R. M. (1974). Tear lactoferrin: a bacteriostatic and complexing protein. *Invest. Ophthal.*, **13**, 550.

BRON, A. J. (1973). A simple scheme for documenting corneal disease. *Brit. J. Ophthal.*, **57**, 629.

EASTY, D. L. (1977). Manifestations of immunodeficiency diseases in ophthalmology. *Trans. Ophthal. Soc. U.K.*, **97**, 8.

EASTY, D. L. (1978). Allergic disorders of the eye. *Practitioner*, **220**, 581.

EASTY, D. L. (1980). Infections of the eye. *Practitioner*, **226**, 593.

EASTY, D. L. (1981). Allergic diseases of the eye. In: *Immunological and Clinical Aspects of Allergy*. Ed. M. H. Lessoff. Lancaster: M.T.P. Press.

EASTY, D. L., BIRKENSHAW, M. and MERRETT, T. (1980). Immunological investigations in vernal eye disease. *Trans. Ophthal. Soc. U.K.*, **100**, 95.

RODRIGUES, M. M., ROWDEN, G., HACKETT, J. and BAKOS, I. (1981). Langerhans cells in the normal conjunctiva and peripheral cornea of selected species. *Invest. Ophthal. & Vis. Sci.*, **21**, 759.

WACKER, W. B., DOMOSO, L. A. and KALSOW, C. M. (1977). Experimental allergic uveitis. Isolation, characterisation and localisation of a soluble uveopathogenic antigen from bovine retina. *J. Immunol.*, **119**, 1949.

ZINN, K. M. (1973). Ocular fine structure for the clinician. In: *International Ophthalmological Clinics*. Boston: Little, Brown & Co.

CHAPTER FOUR

Virology of the Herpesviruses

It is a measure of the success of herpesviruses as parasites that they are extremely widespread throughout the animal kingdom, that they frequently remain associated with the host throughout life, and that many of them achieve the sophisticated stage of parasitism whereby they do not cause clinical disease throughout this lifelong infection. The four members of the group which naturally infect humans, the Epstein-Barr virus, cytomegalovirus, herpes zoster and herpes simplex, show all these characteristics as well as the propensity in some circumstances to cause severe and even fatal disease.

All four are typical of the herpesvirus group in their morphology, which remains a major feature used in their classification. In all, the viral capsid is enclosed within an envelope and itself contains the core of DNA. Antigenically however they are not closely related, and show no serological relationship with each other. As a result they have been assigned to four groups within the herpes viruses. This juxtaposition of similarities and differences is continued in their biological characteristics. All produce lifelong infections but the pathology (if any) that results varies widely, due to the fact that the four viruses infect and remain latent in very different cells and tissues within the body.

Epstein-Barr virus usually gains entry into the body via the throat. When infection is acquired in young children it is asymptomatic; latent infection is established in B-lymphocytes and some people become infectious carriers so that the virus can be very widely disseminated throughout a population without causing any apparent illness. However, when infection is delayed, the disease infectious mononucleosis results in about 50 per cent of individuals (Chapter 13). Virus multiplies in B-lymphocytes and probably epithelial cells in the lymphatic tissue of the nasopharynx, and is disseminated throughout the body presumably in B-lymphocytes. The characteristic mononucleosis, enlargement of lymph nodes and much of the general pathology result from the host's immune reaction via the T-lymphocytes against the infected B-lymphocytes. As the acute phase of the disease progresses antibodies are formed against a variety of viral antigens, the number of productively infected B-lymphocytes falls to very low levels, and the illness resolves. However, latent infection remains in the B-lymphocytes. During latent infection, the viral DNA exists as an integrated part of the DNA of the host cell and also as extrachromosomal DNA. A small proportion of lymphocytes continue to produce virus, and in Western societies about 20 per cent of latently infected people shed infectious virus from the oropharynx. In immunosuppressed individuals this proportion is increased to about 50 per cent but recurrence of clinical disease associated with the continuing infection is not seen.

Cytomegalovirus infection produces vastly different clinical responses, depending on the circumstances. In adults, infection (it is thought via the throat) is usually asymptomatic but various disease states including hepatitis, pneumonia and 'cytomegalovirus mononucleosis' have been associated with the agent (Chapter 13). Virus is excreted particularly in the urine and saliva, and the infection is probably lifelong. Latent infection is established in the lymphocytes but may be widely disseminated. The importance of the virus is magnified greatly in two particular circumstances. In individuals undergoing immunosuppression, for instance after organ transplantation, the infection can be troublesome, particularly since it is often carried in the kidney and can cause degeneration and loss of function of the transplanted tissue. The virus can also infect the fetus *in utero* (Chapter 12). In this situation the infection can lead to malformation or death; on the other hand it can again be asymptomatic. The very wide spectrum of clinical signs in infants infected at birth with cytomegalovirus suggests that the virus can infect tissues throughout the fetus.

Herpes zoster virus causes varicella, the widespread childhood disease, and zoster when the infection is reactivated; hence the alternative name, varicella zoster virus. In varicella, infection of the nasopharynx precedes haematogenous spread of virus to the skin where further multiplication occurs before and during the rash. Either from the skin or from the blood-stream, the virus invades the nervous system and can establish latent infection in any of the dorsal root ganglia. However, the extent of spread of latent infection through the nervous system is not known. After recovery from varicella the majority of individuals show no further clinical disease though it is assumed that the majority, if not all, carry the virus. That this excellent control of the continuing infection is mediated by the immunological response is suggested by the association of recurrent clinical disease—herpes zoster—with immunosuppression or immunodeficiency, though these are of course not prerequisites for its development. The skin lesions, similar in their pathology to the rash of varicella, are usually restricted to one dermatome, usually of the thorax. However, other parts of the trunk or the head may be the affected site and in the latter case the eye can be involved.

The Herpes Simplex Virus

Virology.—Herpes simplex viruses (HSV) are one of the most common causes of infection in man. There are two distinct serotypes (HSV-1 and 2) which are transmitted along different routes. HSV-1 is transmitted by direct contact between skin surfaces and mucous membrane, and generally affects areas above the waist, the maximum frequency occurring during childhood. HSV-2 is transmitted by venereal routes or from a maternal genital infection to the newborn. HSV-2 infection therefore occurs during adolescence or young adulthood and involves body surfaces below the waist, primarily affecting the genitals.

Herpes simplex viruses consist of four major components, a centrally located core surrounded by three concentric structures, capsid, tegument and envelope (Figures 4.1 and 4.2). The core contains DNA coiled around proteins arranged in the form of a barbel. The capsid contains 162 capsomeres and forms an icosahedral structure which measures about 100 nm. The tegument is composed of fibrillous material and lies between the capsid and the envelope. The envelope is derived from nuclear and other cell membranes, and confers an external particle diameter of 150-200 nm. The envelope is composed of lipid, which makes the virus susceptible to lipid and ether solvents, and proteins, which are similar to those found in the membranes of infected cells, so that immunological mechanisms which are set up to destroy the virus may also act against the cell. There are at least 49 proteins specified by the virus, 33 of which are present in the virion. The variations in protein structure within

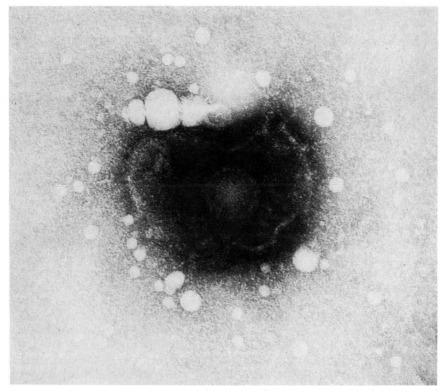

Figure 4.1. Electron micrograph of herpes simplex virus, showing the enveloping membrane and centrally placed capsid. (× 132 600; Courtesy, Dr. Susan Clarke.)

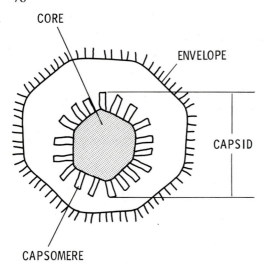

CORE

ENVELOPE

CAPSID

CAPSOMERE

Figure 4.2. Sectional diagram to demonstrate the basic morphological structure of the herpes viruses.

various strains of either type 1 or 2 HSV may influence immune responses, serodiagnosis and disease severity.

DNA of HSV-1 and HSV-2 are double-stranded linear molecules 99 ± 5 million daltons in molecular weight (Table 4.1). *In vitro* it is possible to infect cells with naked DNA, free of virus proteins, and to demonstrate defective DNA in some strains of HSV, which is of possible relevance to the oncogenic potential of HSV. HSV-1 and 2 show different responses to exposure to a high temperature, HSV-2 being more labile at 39° than HSV-1. There are also differences in susceptibility to antiviral agents, which therefore affects therapy. Fever is known to reactivate HSV-1 recurrence but is not thought to be an important trigger of recurrence in HSV-2 infection. The viruses are also labile at low pH and they can be recovered from the gastro-intestinal tract. It is unlikely that either HSV-1 or HSV-2 would remain infectious for any duration outside the human body.

New approaches have now been developed to determine the nature of the herpes viruses by the analysis of herpes virus DNAs. DNA double strands can be separated into complementary single strands by treatment with heat or alkali, a process which can be reversed. Where repeated and simultaneously inverted sequences of nucleic acid occur in the double strand, parts of the single strand will be complementary to each other and may self-anneal, forming one or several loops which can be visualised with the electron microscope. Using such techniques, a search has been carried out for homology between different viruses when these viruses are mixed and incubated under annealing conditions. Complementary regions of single strands may hybridise. The use of radioactively labelled DNA allows detection of the hybrid double strands. On a basis of molecular data of this sort, arising from sequence homology or genome arrangement and length together with the biological properties of the virus, a new subgrouping of herpes viruses has recently been

TABLE 4.1

DIFFERENCES BETWEEN HERPES SIMPLEX VIRUSES, TYPES 1 AND 2

	Type 1	Type 2
Clinical	Infects non-genital sites	Infects genital sites primarily
Latency	Primary involvement of the trigeminal ganglion	Primary involvement of the sacral ganglia
Transmission	Via non-genital route	Via a genital route
Disease in animal model (rabbit) of keratitis	Early epithelial disease without the appearance of stromal disease	Delayed appearance of epithelial disease, with elevation of the edges using SEM. Increased risk of stromal disease
	Virus isolated up to 16th day	Virus isolated at 31st day in low titre
Biochemical and Biophysical		
DNA guanine and cytosine (Mol %)	67	69
Homology of viral DNAs proteins	Around 50% unique capsid proteins; differences in thymidine kinase	
Heat stability	more stable	more labile
Biological		
Chick embryo chorioallantoic membrane	small pocks	large pocks
Tissue culture	Differences between types in their ability to propagate, their cytopathic characteristics or plaque size and susceptibility to antiviral drugs in certain cell-culture lines.	

Adapted from Nahmias and Visintine (1976).

adopted. Thus, viruses which have similar DNA size and arrangement fit well into subfamilies called alpha, beta and gamma. Subfamily alpha contains the herpes simplex virus group containing HSV-1 and 2, and Herpes B virus. Subfamily beta contains the cytomegalovirus group, while subfamily gamma contains the lymphoproliferative group with the EB virus (Table 4.2).

A second fundamental technique has been developed which has directed attention at strain differences between viruses. It involves the use of bacterial endonucleases, restriction enzymes the action of which is directed towards a certain sequence within a DNA double strand. These enzymes cleave DNA into well-defined fragments dependent on the occurrence of a specific recognition sequence. Fragments are formed which may be separated by electrophoresis through an agarose gel, where they form bands in positions which are related to their size (Figure 4.3). This has allowed the development of a variety of new approaches towards the formulation of functional maps of viral genomes. Investigations have shown not only that HSV-1 and 2 can be discriminated by the technique, but also that different strains of HSV-1 can be

TABLE 4.2

CLASSIFICATION OF HERPES VIRUSES

Subfamily Alpha	*Herpes simplex virus group*
	HSV-1
	HSV-2
	Herpes B virus
	Bovine mamillitis virus
	Equine abortion virus
Subfamily Beta	*Cytomegalovirus group*
	Human CMV, and possibly other mammalian cytomegaloviruses
Subfamily Gamma	*Lymphoproliferative virus group*
	EB virus
	EBV-like simian viruses
	Herpesvirus saimir
	Herpesvirus ateles
Orphan (perhaps Delta)	Varicella zoster virus, and probably related simian viruses.

identified. It is apparent that there are a large number of herpes simplex strains circulating in the human population. Neumann-Haefelin and Sundmacher (1981) found that there was a considerable heterogeneity of strains in corneal isolates from a large population of infected patients. Studies of neurovirulence in mice and the biochemical analysis revealed considerable differences between individual strains. However, no correlation was found to exist between biological and biochemical strain characteristics and clinical features of the disease process.

Laboratory diagnosis.—Morphological techniques can be used to demonstrate intranuclear inclusions and multinucleated giant cells in smears of cells which have been fixed in 90 per cent alcohol, obtained by scraping the base of herpetic vesicles or ulcers of the skin or mouth, or from scrapings of the conjunctiva or cornea. The inclusions are characteristic of herpesviruses including HSV and VZV. Intranuclear inclusions are less readily apparent in Giemsa-stained smears, and Papanicolaou-stained smears show the changes more clearly.

There are an increasing number of serological tests which can be carried out, and it is possible that eventually it will be possible to identify strain differences using more sophisticated technology. Neutralisation, complement fixation, passive haemagglutination, complement-mediated cytolysis and in direct immunofluorescent tests can be employed. The enzyme-linked immunosorbent assay (ELISA) is likely to become useful in the measurement of antibody in small amounts of fluid, such as tears. Antibody to HSV-1 and HSV-2 can be determined by more specialised serological techniques, such as microneutralisation, kinetic neutralisation, multiplicity analysis, and inhibition passive haemagglutination tests. Primary infection is suggested by a four-fold rise in titre between the acute and convalescent serum obtained one week or

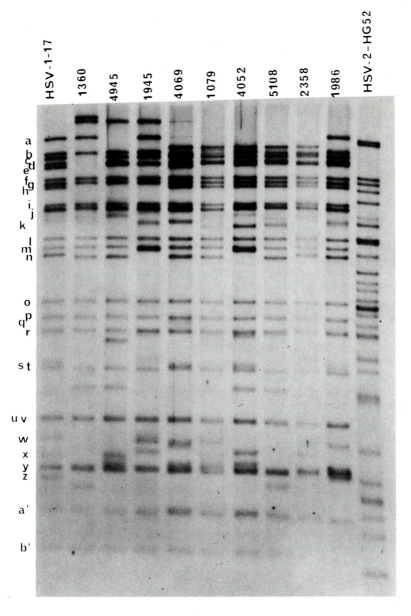

Figure 4.3. Agarose gel electrophoresis patterns following endonuclease restrictase cleavage digest of HSV isolate DNA. Nine HSV-1 facial-lesion isolates are compared with standard type 1 strain 17 on the left, and HSV-2 strain HG 52 on the right. (Courtesy, Professor J. H. Subak-Sharpe and Dr. Stafan J. Chaney.)

more later. The difference in titres during and following recurrence is less clear. Microassays for identifying HSV antibody in tears have been reported by Darougar and Forsey (1981).

Specimens for virus isolation should be frozen at −70°C until processed. Transport medium has facilitated the movement of specimens, since the swab with which the specimen is obtained, when placed in medium, can be stored and transported at ambient temperature. Herpes simplex virus can be isolated readily in tissue-culture systems, and a pathognomonic cytopathic effect is detected rapidly within one to three days. Specific identification of HSV and its antigenic types can be obtained by neutralisation or immunofluorescence. The latter can be used for rapid identification and direct typing of clinical specimens. These tests have been used in the past for diagnosis of HSV infections in brain biopsies taken from patients suspected of suffering herpes encephalitis.

The virus can be easily demonstrated in vesicular fluid, biopsy or autopsy specimens, or tears, using electron microscopy which may reveal enveloped or non-enveloped particles. Using this technique, HSV cannot be distinguished from other herpes viruses such as cytomegalovirus or varicella zoster. The use of specific antibody labelled with ferritin or horseradish peroxidase will allow a clear-cut identification.

Methods for typing of HSV-1 and 2 are rapidly becoming more sophisticated, using monoclonal antibodies, restriction endonuclease viral DNA analysis, and drug sensitivity (Zimmerman et al., 1983). Monoclonal antibodies can detect and type the virus in a rapid test procedure in both isolates and in direct smears if a sufficient number of infected cells is available. The development of selective antiviral drugs such as bromovinyl deoxyuridine will intensify the need to type patient smears or isolates rapidly and accurately for effective therapy in serious disease.

In the next chapters the major herpes viruses which affect the eye, the herpes simplex virus and herpes zoster virus, will be discussed. The ocular effects of the cytomegalovirus and the EB virus are discussed in Chapters 12 and 13.

REFERENCES

DAROUGAR, S. and FORSEY, T. (1981). A micro-immunofluorescent test for detecting type-specific antibodies to herpes simplex virus. In: *Herpetic Eye Diseases*, p. 183. Ed. R. Sundmacher. Munich: J. F. Bergmann Verlag.

NAHMIAS, A. J. and VISINTINE, A. M. (1976). Type 2 herpes simplex virus infections. *Survey Ophthal.*, **21**, 115–120.

NEUMANN-HAEFELIN, D. and SUNDMACHER, R. (1981). Herpesviruses—common properties and heterogeneity. In: *Herpetic Eye Diseases*, pp. 3–13. Ed. R. Sundmacher. Munich: J. F. Bergmann Verlag.

ZIMMERMANN, D. H., MUNDON, F. K., CRUSON, S. E., HENCHAL, L. S., DOCHERTY, J. J. and O'NEILL, S. P. (1983). Typing of herpes simplex virus types 1 and 2 in clinical isolates by the use of monoclonal antibodies, restriction endonuclease viral DNA analysis, and sensitivity to the drug (E)-5-(-2-bromovinyl)–2'-deoxyuridine. In: *International Herpesvirus Workshop, Oxford*, p. 96.

CHAPTER FIVE

Latency and Recurrence in Herpes Simplex Virus Infection

W. A. BLYTH

THE mouth is usually the site of primary infection with type 1 HSV. Although the infection is often mild or even asymptomatic, severe gingivostomatitis with associated lymphadenitis can develop. The infection is usually acquired in early childhood and traditionally has been extremely common, with over half of populations affected. However, the infection is now somewhat less common, particularly in socio-economic classes 1 and 2 of western societies. Recurrent disease varies in its frequency in different individuals and may decrease with age. Virus is shed in the mouths of 2–5 per cent of asymptomatic carriers with or without a history of disease, so that the epidemiological cycle is hard to break. From primary infection in the mouth the latent infection is carried in the trigeminal ganglion.

The frequency of infection with HSV has meant that subsequent recurrent infections with type 1 at different sites (most usually the eye) or with type 2 venereal infection of the genitalia have usually been in 'immune' hosts. However, if the epidemiology of infection is changing so that more people suffer their primary infection in the eye for instance, the severity of disease seen in such cases may increase. Studies in mice and rabbits with ocular herpes infection indicate that the protection afforded by previous primary infection might mitigate against the chances of further infection from another source.

To discuss the mechanisms underlying latent infection and recurrent disease it is necessary to rely largely on evidence from animal models of the disease, predominantly mice, rabbits and guinea-pigs. Moreover, models of recurrent disease are established only for infection in the skin. When this evidence has been considered, the closeness of analogy to the human disease will be assessed, as will the similarities and possible differences in the disease as it affects the skin and the eye.

Primary Infection

To establish infection with HSV the virus must be injected into the tissue or the surface must be damaged, for instance by scarification. Virus introduced fractionally after scarification does not take. During the days following inoculation, virus multiplies predominantly in epithelial cells but it can invade the deeper surrounding tissue. Peak virus titres are reached 3–4 days after introduction into the skin, and both here and in the eye, after conjunctival or corneal entry, active disease ceases within two weeks. Severity of clinical signs is related to dose of virus and to the extent of damage induced at the inoculation site, but lack of such signs does not imply that infection did not occur. The usual signs in the skin are inflammation, vesicle formation and ulceration, leading to scabbing. With HSV type 1 there is no evidence for blood-borne spread of virus to other tissues, though some virus or viral antigens must reach the lymph nodes to initiate the immune response, but with type 2 there may be such spread. As far as is known, according to experimental evidence, the virus (type 1) is cleared from the skin or eye of mice and rabbits when the primary lesions heal but there is some evidence of chronic or latent infection in the skin when guinea-pigs are infected in the foot pad (Scriba, 1977).

Spread of Infection to the Nervous System and Establishment of Latency

HSV can be isolated from the related sensory ganglia very soon after its inoculation into the skin or eye. Indeed with a large inoculum (10^7 plaque-forming units of virus), virus from the inoculum itself can be found in the ganglion; multiplication at the periphery is therefore not essential for invasion of the nervous system. In one experimental study amputation of the infected limb two days after inoculation of virus into the footpad did not stop establishment of latent infection in the dorsal root ganglia. Virus gains entry into the axon presumably via the sensory nerve endings in the skin and is carried by retrograde axonal flow to the cell body of the neuron in the ganglion. Travel of virus up the nerve could also occur by multiplication in Schwann cells and cell-to-cell transfer along them, but the observed speed of travel shows that this route is irrelevant to the establishment of infection in the nervous system.

During primary infection in peripheral tissue there is also productive infection in neurons of the sensory ganglia. Peak virus titres are found 4–6 days after inoculation and infectious virus can not usually be found later than 10–14 days after inoculation. It is likely that neurons productively infected with HSV inevitably die, so that these individual cells clearly cannot become latently infected. There is now evidence that productive infection in the ganglion, far from being necessary to the establishment of latent infection, might under some circumstances hinder its development (Sekizawa *et al.*, 1980). In this study mice were treated with anti-HSV serum during primary infection induced by inoculating the scarified cornea with HSV type 1. In those animals most successfully treated no infective virus could be isolated from the trigeminal ganglion during primary infection, but the incidence of latent infection was higher than in animals treated with normal serum. It is likely, therefore, that when a virus particle reaches the neuron cell body either the virus replicates and kills the cell, or replication does not start and the viral DNA remains latent in the cell, integrated into the DNA of the host or as extrachromosal DNA.

Latent HSV infection is, of course, not restricted to the sensory ganglia. In humans the virus has been isolated from the ganglia of the sympathetic system, and in mice infected by the intra-ocular route the superior cervical ganglion is frequently infected (Price and Schmitz, 1979). Even in mice infected in the skin of the ear this ganglion can occasionally become infected. More important perhaps is that after infection in the skin, HSV type 1 can be isolated from the brain stems of mice without signs of neurological disease and, during latent infection, sequences of viral DNA have been identified in the brain stems of mice infected intra-ocularly (Cabrera et al., 1980). In assessing this evidence it should be noted that in mice, strains of HSV type 1 are neurovirulent, so that doses of virus greater than about 10^5 plaque-forming units injected into the skin cause fatal encephalitis in a considerable proportion (often 10–80 per cent) of the animals. With HSV type 2 the fatal dose is usually at least 100-fold less than with type 1.

Productive infection with a virus such as HSV is simply defined. When cells are disrupted immediately after tissue is removed from the host and the suspension is inoculated on to susceptible cell cultures, the virus can be isolated. During latent HSV infection, however, no virus is found by this technique. Only if tissue is cultivated in vitro as an organ culture for some days or even weeks can the virus be isolated. Often the organ culture (frequently of one or more sensory ganglia) is grown for four days before being disrupted and seeded onto indicator cell cultures for virus growth. Such techniques never have absolute sensitivity of course so that interpreting negative results is difficult. For instance, it was noted previously that infective HSV could not be isolated from ganglia by immediate disruption of cells later than about two weeks after infection. In one study, however, where especially sensitive indicator cells were used to detect virus growth, low levels of infective virus were found in sensory ganglia from a high proportion of mice for longer than this two-week period, and the incidence of virus isolation decreased only slowly over a period of some months (Schwartz et al., 1978). If this observation can be confirmed it raises the possibility that chronic productive infection continues during the early phase of latent infection. Alternatively, this virus might arise from frequent reactivation from the latent state (see below); a choice cannot yet be made between the two interpretations.

Control of Latency

It could be argued that a latent infection requires the most intimate relationship that can exist between a virus and host cell and that by virtue of the establishment of this relationship the virus is brought under the control of the cell metabolism. When the specialised nature of the neuron is considered (for instance the complete repression of cell division) control of a DNA virus might even be automatic. However, in practice the control of HSV by the host is clearly not complete and there are many other mechanisms that might affect the relationship. The immune response against HSV includes production of antibodies that neutralise viral infectivity. The titre of these antibodies remains high throughout life even in the absence of recurrent disease, which suggests periodic production of viral antigens to provide continuing stimulus to the immune system. In some experimental systems such antibody can prevent replication of HSV in the ganglion. For instance when latently infected ganglia in millipore chambers were implanted into the peritoneal cavity of normal mice, infective virus developed. However, if the recipient mice were treated with antiserum against HSV or were themselves latently infected, no such virus appeared (Stevens and Cooke, 1974). Under natural circumstances the picture cannot be so simple since, in the study cited previously where mice were treated with antiserum during primary infection, latent infection continued under control when all detectable antibody in their *serum* had disappeared (Sekizawa *et al.*, 1980). In a further study, antibody administered passively to mice during primary infection limited *spread* of infection in the nervous system but not establishment of the latent infection (McKendall *et al.*, 1979). Perhaps more important, agammaglobulinaemic patients are not especially susceptible to overwhelming HSV infection.

The cellular immune system is also stimulated by HSV infection. Cytotoxic T-lymphocytes appear in the draining lymph node early in experimental infection, but their presence is transient (Nash *et al.*, 1980). On the other hand, lymphocytes that undergo transformation in response to HSV antigens are present for long periods. Some studies in humans suggested that a temporary specific depression of CMI was associated with recurrent herpes simplex but these reports need confirmation before they can be assessed (Babiuk and Rouse, 1979). Results from immunosuppression both experimentally and in humans are complex. In one experimental study recurrent herpes was not induced by various immunosuppressive agents but in another its incidence was increased (Blyth *et al.*, 1980*a*). When the variety of agents, different dosages and periods of treatment and underlying disease are considered, it is hardly surprising that experience with human patients has been varied. In some studies recurrent herpes simplex has been frequent, in others it has hardly appeared. However, one thing is agreed; that if recurrent herpes appears in immunosuppressed patients the lesions are likely to be severe and extensive. It may not be too bold to suggest that the host's immune response may not provide the overriding mechanism by which latency is controlled. However, it undoubtedly is important in recovery from productive infection.

Reactivation of Infection in the Nervous System

Infectious HSV can be isolated from affected ganglia of very small proportions of latently infected mice (0–10 per cent in different studies). This probably represents the spontaneous recurrence of productive infection, i.e. reactivation of the latent infection. The mechanisms governing this reactivation are not known, but the incidence of isolation can be dramatically increased by various stimuli. These include administration of cyclophosphamide, pneumococcal infection, section of the nerves distal to the ganglia, and trauma to the ganglia. Some authors have suggested that the cyclophosphamide acts by immunosuppression, but at the very high doses found necessary for this effect (up to 200 mg/kg) this cannot properly be assumed. The last two techniques induce direct changes within the ganglion, and the chromatolysis in neurons after nerve section, with its attendant dramatic effect on the cellular metabolism, might be particularly significant in the release of virus from the latent state. These results have led to the view that the ganglia are the main site of latent infection. However, this view must be treated with caution; there is already some evidence that virus spreads to the brain (in mice) (Cabrera *et al.*, 1980; Kastrukoff *et al.*, 1981), and it may be that the ganglia assume a position of importance in HSV infection only because virus replication is most easily reactivated from this site.

Development of Recurrent Disease

By interpreting the experimental results on reactivation of infection in the ganglion, some authors have suggested that recurrence of herpes simplex involves the following steps: stimulation in the nervous tissue resulting in production of infectious virus, transfer of virus along axons to the periphery, and multiplication of virus in epithelial cells to produce a lesion. In this sequence it is implicit that the major site of control of the infection is in the ganglion and that, if virus escapes from this control (and invades peripheral tissue) a lesion results (Merigan, 1974).

However, it is difficult to find evidence for this sequence. Clinical lesions at the periphery have not been recognised in animals subjected to the stimuli known to reactivate virus in the ganglion. This was particularly apparent in latently infected rabbits in which trauma was induced by insertion of a needle into the trigeminal ganglion. Although infectious virus was isolated from the eye secretions of about 80 per cent of these animals, no clinical signs in the eye were noted (Nesburn, 1976). There are many other reports of shedding of infectious HSV in eye or mouth secretions without obvious clinical signs and, by organ cultivation *in vitro*, the virus has been grown from the skin of latently infected but clinically normal mice. These animals were infected in the skin of the pinna, and skin from this area was cultured. Thus it is clear that the presence of HSV in skin or secretions is insufficient to cause recurrent clinical lesions, and 'controls' other than those in the nervous system must be overcome before disease develops. It is very probable that reactivation of infection in the nervous system is an important step, but its relationship to induction of recurrent disease in a target organ is not yet understood.

In humans it is characteristic of recurrent herpes labialis that lesions are apparently induced by a variety of stimuli. These vary widely: some primarily affect the skin, such as sunburn or other minor trauma, others have both a central and a local effect, such as upper respiratory tract infections (with local inflammation around the nose as well as systemic effects); in others, such as menstruation and emotional stress, the site of action could be anywhere in the body. Experimentally, only procedures that primarily affect the skin by causing inflammation have so far induced recurrent disease in the skin. These include irradiation by UV light, trauma (produced by stripping the skin with cellulose tape) and application of various chemicals to the skin. All are applied in the area of original infection by the virus and recurrent disease takes a form similar to that in humans. Vesicles develop, they are infiltrated by cells and the lesions can form ulcers before scabbing and healing follow. All the stimuli that induce such disease damage cells in the epithelium, and all induce repair mechanisms in the skin cells. This action in the skin does not of course preclude effects elsewhere, for instance in the nervous system through alterations at the nerve endings in the skin. Indeed there is already some evidence that trauma in the skin can lead to the appearance of an increased incidence of infectious virus in the ganglia. There are a number of studies which have produced good evidence of virus reactivation in the eye but have not shown true disease recurrence at a clinical level. A number of stimuli have been tested in experimental animals; Nesburn (1976) showed that topical injection of adrenaline, electrical shock and trauma to the trigeminal ganglion produced shedding of herpes simplex virus in tears in previously infected eyes. Kwon et al. (1981) induced shedding by using iontophoresis to increase corneal adrenaline concentration, and at the same time were able to show reactivation in the trigeminal ganglion. Willey et al. (1983) have been able to demonstrate reactivation in mice by adrenaline iontophoresis. From consideration of such results and other evidence in both humans and animals the following scheme has been proposed to explain the development of recurrent herpes simplex.

Virus 'escapes' intermittently from the latent state in neurons in the ganglia so that a productive infection develops with eventual death of the neuron. On occasions, such virus travels down axons potentially to invade cells for instance in the skin, salivary gland, or lacrimal gland. Here the virus particle is disposed of, for example by polymorphonuclear leucocytes or macrophages (particularly if it is opsonised by antibody), or it invades a cell. Indeed it is possible that it is delivered directly into a cell by transfer across the membrane of a nerve ending. If the cell supports virus replication it is liable to recognition and destruction by cell-mediated mechanisms by virtue of the viral antigens expressed in its membrane. Alternatively the cell's metabolic state in an organised tissue might render it non-permissive for virus replication even in the absence of efficient immunological control. In either case the infection would not develop. Only on relatively rare occasions do conditions favour virus replication to the extent that a clinical lesion develops in spite of established control mechanisms. In skin it appears that these conditions are met during an inflammatory reaction and regeneration after injury. The epithelial cells are then metabolically altered, and pharmacological changes then occurring are known to suppress some local immunological responses. This development of recurrent lesions is controlled by mechanisms operating in the skin as well as those that control viral latency in the neuron (Figure 5.1; Hill and Blyth, 1976).

Effect of Treatment on Latent Infection and Future Recurrent Lesions

It is possible that during recurrent disease the infectious virus in peripheral tissue can act as a source for further invasion of the nervous system, perhaps with establishment of new foci of latent infection. The evidence now available, though scant, suggests that even if this occurs it is not necessary for continued latent infection. With potent antiviral drugs now available to treat both primary and recurrent herpes simplex infections such theoretical considerations become important in considering a strategy for therapy. If experimental primary infections are successfully treated there is undoubtedly less replication

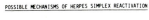

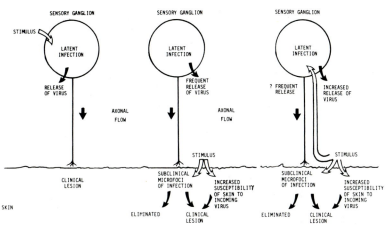

Figure 5.1. On the left the 'ganglion trigger' theory requires that an occasional stimulus (so far undefined) acts directly on neurons in the ganglia to release virus from latency. Virions travel via the axon to the periphery where they replicate to cause a lesion. The latent infection is controlled in the nervous system.

In the centre the 'skin trigger' theory suggests that virus is frequently released from latency (perhaps without stimulus or by minor physiological changes), travels axonally to the periphery and is then usually eliminated. Only if a stimulus affects the peripheral tissue to provide favourable conditions for virus replication does a lesion develop. Recurrent disease is controlled in the peripheral tissue.

On the right the combined (and most plausible) theory suggests that stimuli applied to peripheral tissue (e.g. trauma or UV light) acts both locally and in the nervous tissue. Lesions result only if conditions favour replication of virus in both sites, and control mechanisms act both centrally and at the periphery.

of virus in peripheral tissue, and it is reasonable to assume that less virus is therefore available to establish infection in nervous tissue. With such treatment less infective virus can be isolated from ganglia during the primary infection, and in some studies a lower proportion of mice showed latent infection in the ganglia (Field *et al.*, 1979). However, the inverse relationship between the amount of infective virus found during primary disease and the incidence of latent infection in animals treated with antiserum against HSV (cited previously) gives cause for concern that treatment of primary disease may not always be entirely beneficial.

Recurrent herpes simplex can be prevented in experimental studies if systemic or local treatment with, for instance, Acyclovir is started before the skin is damaged to elicit lesions (Blyth *et al.*, 1980*b*). Alternatively, the severity of clinical lesions can be lessened if local treatment is started when inflammation first develops. However, such treatments do not affect the chance that recurrent disease will develop after later occasions when the skin is damaged without treatment, nor do they alter the incidence of isolation of virus from ganglia cultured *in vitro* some time after treatment has been stopped. Thus it seems likely that treatments so far tested do not affect the latent infection.

Comparison between Species and between Anatomical Sites

Results from experiments in animals allow some detail to be added to the pattern of disease production by HSV and to discussion of a likely sequence of events underlying the clinical disease. Where comparison is possible with observations on the disease in humans, the chain of events is so similar as to suggest that the infections in animals are reasonably close models of the human disease and that interpretations drawn from the one might well apply to the other. Some important points cannot yet be compared however. One such is the question of the dissemination of the latent infection (or even productive infection) within the central nervous system. There is some preliminary evidence to suggest that in humans, as in mice, viral DNA occurs in brain tissue (Sequiera et al., 1979), but this needs confirmation. There is also indirect epidemiological evidence linking a variety of psychiatric abnormalities with carriage of HSV, but this too is difficult to assess (Cleobury et al., 1971). Further understanding of the development of herpetic encephalitis in humans, and possibilities for its treatment, must probably await more evidence on this important point. Similarly, more knowledge of the mechanisms and relative importance of controls of the infection operating in the nervous system and in peripheral tissue might allow new approaches to treatment or prevention of recurrent disease. In this context vaccines are being developed, but clinical use is probably some time away.

Comparison of recurrent herpes in the skin and the eye poses some fascinating questions. In true primary ocular infection the virus must obviously originate from some other person. However, in initial ocular infection in someone carrying the virus, the origin of the infecting virus is open to question. Since virus can be shed in saliva, this may provide an exogenous source for infection when labial lesions are absent, but the inoculum could also arise from the nervous system of the patient. This last possibility, for which there is already experimental evidence, requires that neurons providing axons to ophthalmic tissues become latently infected as a result of lesions in or around the mouth, and clearly implies spread of latent infection within the nervous system of humans.

The pathogenesis of recurrent lesions also poses questions. The absence of clinical signs when HSV can be isolated from eye secretions suggests that local control mechanisms must be overcome for keratitis to develop. On the other hand disease might result only if virus is delivered directly from nerve endings to epithelial cells in the conjunctiva or cornea so that virus in secretions might be irrelevant. Stimuli that induce recurrent ophthalmic herpes are not nearly so well defined as those acting on the skin. Indeed, with the possible exception of fever their presence might even be questioned. Only with information on some at least of the areas of doubt will it be possible to use the new therapeutic agents most effectively. With such information however it may be possible to avoid the development of recurrent lesions instead of merely treating each episode of disease as it arises.

REFERENCES

BABIUK, L. A. and ROUSE, B. I. (1979). Immune control of herpesvirus latency. *Canad. J. Microbiol.*, **25**, 267–274.

BLYTH, W. A., HARBOUR, D. A. and HILL, T. J. (1980a). Effect of immunosuppression on recurrent herpes simplex in mice. *Infection & Immunity*, **29**, 902–907.

BLYTH, W. A., HARBOUR, D. A. and HILL, T. J. (1980b). Effect of Acyclovir on recurrence of herpes simplex skin lesions in mice. *J. Gen. Virol.*, **48**, 417–419.

CABRERA, C. V., WOHLENBERG, C., OPENSHAW, H., REY-MENDEZ, M., PUGA, A. and NOTKINS, A. L. (1980). Herpes simplex virus DNA sequences in the central nervous system of latently infected mice. *Nature*, **288**, 288–290.

CLEOBURY, J. F., SKINNER, G. R. B., THOULESS, M. E. and WILDY, P. (1971). Association between psychopathic disorder and serum antibody to herpes simplex virus (Type 1). *Brit. Med. J.*, **1**, 438–439.

FIELD, H. J., BELL, S. E., ELION, G. B., NASH, A. A. and WILDY, P. (1979). Effect of acycloguanosine treatment of acute and latent herpes simplex infections in mice. *Antimicrob. Agents & Chemother.*, **15**, 554–561.

HILL, T. J. and BLYTH, W. A. (1976). An alternative theory of herpes simplex recurrence and a possible role for prostaglandins. *Lancet*, **1**, 397–399.

KASTRUKOFF, L., LONG, C., DOHERTY, P. C., WROBLEWSKA, Z. and KOPROWSKI, H. (1981). Isolation of virus from brain after immunosuppression of mice with latent herpes simplex. *Nature*, **291**, 432–433.

KWON, B. S., GANGAROSA, L. P., BURCH, K. D., DE BACK, J. and HILL, J. M. (1981). Induction of ocular herpes simplex virus shedding by iontophoresis of epinephrine into the rabbit cornea. *Invest. Ophthal. & Vis. Sci.*, **21**, 442–449.

MCKENDALL, R. R., KLASSEN, T. and BARINGER, J. R. (1979). Host defences in herpes simplex infections of the nervous system: Effect of antibody on disease and viral spread. *Infection & Immunity*, **23**, 305–311.

MERIGAN, T. C. (1974). Host defences against viral diseases. *New Engl. J. Med.*, **290**, 323–329.

NASH, A. A., QUARTEY-PAPAFIO, R. and WILDY, P. (1980). Cell mediated immunity in herpes simplex virus-infected mice: Functional analysis of lymph node cells during periods of acute and latent infection, with reference to cytotoxic and memory cells. *J. Gen. Virol.*, **49**, 309–317.

NESBURN, A. B. (1976). Effect of trigeminal nerve and ganglion manipulation on recurrence of ocular herpes simplex in rabbits. *Invest. Ophthal.*, **15**, 726.

PRICE, R. W. and SCHMITZ, J. (1979). Route of infection, systemic host resistance and integrity of ganglionic axons influence acute and latent herpes simplex virus infection of the superior cervical ganglion. *Infection & Immunity*, **23**, 373–383.

SCHWARTZ, J., WHETSELL, W. O. and ELIZAN, T. S. (1978). Latent herpes simplex virus infection of mice—infectious virus in homogenates of latently infected dorsal root ganglia. *J. Neuropath. Exp. Neurol.*, **37**, 45–55.

SCHRIBA, M. (1977). Extraneural localisation of herpes simplex virus in latently infected guinea pigs. *Nature*, **267**, 529–531.

SEKIZAWA, T., OPENSHAW, H., WOHLENBERG, C. and NOTKINS, A. L. (1980). Latency of herpes simplex virus in absence of neutralising antibody: model for reactivation. *Science*, **210**, 1026–1028.

SEQUIERA, L. W., JENNINGS, L. C., CARRASCO, L. H., LORD, M. A. and SUTTON, R. N. P. (1979). Detection of herpes simplex virus genome in brain tissue. *Lancet*, **2**, 609–612.

STEVENS, J. C. and COOKE, M. L. (1974). Maintenance of latent herpetic infection: apparent role of antiviral IgG. *J. Immunol.*, **113**, 1685–1693.

WILLEY, D. E., NESBURN, A. B. and TROUSDALE, M. D. (1983). Reactivation of latent ocular herpes simplex virus infection in mice by epinephrine iontophoresis. In: *International Herpesvirus Workshop, Oxford*, p. 178.

CHAPTER SIX

Immune Responses to Herpes Simplex Virus

ALTHOUGH there have been many advances in the control of virus disease by the development of vaccines, during the last two decades there has been considerable interest in the way the host defends itself against viral infections, particularly in relation to latent infection (Notkins, 1974). It is because of the realisation that the herpes simplex virus may be important in other diseases such as carcinoma of the cervix uteri that scientific interest has been directed into the investigation of the immune responses against the virus *in vitro* and *in vivo*, using animal models. In this section the information so gathered will be discussed, and the immune reactions which have been reported in humans following various types of herpetic disease will be described.

In vitro Investigations

It has long been realised that a number of viruses remain infectious in the presence of neutralising antibody. This focused attention on the role of cell-mediated immune defence mechanisms in the recovery from certain viral infections (Allison, 1972). It became apparent that the mechanism by which the immune system responds against the invading organism to successfully defend the host depends upon the way in which the virus spreads from one cell to another (Lodmell *et al.*, 1973). Thus, three different routes may be involved: firstly, an extracellular route, when near or distant cells can be infected; secondly, viruses can spread directly to contiguous cells without being exposed extracellularly to antibody; and thirdly, the virus or viral genome can pass to daughter cells during cell division. These types of spread are referred to as types 1, 2 and 3.

The herpes group of viruses spread from cell to cell by type 2 routes. Theoretically, the host defences could interrupt the spread of virus by one of three methods (Notkins, 1974): the cells could be destroyed, the intercellular connections could be ruptured, or contiguous uninfected cells could be destroyed so that the virus would need to travel by the extracellular route to reach target cells for further viral replication. A number of viruses induce the appearance of new antigens on the surface of infected cells, and the interaction of antibody and complement with these antigens may result in cell destruction (Brier *et al.*, 1971). However, cell-mediated immunity probably plays a more important role in stopping cell-to-cell spread. Several observations have pointed to this possibility. It is known that viral antigens stimulate specifically sensitised lymphocytes (Rosenberg *et al.*, 1972). *In vitro* incubation of specifically sensitised lymphocytes with virus-infected cells can result in cell destruction. This is due either to the action of specifically immune lymphocytes on the infected cells, or to the production of biological mediators from the stimulated lymphocytes which might destroy both infected and uninfected cells (lymphotoxin), inhibit viral replication (interferon) and attract inflammatory cells to the site of the infection.

In HSV infections there may be persistence of the virus in the tissues, presumably because immunological destruction of the infected cells occurs after newly synthesised virus has spread to contiguous cells and, more importantly, by reason of its neurotropic potential, has entered and ascended the sensory neuron and reached the posterior root ganglion where it may exist in latent form. However, prevention of virus spread has connotations in the case of HSV, where containment of an infection cannot be explained by simple rejection of altered cells. Thus, although it is known that HSV-infected cells can be destroyed by anti-HSV antibody and complement, there are varying reports of the effect of such a combination on the spread of virus from cell to cell (Lodmell *et al.*, 1973). This is because spread of HSV occurred to contiguous cells before the cells initially infected were destroyed. The cell-to-cell spread was therefore one step ahead of the antibody-mediated immune attack, and so the infection persisted. Similarly, the rapidity of the spread suggested that specifically immune lymphocytes would have little chance of overcoming the infection before the virus had spread to the contiguous cells. Lodmell *et al.* (1973) have suggested that non-specific inflammatory cells might destroy surrounding uninfected cells by the release of biological mediators, thus severing the connection between infected and uninfected cells and halting the infection. Lodmell and his associates found that the combination of macrophages, specific antibody and complement *in vitro* could inhibit and cure the infection, whereas either macrophage or antibody with complement alone were not able to do this, although the rate of spread was reduced. It was therefore proposed that there was an initial phase of specific antigen recognition consisting of the interaction of antibody and complement with virus and the virus infected cell, associated with the stimulation of immune lymphocytes by viral antigens. The resulting lymphoblastic responses generated biological mediators chemotactic for inflammatory cells. A non-specific phase would consist in this inflammatory cell attraction to the site of virus activity, where the action would be exerted on both infected and non-infected cells in the immediately contiguous cells. In addition, lymphotoxin and interferon would help to contain the infection by inhibition of viral replication or by breaking connections between adjacent cells. This inflammatory attack would destroy cells so that virus would become extracellular and thus be neutralised by antibody.

Influence of Antibody

Intracellular virus is not accessible to antibody, and since HSV may be able to spread directly from cell to cell, it has been suggested that lysis of infected cells is necessary for elimination of an infection. This is supported by the work of Lodmell *et al.* (1973) in which spread of infection occurred despite the presence of high antibody concentrations in the culture medium. In general, homotypic antibody may protect against subsequent viral challenge, but does not appear to be essential for recovery from infection after it has commenced. Thus, in 1930, Andrewes noted that the incorporation of antibody into the medium used to nourish explants infected with HSV did not prevent the development of viral induced intranuclear inclusions. Black and Melnick (1955) observed growth of virus in tissue cultures in the presence of antibody. Later, other workers showed that HSV plaques would also grow despite the incorporation of antibody in the medium (Wheeler, 1960; Lodmell *et al.*, 1973; Hoggan *et al.*, 1961; Christian and Ludovici, 1971). To explain these observations the intercellular bridge theory was proposed, which stated that established plaques continued to grow despite the presence of antibody because the virus spread between adjacent cells through intercellular bridges (Hoggan *et al.*, 1961; Christian and Ludovici, 1971). Despite such proposals and findings, other workers have reported that immune serum in an agar overlay could cause a significant reduction in plaque size (Ennis, 1973; Ennis and Wells, 1974), a finding which cast doubt on the intercellular bridge theory. Pavan and Ennis (1977) have shown that established type 1 HSV plaques were eliminated by antibody. Antibody had to remain in contact with infected cells for several days to have a maximum effect. This did not prevent the production of viral-induced antigens in a cell when applied after the cell was infected, but did prevent the transmission of infection to contiguous cells. Strains which were resistant to elimination by antibody formed syncytia, and did not grow to significantly higher titres than non-resistant strains. Resistant strains were as easily neutralised by antiserum as non-resistant strains.

Treatment of herpes simplex virus-infected cells with virus antiserum, with or without complement, yielded reduced infectious extracellular virus (Skinner *et al.* 1975/76). This was shown to be due to an immune alteration of the cell membrane which inhibited release of virus particles from the infected cells, and not due to neutralisation; both type-common and type-specific antigens of herpes simplex virus were involved. Skinner *et al.* (1975/76) suggests that the phenomenon plays an important role in immunological control of virus infection in the whole animal. *In vivo* the effects would be greatly magnified because the infected cells would be exposed to antibody in the presence of complement for the duration of the infective process, so that the transmission of infectious virus to susceptible nearby or distant cells would be reduced.

Increasing knowledge on the importance of antibody against HSV for herpetic infections prompted Knoblich *et al.* (1983) to study antibody formation in HSV-1- and HSV-2-infected mice. Neutralising IgM antibody synthesis was detectable from day 5, and IgG formation occurred from day 10. Female mice produced more antibody than males, and drugs with anti-androgenic activity enhanced antibody formation both in females and males, indicating the influence of the sex steroids on antibody production. Injection of silica enhanced antibody formation, and because of this it is conceivable that macrophages suppress antibody formation. Indomethacin enhanced antibody formation, which points to the macrophages secreting prostaglandins as possible mediators of this suppression. Knoblich et al. 1983) concluded that HSV-1 and 2 interact differentially with some cellular compartments necessary for antibody formation against HSV. It is possible that certain mouse T-cells are destroyed by infection with HSV-2 but not HSV-1.

In summary, antibody prevents further spread of extracellular virus, and probably neutralises whole virus particles which have been released following cytolysis by immunocompetent cells. The in vitro tests show that new plaques do not form in tissue culture in the presence of specific antibody. The reports concerning the influence of antibody on the size of plaques in culture are rather conflicting. This seems to be related to the presence or absence of complement in the test system. It is clear that other important mechanisms exist to control the spread of infection, and there is good evidence that cell-mediated immune mechanisms play a part in this control.

Influence of Cell-mediated Immunity

The importance of cellular mechanisms in the in vivo control of virus infection with HSV was demonstrated by Ennis (1973), who showed by plaque-size reduction that sensitised spleen cells together with antibody were able to control the spread of herpes simplex virus. Specifically immune lymphocytes can also directly lyse HSV-infected cells. T-cell-mediated cytotoxicity against herpes simplex virus-infected target cells was investigated by Pfizenmaier et al. (1977), who found that T-lymphocytes taken from mice infected with HSV were cytotoxic.

Antibody-dependent, cell-mediated cytotoxicity may be mediated by a number of cell types (Grewal et al., 1977). Polymorphonuclear leucocytes and macrophages, together with lymphocytes, may act against antibody-sensitised virus-infected cells. Polymorphonuclear leucocytes are more effective in preventing in vitro spread of virus on a cell-to-cell basis, and it is possible that polymorphs are important in limiting early spread of the herpes simplex virus.

The interaction of immune T-lymphocytes with HSV antigens results in their proliferation (Shillitoe et al., 1977) with the production of lymphokines, including macrophage migration inhibition factor, chemotactic factor and immune interferon. Antigen-antibody complexes have also been shown to induce some of these responses (Fujibayashi et al., 1975). The interferon would inhibit viral replication in nearby susceptible cells while the other factors would amplify immune responses. The experimental measurement of in vitro lymphocyte proliferation and lymphokine production has been useful in research for assessing the degree of cell-mediated immunity to HSV antigens of an individual at the time of sampling. On the other hand there is some evidence that HSV can have inhibitory effects on cell-mediated immune responses. The virus can multiply in T-lymphoblasts in vitro (Westmoreland,

1978), and infectious HSV can inhibit mitogen- and antigen-induced lymphocyte blastogenesis, probably by infecting the lymphoblasts (Plaeger-Marshall and Smith, 1978). At the same time there is evidence that human monocyte chemotaxis can be depressed (Kleinerman *et al.*, 1974).

ANIMAL STUDIES

Antibody Responses

HSV contains numerous antigens consisting of various proteins, some of which are situated on the surface envelope but most of which are formed in the various stages of development of the virus in the nucleus or cytoplasm. When antigens are released from the cell infected with live virus, they excite a wide range of antibodies which may be complement-fixing, precipitating or neutralising. Neutralising antibody may appear as early as the third day after infection in experimentally infected rabbits, but this antibody usually requires the presence of complement for its detection. Serological responses to primary infection with HSV are complicated, and are dependent upon many factors, including the dose of live virus, its type, and its virulence. Lerner *et al.* (1974) investigated the influence of five strains of HSV-1 and two strains of HSV-2 in rabbits. Type-specific and heterologous antibody responses were determined. Homotypic complement-requiring neutralising antibody was elevated above conventional neutralising antibody in the presence of positive antigenic stimulation, and usually indicated a primary immune response. This situation was maintained up to 21 days. The complement-requiring antibody was IgM subclass at 7 and 14 days, and became included in the IgG subclass at 21 days. Passive haemagglutinating antibody appeared earlier and in higher titre than neutralising antibody. This therefore is not a measure of neutralising antibody. It has been shown that HSV-1 and HSV-2 can be differentiated by serological techniques (Nahmias and Dowdle, 1968; Nahmias *et al.*, 1969).

Cell-mediated Immunity

Cell-mediated immunity has been considered to be an important factor in the defence against certain viral infections since 1970 (Glasgow, 1970). The development of a number of *in vitro* systems for the study of the role of CMI in other diseases led to increasing interest concerning its role in virus diseases. Rosenberg *et al.* (1972) reported on lymphocyte transformation studies using herpes simplex antigen on cells taken from infected rabbits. Lymphocytes from infected rabbits were stimulated as much as 30-fold, whereas lymphocytes taken from controls were unaffected. Sensitisation occurred 3 days after initiation of infection, and could be detected up to 120 days later. Infectious virus, in comparison with inactivated virus, produced less lymphocyte transformation. It was considered that the transformation of sensitised lymphocytes by viral antigens appeared to be a simple, highly specific and quantitative *in vitro* technique for the study of cellular immune response to viral infections. Soluble viral antigens produced a two-fold stimulation, whereas the partially purified virus and density-gradient-purified virus produced 13- and 26-fold stimulation respectively. Several important factors emerge from the work of

Rosenberg *et al.* (1972) which are helpful when undertaking studies into CMI in either animals or humans. Thus, it is important to eliminate soluble factors in the crude virus pool that might be cytotoxic to lymphocytes. To achieve sufficient quantities of viral antigens to produce maximal stimulation, the crude virus should be concentrated and purified. Since certain viruses can replicate in macrophages or lymphocytes, and since macrophages may facilitate the stimulation of lymphocytes, infection of either of the cell types might depress the ability of the antigens to stimulate lymphocytes.

Rosenberg and Notkins (1974) reported that the physical state of the virus and whether the virus is combined with antibody are crucial determinants of the type and magnitude of the immune response. Infectious virus induced both humoral and cellular responses, while animals inoculated with UV-inactivated virus failed to develop humoral immunity, but did develop cell-mediated immunity similar to that obtained with infectious virus, but the magnitude of the response was lower. It was also found that antigens of HSV enhance lymphocyte stimulation if they form complexes in the presence of excess antigen or at equivalence, but inhibit lymphocyte stimulation in the case of antibody excess. In contrast, when cell-bound viral surface antigens were incubated in the presence of antibody, lymphocyte stimulation was depressed. It therefore appears that the state in which the virus is presented to sensitised lymphocytes is important in determining whether or not stimulation will occur. It seems that lymphocytes or macrophages can more readily make contact with, phagocytose or process virus-antibody complexes that are in the fluid phase than they can with those fixed to cell membranes.

The role of cell-mediated immunity in the resistance of mice to subcutaneous herpes simplex virus infection was investigated by Oakes (1975 *a, b*), following the use of immunosuppressive doses of antilymphocyte sera or antithymocyte sera. Subcutaneous infection of these mice led to the spread of virus from the site of the inoculation to the central nervous system. Neutralising antibody could not be detected in the sera of treated mice after HSV inoculation. Passive transfer of antibody to treated mice did not restore resistance to subcutaneous HSV infection, but adoptive transfer of HSV-sensitised spleen cells did provide significant protection against infection. Similar findings were reported by Rager-Zisman and Allison (1976) using cyclophosphamide. The development of fatal infection in immunosuppressed mice could be curtailed after transfer of specifically immune spleen cells, while passively transferred antibody had no effect. Significant protection was also achieved when normal spleen cells plus immune serum was administered simultaneously. The results indicated that protection against this virus infection is predominantly T-cell dependent, and suggested that antibody-dependent cell-mediated protection may also be operative *in vivo*.

Although it has been shown that herpes simplex virus is predominantly neurotrophic, as has already been indicated, the virus may also productively infect human lymphocytes. It has been shown that HSV is replicated in mitogen-stimulated human T-cells as defined by monoclonal antibodies (i.e. OKT 3, OKT 4 and OKT 8). Munk *et al.* (1983) have produced evidence suggesting that these lymphocyte subsets express Ia antigen on their surface, which expose specific receptor areas for HSV. A receptor function for Ia antigen itself seems unlikely but the antigen may serve as a marker for the susceptibility of human lymphocytes to HSV infection.

Herpes simplex virus type 1, strain KOS, encodes at least 4 different glycoprotein antigens. These antigens are exposed on virion envelopes and surface membranes of infected cells. Glorioso et al. (1983) have shown, using limiting dilution analysis, that cytotoxic T-lymphocytes recognise type-specific determinants associated with glyoprotein and that these determinants may partially overlap with sites recognised by virus-neutralising antibodies.

The influence of T-cell subsets on herpes simplex virus infection in laboratory animals has been investigated (Jayasuriya et al., 1983; Altmann and Blyth, 1983). HSV-specific suppressor T-cells with a requirement for prostaglandin synthesis limit the pathogenicity in HSV-1 infection in mice, in the CNS and in zosteriform cutaneous spread. Altmann et al. (1983) conclude that delayed-type hypersensitivity responses contribute to the pathogenesis of HSV-induced disease.

Identification of HSV in Corneal Epithelium and Stroma in Laboratory Animals

It has often been argued that stromal disease either is a manifestation of a hypersensitivity phenomenon or represents the penetration and proliferation of the live virus into the stroma. This is because locating the virus in corneal stroma has not been easy, though a number of techniques have been employed in discovering its presence.

In epithelial disease, there has been little difficulty in identifying virus. Kaufman (1960) reported that the diagnosis of herpes simplex keratitis could be made from corneal scrapings using fluorescein-labelled antibody within 1½ hours of collection of a specimen. Pettit et al., (1964) confirmed the value of fluorescent antibody techniques in the diagnosis of herpes simplex keratitis. Smears taken from laboratory animals with experimental epithelial disease showed large, brightly staining intranuclear inclusions and cytoplasmic fluorescence, which was marked around the nucleus and at the cell margin. Smears taken from human cases with herpetic keratitis gave a picture similar to that found in the experimental animal. A positive fluorescent antibody technique showed good correlation with virus isolation by culture in both animals and man. The location of the stain also correlated with the distribution of virus particles in the cytoplasm and the nucleus of the epithelial cell in the rabbit cornea. Uchida and Kimura (1965) demonstrated specific localisation of herpes simplex antigen in the conjunctiva of rabbits with primary experimental kerato-conjunctivitis. Viral localisation was noted in the cytoplasm as well as in the nuclei of conjunctival epithelial cells.

Tanaka and Kimura (1967), using similar techniques, were able to demonstrate herpes simplex virus antigen in the stroma of experimentally infected rabbits. The virus appeared to be in the keratocytes, as supported by electron microscopy. Fluorescein antibody stain was identified in the outer fifth of the stroma underlying an epithelial lesion at day four. Flat sections showed the FA-stained areas to be in the stromal cells between the lamella. At 7 and 10 days after inoculation, corneas showed extensive staining which extended far beyond the areas of epithelial involvement. Sections studied by EM confirmed that virus particles had extended into the stroma. In one eye which had been inoculated by a scratch method, virus particles were present in cells which appeared to be polymorphonuclear leucocytes, monocytes and keratocytes. The use of these techniques, therefore, confirms the view that the keratocytes are invaded by virus, which thereupon proliferates in the cell and possibly spreads to the extracellular environment.

Peroxidase-labelled antibody was employed to localise herpes simplex virus in the corneal epithelial cells maintained in culture (Shabo *et al.*, 1973). With light-microscopy, intranuclear and paranuclear staining was noted in cells infected with the virus; this was confirmed with electron-microscopy, which is able to detect specific virion labelling. Thus it was possible to study infected cells at both light- and electron-microscopy levels with the same antibody conjugate.

Dawson *et al.* (1966) demonstrated for the first time that infection could be induced in deep ocular structures with HSV. Rabbit ocular tissue was investigated by light- and electron-microscopy and after infecting the corneal epithelium with a strain of herpes simplex virus which regularly produces lesions in the stroma. Specimens of tissue were then taken from the central cornea and the corneal scleral junction. Particles with the characteristic morphology of herpes simplex virus were found in the corneal epithelial cells and in the nerves at the limbus. Within the nucleus of one Schwann cell there were characteristic herpes particles bounded by a single membrane ('naked virus particles') about 75–100 nm in diameter and containing a dense central nucleolid. Other particles present in the cell membrane were similar in structure to the nuclear particles, but possessed a second limiting membrane or envelope. Infection of the limbal nerves was detected 48 and 72 hours after inoculation. However, there was no evidence of viral particles in the stromal keratocytes.

Several studies have reported the localisation of herpes simplex antigen in more detail with the increasing sophistication of electron-microscopical technology. Ultrastructural localisation of herpes simplex virus antigens on rabbit corneal cell cultures was carried out using sheep antihuman IgG and antihorse ferritin hybrid antibodies (Henson *et al.*, 1974). HSV antigens were demonstrated on the surface of infected cells and on extracellular virus. In disrupted infected cells, label was also found along many of the intracytoplasmic membranes and nuclear membranes. HSV-induced antigens are associated with and widely distributed along surface and internal membranes of infected cells.

The ultrastructural localisation of HSV antigen in cells of the rabbit cornea by immunoferritin techniques is now thought to be complicated by failure of the reagent to diffuse through cell membranes and dense collagen surrounding the keratocytes of the tissue. Metcalf and Helmsen (1977) in reviewing their own observations using these techniques suggest that there are many similarities of antigen production in HSV-infected corneal cells in tissue culture and in the infected cornea. They were able to confirm that viral antigens were incorporated into surface membranes of infected corneal cells in animals with experimental herpetic keratitis. Antigen was also demonstrated in the cytoplasm and nuclei of infected cells and in association with the outer nuclear membrane.

Clinical Disease in Laboratory Animals

The rabbit has often been the animal of choice in experiments concerning herpes simplex infection of the eye, because of its large cornea and the ease with which it can be manipulated. The clinical course of the primary disease in rabbits had been documented by Pavan-Langston and Nesburn (1968), where the disease was followed over a period of fifteen days. Tear film cultures were taken, and the lacrimal, Harder's nictitans glands, the conjunctiva and the three corneal layers were cultured for virus. The relative amounts of virus in the corneal layers and conjunctiva were determined by plaque count. The data gathered was correlated with the clinical study of acute herpetic keratoconjunctivitis. The studies showed an unexpected order of events. Within four to six hours after inoculation of the untraumatised eye, HSV could no longer be cultured, probably because it had entered an eclipse phase and was no longer in an infectious form. After ten hours virus could once again be isolated, in small amounts at first but increasing to a maximum at 16 hours. Positive lacrimal-gland and conjunctival cultures were obtained up to the fifth day, after which there were no further isolates from conjunctiva or gland, although virus isolates could be obtained from the tear film. It was also found that viral invasion of the cornea conformed with previous reports that HSV invades all corneal layers in acute primary keratitis, and that the onset of corneal oedema is temporally related to the appearance of infectious virus in the stroma and the endothelium. Infectious virus abruptly disappeared from the cornea after day seven.

Several studies have been made of the effects of HSV-1 and HSV-2 in ocular disease in rabbits. Oh *et al.* (1972) reported that type 2 strains of HSV produced more severe lesions than type 1 strains. Other investigators had previously noted differences in the ocular disease induced experimentally in rabbits by different strains of HSV. Small-plaque variants were less capable of producing keratitis than large-plaque variants, and Wheeler (1964) showed that the HF strain caused a more severe keratoconjunctivitis than the HPF strain. Maloney and Kaufman (1965) noted that some strains became more widely disseminated in the ocular tissue than others. Type 1 strains cause superficial keratitis that heals rapidly without corneal scarring, whereas type 2 strains produce extensive deep stromal keratitis resulting in corneal opacification, total pannus and scarring. Stevens and Oh (1973) showed that there was persistent epithelial loss and marked epithelial hyperplasia in type 2 infection, in contrast to type 1 disease where there was rapid recovery from the infection with good epithelial regeneration and a lack of epithelial hyperplasia. The stromal infiltration of inflammatory cells in type 2 infected eyes was deeper and more severe than in type 1 infection. Infiltration of the endothelium, iris and choroid by inflammatory cells was more frequently found in type 2 infected eyes. Virus was recovered in high titres in type 1 infections, but ocular inflammation did not persist beyond the 15th day after inoculation. In contrast, in type 2 infections, the virus was recovered in lower titres, while the inflammation was severe and persistent through day 31.

Wander *et al.* (1980) have suggested that it is possible that the different clinical patterns of herpetic ocular disease may be attributed at least partially to the differing biological behaviour of specific strains of HSV. The anterior-segment disease induced by seven different strains was compared following corneal inoculation. It was found that different disease patterns were produced by each strain.

Scanning and transmission EM studies were carried out by Spencer and Hayes (1970), and the appearances were correlated with clinical disease. A sharply demarcated central zone of ulceration containing many degenerating epithelial cells was noted, possibly derived from the bordering cells and from the basal layers. These had a rounded configuration and averaged 10 μm in diameter. Transmission EM of the cells showed particles resembling herpes simplex virus between cells and their nuclei and cytoplasm. Adjacent zones of epithelium presented a depressed appearance with scalloping of individual cells. The configuration of the outer margins of the lesions resembled that of the border between zones of ulceration and scalloped cells.

When the lesions induced in the experimental animal by type 1 and 2 were compared (Hollenberg et al., 1976), scanning EM demonstrated similar morphology in most respects, those due to type 2 virus showing elevated edges. In both HSV-1- and 2-induced lesions, infected epithelial cells first separated from neighbouring cells, becoming globular and finally detaching to leave a central excavation. During healing following HSV-1 infection, normal epithelial cells invaded the central crater from all sides to cover damaged cells and reconstitute the epithelial surface.

One of the complications which may occur in herpes simplex keratitis is stromal ulceration, which may lead to scarring with irregularity of the corneal surface, formation of a descemetocele, or rarely, to corneal perforation. With the injudicious use of topical steroids, such complications become pronounced. McCulley et al. (1970) demonstrated collagenolytic activity in the epithelium of rabbit corneas experimentally infected with herpes simplex virus in trephined corneal explants. Control epithelial explants demonstrated minimal to no collagenase activity. This finding may offer one explanation for destructive disease involving the stroma, although there are many other factors acting to produce tissue damage of this nature.

Local and systemic responses to epithelial and stromal herpes simplex keratitis have been examined by a number of workers. Experimental work on specific immunity in relation to HSV infection of the cornea has demonstrated that infection of one eye can protect that same cornea from re-inoculation of the virus (Hall et al., 1955; Okumoto et al., 1959). The extent of resistance shown by a previously uninfected eye, following immunisation at a distant site was less clear, there being a negligible protection in some reports (Hall et al., 1955; Pollikoff et al., 1972), while others found evidence of some protection (Ey et al., 1963). Carter and Easty (1981) investigated the influence of previous cutaneous infection by the same strain of HSV in rabbits on the severity of epithelial disease, by employing the technique devised by Jones and Al Hussaini (1963), where microtitrations of log dilutions of virus suspensions are inoculated into corneas at multiple sites (Figure 6.1). The method was originally employed in the investigation of antiviral therapy, but it can be usefully adapted in the evaluation of the influence of systemic immune responses on the spread of virus in the corneal epithelium. Observations made

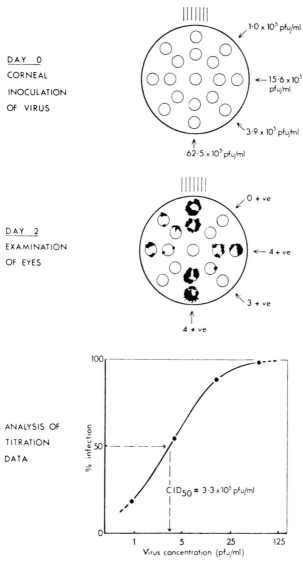

Figure 6.1. Diagrammatic presentation of the Jones–Al-Hussaini technique of multiple trephination of the corneal epithelium using log dilutions of virus suspensions.

after a period of 48 hours allows the construction of a dose response curve, and subsequent changes in the extent of virus proliferation can be measured using densitometry on scale drawings made of the epithelial lesions (Markham *et al.*, 1977). Previous live virus infection in the skin induces an immune response which inhibits virus proliferation and spread in the epithelium,

demonstrable as dose response curves at two days, which indicate that there
is significant inhibition of viral proliferation (Figure 6.2). Previous infection of
one eye causes both protection of itself and of the opposite eye to a lesser
extent. Virus disease of the corneal epithelium induces systemic changes in
serum antibody, and at the same time, cell-mediated immunity shows a
positive response, which appears significantly earlier in secondary corneal
inoculation than in primary disease. Although it is probable that systemic
immune responses do not necessarily mirror the events occurring locally in the
vicinity of the eye, there is a correlation between the initiation of healing in
the corneal disease (Figure 6.3) and the onset of cell-mediated immune
responses, occurring at day 8 in rabbits with primary disease, and at day 6 in
animals with secondary disease. Complement-fixing antibody did not appear
in the serum until after the ulcers had shown evidence of resolution. It is
therefore possible that the activation of mechanisms operating locally to halt
the spread of corneal infection correlates with the systemic lymphocyte
transformation response. The increased protection observed in previously
infected eyes could be due to specific immune processes or, alternatively or in

VIRUS DOSE-RESPONSE CURVES FOR CORNEAL INOCULATION

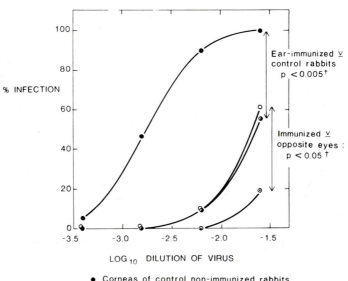

Figure 6.2. Virus dose response curves in immune and non-immune
rabbits, and in rabbits in which one eye had been previously challenged
with a primary infection of herpetic keratitis. (Courtesy, Editor of the
British Journal of Ophthalmology.)

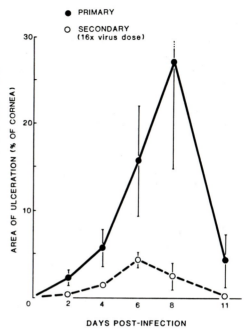

Figure 6.3. Areas of corneal ulceration in non-immune and immune rabbits in non-specific units measured by densitometry. Healing started two days earlier in the immunised group, which correlated more closely with cell-mediated responses than humoral responses. (Courtesy, Editor of the *British Journal of Ophthalmology*.)

addition, to non-specific effects of the earlier infection. These mechanisms might involve the presence of specific antibody in the cornea or tears, increased numbers of specifically immune lymphocytes or K-cells, the presence of macrophages, the production of immune interferon, or the persistence of residual inflammatory changes in the local environmental tissues of the corneal surface.

Mechanisms for ocular protection and re-infection of the eye have been investigated by Dawson and his associates (1978). Following initial infection with herpes simplex virus, neurons of the trigeminal and ocular autonomic ganglions are infected and act as a primary reservoir for recurrent virus shedding and re-infection of the eye, both in man and rabbits. In a rabbit model it was determined that the virus strain specificity or previous site of infection were both important in protecting against ganglionic infection following challenge, of the eye of previously infected animals. Infection of the cornea with a homologous strain of HSV led to ganglion infection only rarely in rabbits whose primary infection had been either on the lower lid or the eye. When rabbits whose primary infection had been in the eye received ocular challenge in the same eye with a different strain of herpes simplex virus there was a significantly more frequent infection of the trigeminal and superior cervical ganglions. This superinfection occurred even though both strains were type 1 HSV. It was concluded that patients with previous herpetic orofacial lesions who develop eye disease caused by the same strain of herpes simplex virus would be less likely to develop latency in the ganglion concerned.

There has been a certain amount of controversy about the influence of immunity on the spread of virus in the nervous system, it being held by some that once a primary infection has occurred, there is little likelihood of a further infection with another strain of virus (Klein, 1983). However it has recently been reported that multiple strains of latent HSV-1 may be detected within individual human hosts (Lewis *et al.*, 1983). Thus in at least some cases, individuals may harbour more than one strain of latent HSV within the same ganglion or in separate neuroanatomical sites. It therefore seems that these multiple strains arise from exogenous superinfections or by simultaneous infection with more than one strain of HSV.

The influence on ocular disease of previous infection at another site in mice has also been investigated by Tullo *et al.* (1982). The ear was infected one month before secondary inoculation of the contralateral eye, using the same strain of HSV. When compared with primary eye disease, it was necessary to increase the dose of the inoculum 100-fold (i.e. 2 logs) in order to induce a keratitis. The clinical signs appeared more rapidly in the secondary infection, were more localised and were largely reversible. Washings of the eye for virus culture indicated that virus was cleared from the tear film more rapidly in secondary infection (Figure 6.4). Interestingly, corneal sensation was greatly reduced in primary infected mice, but for a transient episode only in secondary infection (Figure 6.5). Evidence for latent virus following organ culture of the dermatomes of the trigeminal ganglion was much less following secondary infection, with little evidence of spread to the brain stem, or to ganglia in other dermatomes. Whether the anaesthesia is a manifestation of the involvement of the complete sensory neuron, or whether it is a result of peripheral damage, with secondary effects on the sensory receptors in the cornea, is unclear, particularly in view of the severe corneal damage which occurs following primary disease where the anterior segment is considerably altered in the long term.

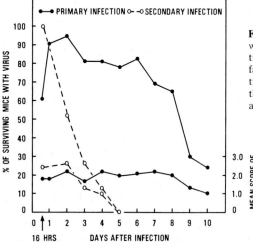

Figure 6.4. Virus isolation from eye washings in primary and secondary infection in corneae of mice. There is a rapid fall off of productive virus following infection in immune animals. The variation in the mean score of virus in eye washings is also shown. (Courtesy, Editor of *Archives of Ophthalmology.*)

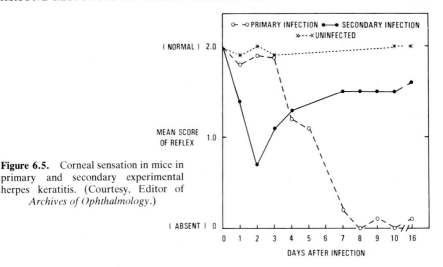

Figure 6.5. Corneal sensation in mice in primary and secondary experimental herpes keratitis. (Courtesy, Editor of *Archives of Ophthalmology*.)

Following corneal inoculation in mice, Tullo *et al*. (1982) have demonstrated spread of virus to involve the brain stem and other dermatomes of the trigeminal ganglion of the same side. Inoculation of skin supplied by the mandibular division of the Vth nerve results in the establishment of latency in the first division. Spread may also occur via the sympathetic nerves to the superior cervical ganglion, where latency is also established. It is possible that a pattern of latent virus is established following primary disease, which recurrent disease does not necessarily reflect, in that it may occur in sites other than those involved during the primary attack.

HSV-1 latency has been studied in mice after corneal and lip inoculation, and tongue inoculation (hypoglossal model) (Openshaw and Sekizawa, 1983). With tongue inoculation virus was isolated from pure motor hypoglossal nerve fibres at the acute stage of infection. Inflammatory cells were clustered at the point of nerve exit from the mudulla and viral capsids were demonstrated at the same exit area in motor neurons and astroglial nuclei. HSV antigens were present in the large motor neurons of the brain stem hypoglossal nuclei. After corneal inoculation, virus was isolated from the optic nerve in a proportion of animals at the acute stage of infection. At the latent stage, ocular explants yielded virus in 26 per cent of eyes. It was possible to induce recurrence by the use of epithelial irritants in the cornea and elsewhere only if the irritant was applied at a former site of infection. It was concluded from this study that HSV-1 can penetrate the neuromuscular junction and travel directly to the brain in motor axons, and that latency can be established and reactivation be induced in ocular tissue. A further finding was that productive infection in the brain can occur at the latent stage by two mechanisms: reactivation of virus in ganglia and subsequent spread to the brain, and *in situ* reactivation of the virus within the brain.

The importance of the modulating roles of the immune responses and genetic factors on latent virus following foot-pad inoculation was investigated by Al-Saadi and Clements (1983). It was found that there was a difference in the susceptibility of different strains of mice to the formation of latent virus. Interestingly, latent virus was reported in the foot-pad, the frequency of which was also influenced by differing strains of mice.

Humoral and cell-mediated immune responses to HSV antigens were quantitated during the course of primary infection of the rabbit cornea with HSV type 1 (Meyers-Elliott and Chitjian, 1978). T- and B-cells were enumerated and isolated from peripheral blood, pre-auricular lymph nodes and spleen. T-cells were found to be the major population in the lymph nodes and reached maximum numbers at days 6 and 15 following infection. The biphasic response correlated with a positive cellular immune response to HSV antigens by lymphocyte stimulation and to the maximal cytotoxic lymphocyte response to HSV-infected cell targets. T-cell populations were found to reach a maximum in the blood at day 15 post-infection. B-cells constituted the major cell population in the spleen on all days, with a peak at day 15. At this time, neutralising antibody developed. Thus the findings suggested that the rabbit lymphoid tissue has separable lymphocyte populations with functions equivalent to T- and B-cells as defined in murine systems.

The kinetics of lymphocyte transformation in herpes simplex keratitis and the influence of antiviral antibody have been investigated by Meyers-Elliott and Chitjian (1980a). Proliferative cellular responses occurred early in infection and were demonstrated by lymphoid cells from local lymph nodes at day 5, the time at which antibody production was first noted. Peripheral blood and spleen cells were not appreciably influenced at early time periods. Seven months after infection, the presence of autologous serum antibodies enhanced the transformation of stimulated spleen lymphocytes from animals with recurrent disease, results which indicate that antiviral antibodies can affect the cellular immune response in herpes virus infection by modulating the lymphocyte proliferative response to herpes antigens. The inflammatory response to herpes simplex infection of the cornea was studied in athymic and heterozygous mice. The athymic, but not the heterozygous, mice failed to develop necrotising keratitis, and died 13 to 17 days after inoculation. These studies suggest that the immune system protects against dissemination and is involved in the pathogenesis of the necrotising keratitis (Metcalf et al., 1979).

The importance of secretory antibody in the tears of rabbits with experimental ulcerative herpes simplex keratitis was investigated by Centifanto et al. (1970). Topical immunisation of the rabbit conjunctiva and cornea with inactivated herpes simplex virus resulted in the production of herpes-specific IgA antibodies that conferred protection to initial infection with live virus. The antibodies persisted for several months and were found in the tears of the opposite, non-immunised eye. Immunisation also resulted in the production of small amounts of interferon, detected within 24 hours of immunisation. The reason why HSV can be cultured from conjunctiva in spite of the presence of IgA neutralising antibody was thought to be due to 'sensitisation' by IgG antibody. In vitro experiments have shown that persistent or non-neutralisable fractions may be obtained in spite of the addition of IgG to the system, a process which has been called sensitisation. It is possible that sensitisation might account for positive viral cultures both in laboratory animals and the human during ulcerative disease.

Epithelial disease in rabbits was investigated by Pollikoff *et al.* (1972) for the role of interferon or interferon-like virus inhibitor, local and circulating antibody and virus titres, in recovery from initial herpetic keratitis and after re-exposure of rabbit cornea to infection with herpes simplex virus. It was speculated that a link may exist between the decline of virus proliferation and the detection of non-specific, intracellularly acting virus inhibitor, characterised according to certain biological and biochemical properties as interferon. Mechanisms such as the production of antibody and the onset of cellular immunity appeared later, after the decline of the virus inhibitor, and did not appear to play an important role in recovery from primary herpes virus infection. It was concluded that interferon production at the site of the lesion and perhaps in the presence of other non-immune non-specific factors probably played a role in recovery from primary infection. The studies of Carter and Easty (1981) show that there is correlation on a time scale between the onset of healing and cell-mediated immune responses, and it is thought that the activation of these responses is one of a number of factors which co-operate to induce healing (Table 6.1). Where immune responses are normal in that they occur in a host with no impairment of immune protection, there is good evidence that epithelial disease proceeds to resolution without necessarily leading to serious and prolonged stromal or uveal disease. Because of the serious effects which the production of stromal disease may have on the vision of the individual through the risk of developing permanent scarring, there has been considerable interest on location of HSV in the deep ocular tissue and the mechanisms of tissue damage which ensue from its presence.

Immunopathogenesis

In contrast to the epithelium of the cornea, the stroma possesses cells which are fixed and probably have a slow rate of regeneration in the normal state. It can be shown in laboratory animals that HSV antigen may penetrate the stroma as a result of epithelial disease, when there is little clinical evidence of stromal response to these antigens. At the same time, cell infiltration occurs at an early stage of the disease, although it is difficult to demonstrate inflammatory cells in the epithelium. The stroma 'participates' in herpetic keratitis at its earliest stage, and it may be that the front line of defence against the entry of micro-organisms is the early invasion of the superficial stroma with neutrophils. It remains important to try to define the factors which act to prevent virus spread and proliferation, together with the mechanisms, which may be similar or different, inducing lasting tissue damage. Some mechanisms which are theoretically involved in countering proliferation and spread, and those which may cause tissue damage, are demonstrated in Figure 6.6.

In the past the pathogenesis of the stromal lesions of herpes simplex keratitis has been thought to be due to two basic mechanisms; one is that stromal damage was caused by the reaction of viral antigen with immune responses in the host, either humoral or cellular, and was considered to be a hypersensitivity phenomenon; the second was based on the belief that the stromal lesions were the direct consequence of viral multiplication, which resulted in cell death and

TABLE 6.1

MECHANISMS INVOLVED IN COMBATING THE VIRUS PROLIFERATION
IN ULCERATIVE HERPETIC KERATITIS

PRIMARY NON-SPECIFIC REACTIONS
    PMN phagocytosis and killing
    macrophage phagocytosis and killing
    ? mast-cell degranulation
    the complement system
        C3 promotes mast-cell degranulation
           opsonisation by PMN
        C5 promotes chemotaxis of PMN
        C6,7,8 produce cell lysis
    Interferon production

ADAPTIVE SPECIFIC REACTIONS
    primary response with antibody production
        antigen presentation (macrophage)
        clonal selection of population of B-cells
           (influence of helper and suppressor T-cells)
        clonal proliferation IgG- and IgM-producing plasma cells;
           antigen elimination; memory cells
    Secondary response with antibody production
        dependent upon memory cells and existing antibody levels
    Cell-mediated immunity
        cells containing HSV harbour surface antigens so that they have
           self and non-self features, to which T-cells are responsive;
           clonal selection and proliferation; lymphokines; attraction
           and/or activation of non-specific effector cells; lymphokines
           and amplification
    Production of memory T-cells
    K CELLS   Killer cells – effector cells in antibody-dependent,
                   cell-mediated cytotoxicity
    NK CELLS   Natural killer cells

the release of toxic products (Hall *et al.*, 1955; Sery *et al.*, 1966). Irvine and Kimura (1967) designed experiments to test the importance of hypersensitivity by measuring the effect of suppressing it. It was found that total body X-irradiation did not diminish the stromal lesions in a rabbit model, and it was therefore concluded that hypersensitivity did not play a part in the pathogenesis. However, endothelial lesions were observed that seemed to correlate with the time of appearance and the severity of the deep stromal oedema. Virus was cultivated regularly from the endothelium, which suggested that the damage was probably due to the presence of virus within the endothelial cell. Oh (1970) induced microscopic lesions in the endothelium of rabbits following injection of the virus into the anterior chamber. Corneal opacity was produced, with characteristic endothelial lesions and uveitis. The endothelial changes were derangement of endothelial cells, discrete focal lesions (plaques) and diffuse lesions. The diffuse lesions appeared to be directly related to the production of corneal opacity. HSV was readily isolated from the anterior chamber during the peak period of virus multiplication in the infected tissues. This study showed that the cells in the plaques frequently contained eosinophilic

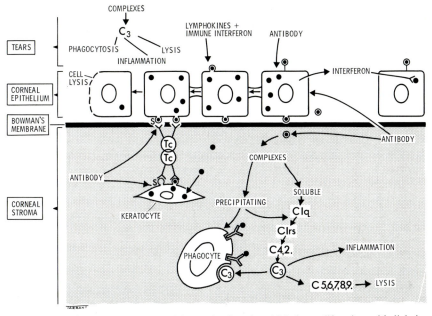

Figure 6.6. Theoretical conception of the mechanisms by which the proliferating epithelial virus is inhibited by adaptive and non-adaptive immune responses. The reactions occurring in the bulbar conjunctiva and the tarsal plates have not been included. The spread of virus from the epithelium into the stroma is represented, and the possible invasion of the keratocyte. Many virus particles become complexed with antibody and may be precipitated, or remain in a soluble form. Where virus is precipitated with antibody it probably becomes phagocytosed. Non-precipitated virus antigen probably excites inflammation via the complement cascade. The actual mechanism by which virus in the epithelium is prevented from spreading from cell to cell is ill understood. Intracellular virus is demonstrated without its capsule in this simple scheme.

intranuclear inclusions, while the diffuse lesions seldom demonstrated inclusions. The results suggested that the plaques represented viral infection of the cells, whereas the diffuse lesions were induced by the action of non-viral mechanisms.

Nagy *et al.* (1978) studied the endothelium in experimental disciform keratitis in rabbits using scanning EM. Benign experimental disciform keratitis was characterised by an intact endothelium, but which was modified by subtle and diffuse morphological changes that were considered to correlate with the diffuse changes reported by Oh (1970). In contrast to the study of Oh, distinct plaques were not seen. SEM in animals with progressive disciform keratitis showed changes such as cellular oedema, cell derangement, and peripheral denudation. The peripheral changes were accompanied by influx of inflammatory cells. The centralised endothelial damage correlated with the severity of the disciform keratitis and anterior uveitis. These findings together with others made in the past, suggest that disciform keratitis may occur in two phases, the initial one being non-specific when the corneal endothelium remains intact with an absence of inflammatory cells in the anterior chamber;

the second phase of early disciform keratitis is accompanied by an acute inflammatory reaction within the anterior chamber. The phase is specific in that there is evidence of HSV antigen specific cell-mediated immune responses in the regional draining lymph nodes (Nagy et al., 1975).

The mechanisms by which antibody may operate to prevent the spread of infection have already been discussed (Meyers and Chitjian, 1976). Such mechanisms are probably effective in controlling virus spread through the corneal stroma, but formation of immune complexes may result in tissue damage, or allow spread of virus further afield through the formation of infectious complexes. Immune rings are occasionally seen in patients with stromal herpes simplex keratitis. Antigen-antibody interactions have been reported to produce damage to the connective tissue stroma of the cornea in specifically sensitised experimental animals, using bovine serum albumin (Sery et al., 1962; Germuth et al., 1962). Meyers and Pettit (1973) described the pathogenesis of corneal inflammation due to herpes simplex virus in sensitised rabbits. Corneal immune rings consisted of local accumulations of inflammatory cells, HSV antigen, host antibody and complement. A linear opacity was produced by injection of HSV and purified HSV antibody simultaneously at opposite sides of the cornea in normal rabbits which had not undergone prior sensitisation. Histopathological studies indicated that inflammatory responses occurred in animals which had been sensitised systemically and locally. HSV antigen, IgG and C3 were demonstrable in identical areas, and their presence was associated with polymorphonuclear leucocytes and collagen necrosis. The components for the humoral induction of immune reactions leading to the tissue damage are present in experimental stromal herpes keratitis in the rabbit. Thus the interaction between antiviral antibody and viral antigens may activate the complement cascade, leading to leucotaxis, and may also stimulate sensitised lymphocytes to liberate mediators of cellular immunity such as lymphotoxin, macrophage migration inhibition factor and other chemotactic agents.

The generation of complement-dependent chemotactic activity was demonstrated by Meyers and Pettit (1974) using the Boyden in vitro assay. It is known that a variety of chemotactic substances act to cause the unidirectional movement of cells toward an attractant, and it is this which has been assumed to be responsible for the accumulation of leucocytes at foci of infection. Such substances include bacteria or bacterial extracts, endotoxin, products of tissue injury, immunologically activated lymphocytes, and antigen-antibody complexes. Chemotaxis is not detectable until the development of increased vascular permeability and protein exudation permits infiltration of polymorphonuclear leucocytes. The PMNs themselves can also generate chemotactic factors from their granules and extracts. Chemotactic factors may be directly chemotactic, or generated from the interaction between other factors, including serum. Serum factors are produced from the complement system and it has been reported that the fifth component of complement (C5a) is activated by cleavage to produce a chemotactic factor. In addition, the complex C5, 6, 7 has been reported to be involved in chemotaxis of leucocytes. Meyers and Pettit (1974) used lucite chemotaxis chambers with upper and lower compartments, separated by a micropore filter. Test material was placed in the lower compartment, fresh PMNs were introduced into the upper compartment, and the chamber was then incubated. The migration of cells through the filter varied according to the production of chemotactic agents in the lower compartment, and the concentration of PMNs could be counted following appropriate staining. The authors found that proliferation of virus in the corneal epithelium during dendritic keratitis resulted in little chemotaxis. During stromal keratitis, when HSV antigen, antiviral antibody, and complement were present in the cornea, significant chemotactic activity was demonstrated. It was concluded from this study, and from the reports of others, that the chemotaxis of PMNs in corneal inflammation following infection with the HSV may result from a number of mechanisms involving cell lysis by herpesvirus-releasing intracellular proteases, the reaction of HSV antigens and cell surface antigens (alone or following their interaction with specific antibody), the release by specifically sensitised lymphocytes of mediators, and nonspecific cell damage releasing proteases and collagenolytic enzymes.

The importance of PMNs in early stromal disease has also been demonstrated by Meyers and Pettit (1973) in sensitised guinea-pigs. The corneal infiltrate following stromal challenge was primarily PMN in cell type, and occurred in animals with delayed type hypersensitivity before circulating antibody was detectable. The reaction at the limbus was polymorphonuclear with the addition of lymphocytes and monocytes. The appearance of plasma cells correlated with the appearance of circulating antibody. The corneal reaction did not appear to be altered however by the appearance of circulating antibody.

The role of PMNs in the development of corneal infiltrates has been further implicated by Meyers-Elliott and Chitjian (1980b). Herpes-infected animals were treated with anti-PMN serum or with chemotherapy to reduce the numbers of circulating PMNs. Depletion of circulating PMNs resulted in nearly complete abrogation of structural injury in the corneal stroma in rabbits. EM studies show that PMNs reached the areas of HSV antigen in the stroma, with damage to the keratocytes and surrounding collagen fibres. In the areas of degenerating keratocytes which were surrounded by degranulating and disintegrating PMNs, the collagen dissolved. In the leucopenic rabbit, collagen destruction was less severe. The findings suggested an immunological cause for the early phase of stromal fibrinoid formation via collagen degradation in herpetic stromal keratitis. The differences in the extent of PMN infiltration correlated well with the amount of eventual scarring and subsequent loss of vision. In spite of the absence of PMNs, vascularisation still occurred in the corneas.

Meyers-Elliott et al. (1980a) have since performed studies in rabbits to characterise stromal herpes simplex virus keratitis, following topical and intrastromal infection of the rabbit cornea with the HF strain of HSV 1, with an aim at correlating the disease manifestations with corneal pathology, viral replication and the presence of HSV antigen in the stroma. In animals receiving topical infection, stromal involvement was frequently seen underlying an epithelial geographic ulcer. In stromal disease, classic disciform keratitis without epithelial disease was seen on the 7th day, and clearing of the stroma occurred by the 21st day after inoculation. Infiltrating polymorphs were found in the stroma and at the limbus between 3 and 15 days in eyes which had suffered either epithelial or stromal inoculation of virus.

The role of cell-mediated immune reactions in experimental models of stromal herpetic keratitis has also been investigated. Williams et al. (1965) found that prior subcutaneous inoculation of rabbits with live herpes simplex virus resulted in significant increase in the incidence of experimental disciform keratitis as compared with animals that had not been pre-sensitised. Swyers et al. (1967) using histological and biomicroscopical observations of the cornea in experimental stromal keratitis showed that there was a close correlation between the development of corneal oedema and the infiltration of lymphocytes that was reached 72 hours after challenge. The observation was consistent with previous studies in guinea-pigs which showed that delayed hypersensitivity to HSV antigens could be passively transferred by cells but not by serum (Lausch et al., 1967). Studies by Metcalf et al. (1976) with experimental stromal keratitis in rabbits indicated that the infiltration is composed of plasma cells, macrophages and lymphocytes as well as polymorphonuclear leucocytes. The observations indicated that the immunological events which occur in the stroma are complicated and that a variety of immunological processes take place in the induction of stromal disease. Metcalf and Kaufman (1976) reported ultrastructural and immunofluorescence studies which lend support to the view that lymphocyte-mediated reactions occur in stromal disease. IF demonstrated the presence of viral antigens in keratocytes, although EM studies did not support this finding. A major infiltrating cell type was the lymphocyte, which was occasionally found in close apposition with a kerato-cyte. Similar findings were made in human corneal discs taken from patients with herpetic keratitis prior to penetrating keratoplasty. Metcalf et al. (1976) state that although the precise mechanism by which immunological pathology occurs is unknown, the presence of viral antigens in stromal keratocytes and the association of lymphocytes with degenerating keratocytes and stromal collagen fibres suggest that a mechanism similar to the one proposed for homograft rejection may operate in the cornea of rabbits and humans with herpetic stromal keratitis.

Sery and Nagy (1977) have pointed out that the use of hyperimmunised animals for the inoculation of corneas with virus in order to reproduce the human situation resulted in a highly artificial situation where the disease process may have little relationship to the human disease process. Previous studies had used a model where a state of hypersensitivity had been induced in rabbits by making periodic injections of viable virus into the stroma of normal animals. Their aim was to induce local hypersensitivity in the cornea, it being assumed that subsequent doses would induce corneal oedema resembling the classical human pathology. No corneal opacities occurred. The 'immune' corneas resisted pathological processes and they retained full clarity (Sery et al., 1966). Subsequently a wide range of virus dosages were assessed with differing strains of virus, and it was discovered that a single small dose of viable H-4 strain herpes virus given intracorneally in normal rabbits produced classical disciform keratitis (Sery et al., 1972). Quantitative examination of the inflammatory cell response of this low-virus-dose model was reported by Sery and Nagy (1977), in order to help explain the complicated pathology associated with the disease. It was found that the ratio of mononuclear to polymorpho-nuclear cells showed considerable variation, the mononuclears being predom-inant in the majority of animals with disciform oedema, while PMNs were predominant in a smaller group. PMNs were absent or scarce in some corneas. It is clear from such reports that the nature of the cellular infiltrate in stromal inflammation varies according to many factors, and that extrapolation to human disease cannot be made without taking into account the many factors which influence this disease process.

There are few reports concerning systemic immune responses to the HSV isolated in the corneal stroma. Nagy *et al.* (1980) evaluated the cell-mediated immune response in the regional lymph nodes taken from rabbits with experimental discrete disciform of the type previously described by Sery and his associates (1972). PHA and HSV antigens were used, and it was found that there was little evidence of impairment in the reactivity of lymphocytes challenged with PHA in animals with disciform oedema. Specific immune reactivity using HSV antigen was found only in those animals that developed concomitant dendritic corneal ulceration in addition to stromal disease, whereas animals with pure disciform keratitis failed to demonstrate a specific immune response in lymphocytes taken from the regional lymph nodes. In terms of a human counterpart of the Sery model of the disease, it would seem difficult to envisage a situation where virus is inoculated into the corneal stroma by some means, such that there is no period of epithelial disease. However, at the same time it is possible to encounter patients with stromal disease in whom both antibody and cell-mediated responses are absent, and in whom there is no other apparent cause for the keratitis. It remains possible that sequestration of virus within the stroma in small quantities could induce local disease without systemic immune responses. Thus in one patient with recurrent attacks of keratitis, HSV was eventually isolated from the epithelium in spite of a continuing absence of cell-mediated or humoral responses. It is therefore possible that there is a human disease parallel to that under current investigation as an animal model by Sery and his associates.

There have therefore been many studies of the immunopathology of the cornea following penetration of virus or its antigen to induce stromal disease, which may have an infinite number of variations. There is good evidence that either antigen or whole virus is able to penetrate stromal cells, and that proliferation may take place within the keratocyte. It has been clearly shown that viral antigens may appear on the cell surface. Once this penetration and proliferation has occurred, mononuclear and PMN cells enter and participate in an inflammatory reaction. Such a reaction is innocent when occurring in other tissues, but becomes a serious disease causing morbidity and incapacity when occurring in transparent corneal tissue.

Strain-specific difference in HSV may account for the variability in disease patterns produced in the rabbit eye, and this is probably true in the human. Although host factors are important in determining the type of disease, it is likely that the strain is relevant. If so, determination of biological differences among strains may explain their variable disease-producing abilities and may eventually lead to new and more selective forms of treatment.

The actual immunological processes which eventually ensue in order to limit virus spread depend on many variables and the understanding of the mechanisms of disease and tissue damage must rest on what is already well known and understood. There are a number of important questions which as yet remain unanswered. It is not clear whether antibody against viral antigens penetrates the corneal stroma in the absence of a local stimulus; IgG has been shown to be present in large quantities and the presence and concentration of specific antibody at the time of viral proliferation in the epithelium would have an influence on the subsequent penetration of virus and induction of prolonged disease. Immune complexes would undoubtedly be formed, and these would subsequently attract PMNs which eventually may produce severe damage. On the other hand, penetration of virus or antigen into stroma which is free of antibody would provoke a different reaction which, it would be anticipated, would be mononuclear at the early stages as it has been shown that the preliminary systemic response occurs in cell-mediated immunity, while the appearance of humoral responses are somewhat delayed. All models of stromal disease are complicated by techniques of inoculation of virus, and because of this the model loses its relation to reality, where the dendritic ulcer leading to stromal disease is often recurrent in nature and is only rarely induced following an episode of trauma. The evidence at present seems to point towards two basic influences in stromal disease; that of viral antigen penetration and intracellular proliferation, and that of a series of immunological sequelae which involve both arms of the immunological system in the protection of the organism against further spread of the virus, together with the multiplicity of mechanisms which act to varying degrees of severity to induce tissue damage. Until the appearance of a model of stromal keratitis which occurs as a consequence of recurrent dendritic ulceration, no real conclusions can be drawn from animal models in relating these systems to the disease process in the human.

Immune Responses in Human Herpes Simplex Keratitis

Background

Immune responses in human HSV disease have been of continuing interest for a number of reasons. Epidemiological studies have been carried out on the frequency of seropositive subjects for HSV in large population samples, and it has been found that this frequency increases with age to reach a plateau at approximately 80 years (Smith et al., 1967). Burnet and Williams (1939) pointed out that there appeared to be a difference in the incidence of antibody to HSV in different social groups. It was found that the incidence was 37 per cent amongst university graduates, 59 per cent amongst non-graduate laboratory workers, and 93 per cent in a group of hospital patients. The comprehensive survey by Smith et al. (1967) showed that there was an age distribution which matched that found in earlier surveys carried out by Holzel et al. (1953) and Buddingh et al. (1953). In an Edinburgh survey there was a high incidence of neutralising antibody in children under six months of age, which fell to 19 per cent at eleven months, to slowly rise again over subsequent decades. The high incidence of antibody in the newborn and very young represents the passive transfer of antibodies from the mother. Most individuals suffer their primary infection in childhood or youth, but with rising standards of living the incidence is likely to fall, thus opening the way for more severe infection in later life, by which time immune responses may be less well marked, with a longer period between initiation of infection and its eventual control.

Although the incidence of seropositive individuals is high, the actual number of subjects who experience clinical disease is much smaller. Scott (1957) found that 64 per cent of a group of children in Philadelphia had specific antibody, although the history of clinical disease was obscure, there being an incidence of herpetic stomatitis of only 1 per cent. It is considered that many subjects become seropositive as a result of subclinical disease, or disease which is not recognised as herpetic in origin.

The observation that recurrent herpes simplex infections occurred in individuals despite the presence of antibody caused a resurgence of interest in other immune mechanisms which might play a role in protection against re-infection, or in causing resolution of established disease.

Several lines of evidence suggest that cellular immunity plays a role in combating HSV infection, especially in relation to cell-to-cell spread. Firstly, HSV infections are more severe in animals with suppressed cell-mediated immunity (Allison, 1972). Second, protection against HSV infections can be transferred to immunosuppressed animals by T-lymphocytes, but not by antibody (Rager-Zisman and Allison, 1976). Third, patients who have been treated with topical or systemic corticosteroid or suffer from recognised immunodeficiency syndromes are subject to more severe corneal or cutaneous herpetic disease. Wilton et al. (1972), in a controlled study of patients with primary and recurrent oral and labial herpes, concluded that susceptibility to recurrent infection may be due to impaired lymphocyte cytotoxicity and production of macrophage migration inhibition factor, in the presence of intact lymphocyte transformation and antibody formation. Russell (1973) showed that patients with recurrent herpes labialis have good CMI response using LT and LMI tests. Russell et al. (1975) showed a similar result using the lymphocyte cytotoxicity test. Antigen-stimulated LT and interferon production were studied in humans after herpetic disease by Rasmussen et al. (1974). A selective increase in interferon production was associated with disease occurrence in some individuals, in the absence of an increase in LT or level of antibody. In certain subjects no interferon response occurred within a period of between 2 and 6 months after disease, and in these individuals lesion recurrence was more common. In immunosuppressed renal and cardiac transplant patients, who are known to suffer from severe herpetic infections (Montgomerie et al., 1969), defective production of interferon by HSV antigen-stimulated lymphocytes was found up to 3 months after transplantation, with a return to normal production in patients who had received transplants 6 months to 6 years previously (Rand et al., 1976).

Sequential changes in cell-mediated immune responses to HSV antigen after recurrent infection were reported by Shillitoe et al. (1977). Lymphocytes of seropositive patients, but not of seronegative controls, responded to HSV by thymidine incorporation, and the supernatant fluids inhibited the migration of guinea-pig macrophages. Lymphocytes from patients with recurrent herpetic lesions responded to HSV by significantly greater thymidine incorporation than seropositive controls, but supernatants did not show an increased macrophage migration inhibition response. One month after the onset of a lesion, the thymidine incorporation to HSV fell to a level of the seropositive controls, and supernatants then induced an increased inhibition of macrophage migration. Lymphocyte responses to *Candida albicans*, purified protein derivative or PHA did not fluctuate according to the presence of a lesion and did not differ from those of the controls. Lymphocyte responses to HSV were unaffected by culture in the presence of serum from seronegative or seropositive controls, or from patients with or without a herpetic lesion. It was suggested that in patients with recurrent herpes labialis, a periodic defect of the migration inhibition response might have allowed the recurrent infection to develop, and that the increased incorporation of thymidine stimulated by HSV *in vitro* was a result of antigenic stimulation from the lesion. Shillitoe *et al.* (1977) reported that lyphocyte responses to HSV in man are mediated by T-cells, by the acquisition of Fc receptors by sensitised cells.

Although it was previously suggested that recurrent herpetic infections could result from inability of the patient's lymphocytes to release migration inhibitory factor after stimulation by HSV (Wilton *et al.*, 1972), the study by Shillitoe *et al.* (1977) indicated that supernatants from patients with active disease inhibited guinea-pig macrophage migration, but the response increased significantly during recovery from infection. An increase in the response and recovery from infection therefore seemed to be related, in contrast to the LT response to specific antigen, which fell simultaneously. It was thought the presence of MIF might be in some way protective against further recurrences of the disease. In a similar study in patients with primary gingivostomatitis, Moller-Larson *et al.* (1978) demonstrated good LT responses which coincided with the onset of recovery.

The mechanisms by which the release of MIF could be protective against recurrent disease is uncertain. In addition to MIF production, other soluble mediators of cell-mediated immunity may potentiate the bactericidal and viricidal functions of macrophages, and in animals macrophages are essential in protection against HSV infection (Hirsh *et al.*, 1970). The soluble mediators of CMI are usually released simultaneously (Rocklin, 1975), and lack of MIF might be associated with absence of other mediators. Interferon can be shown to be reduced prior to the appearance of a lesion (Haahr *et al.*, 1976; Rasmussen *et al.*, 1974). However, production of chemotactic factor and lymphotoxin seems to be normal (Rosenberg *et al.*, 1974).

Cunningham and Merigan (1983) have investigated the production of γ-interferon in the pathogenesis of recurrent herpes labialis. The data suggested that recurrent herpes labialis acts as in *in vivo* stimulus to circulating helper T-lymphocytes to produce interferon. It was speculated that the local tissue macrophages present HSV antigen to helper T-lymphocytes, some of which react by producing interferon and then circulate. The interferon produced appears to be either a direct determinant of frequency of recurrence, or a quantitative marker of other cellular immune events determining frequency.

In a detailed study by O'Reilly *et al.* (1977) patients with herpes labialis and progenitalis were studied for lymphoproliferation, production of LMIF and lymphocyte derived interferon. Virus-specific lymphoproliferative responses were detected in patients with recurrent infection irrespective of the clinical stage of infection. In contrast, transient deficiencies in herpes-specific lymphoid production of LMIF and interferon were regularly documented at the time of, and immediately before, herpes-simplex-induced vesicular eruptions. During convalescence, pronounced production of these mediators in response to antigenic stimulation with inactivated virus antigen preparations was regularly detected.

Other parameters of cell-mediated immunity, such as the lymphocyte cytotoxicity test, have been found unimpaired (Russell *et al.*, 1975), decreased (Steele *et al.*, 1975), or showed fluctuations in accordance with the stage of the disease, with an increase during active disease and a decrease during quiescence (Thong *et al.*, 1975). The production of antigen-stimulated lymphocyte-derived interferon was highest after a recent herpes labialis attack, but showed subsequent decline during convalescence (Rasmussen *et al.*, 1974; Haahr *et al.*, 1976; O'Reilly *et al.*, 1977). Wilton *et al.* (1972) reported an impaired virus-specific production of MIF in patients with active recurrent herpes labialis, which was confirmed by Gange *et al.* (1975) using specific LMIF synthesis in patients with active disease. In contrast, Russel *et al.* (1975) reported increased production of lymphotoxin and monocyte chemotactic factor by HSV-antigen-stimulated lymphocytes in patients with active herpes labialis. A transient deficiency of herpes-specific lymphokine production in the form of LMIF was reported to occur prior to the appearance of vesicular eruptions, and only appeared during the period of convalescence (O'Reilly *et al.*, 1977). Grabner and Jarisch (1979) showed that only a proportion of patients demonstrated production of LMIF 10 days after infection with HSV.

Viral infection itself may either stimulate or depress LT and production of mediators in that such reactions are dose dependent. Immunosuppression by viruses results in loss of lymphocyte responses to unrelated antigens and mitogens (Fireman *et al.*, 1969; Hall and Kantor, 1972; Vesikari and Buinovici-Klein, 1975). Considerable reduction in lymphocyte responsiveness to PHA during a particularly severe attack of cutaneous herpes simplex infection has been seen, which clearly has an overall depressing influence on lymphocyte reactivity. Similarly, in the presence of a reduced viral dose in a primary attack of ocular disease, there was a significant enhancement of specific and PHA LT.

The possible role of PMN leucocytes in the defence against recrudescent herpes simplex virus infection in man has been investigated by Russell and Miller (1978), using ^{51}Cr release assays, to demonstrate whether these cells can damage herpes-simplex-infected target cells sensitised with antiviral antibody. PMN leucocytes were less effective as killer cells than peripheral blood mononuclear cells, but as they are the predominant inflammatory cells within the HSV-1 lesion they may be quantitatively more important. The cytotoxic effects of PMNs and mononuclear cells were significantly reduced by prostaglandin E_1, hydrocortisone and other drugs. It was suggested from the study that antibody-dependent PMN-mediated cytotoxicity may play a role in the human host's defences against recrudescent herpes simplex infection.

Easty *et al.* (1981) reported on a series of investigations into systemic immune responses in patients with either ulcerative disease, stromal disease, or disease found in atopic subjects who seem to be at risk of suffering severe bouts of epithelial disease that may be either primary or recurrent. Serum immunoglobulin and specific antibody levels in the serum demonstrated no group differences. When phytohaemagglutinin (PHA) was used to challenge lymphocytes, group differences were not demonstrated, but when HSV antigen was used in the same groups, there was some reduction in lymphoproliferative response in subjects with severe stromal disease ($p<0.05$). When the two reponses are compared (Figure 6.7) it can be seen that the reduction in mean

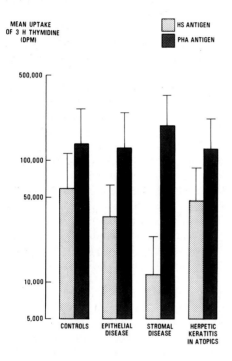

Figure 6.7. Comparison of lymphocyte transformation levels in patients with epithelial disease and stromal disease, and atopics with severe keratitis, using herpes simplex antigen and PHA antigen. In patients with stromal disease there is a depleted response using specific antigen. (Courtesy, Editor of the *British Journal of Ophthalmology*.)

response in specifically stimulated lymphocytes was not mirrored in those challenged with PHA. Similar groups of subjects in the same categories were investigated for macrophage migration inhibition factor (MIF), but no group differences could be found. The studies into specific lymphoproliferative responses following stimulation with HSV antigen confirm earlier studies reported by Easty *et al.* (1973). There are few other reports of investigations into the immune responses following corneal disease of different categories. Grabner and Jarisch (1979) used a direct assay of leucocyte migration inhibitory factor, and reported that cell-mediated immunity to HSV antigen was significantly reduced, as shown by the production of LMIF in patients with primary or recurrent ocular infections, when compared to a control population. However, patients with stromal involvement and anterior uveitis showed significant migration inhibition with HSV antigen, similar to the healthy controls.

Patients with various types of herpetic keratitis have been assessed over a period of time by Easty *et al.* (1981). Primary herpetic keratitis may be associated with a considerable response both in specifically- and PHA-stimulated lymphocytes, while MIF may be produced for a time. In a series of patients with recurrent disease, the specific lymphoproliferative response was increased during the disease, and dropped during the period of convalescence (Figure 6.8). In patients with prolonged stromal disease there was no evidence of a trend which could be correlated with the clinical disease. In atopic subjects with primary disease, the response to both PHA and HSV antigens was unpredictable and failed to correspond to the clinical disease.

The influence of autologous serum on LT in patients has been assessed (Carter *et al.*, 1981; unpublished data). Where lymphocytes were cultured in the presence of autologous serum or serum taken from seronegative controls, it was noticed that the autologous serum enhanced LT. Both in seropositive controls and in patients, there was a depression of LT in the presence of autologous serum in cultures harvested at 7 days. This suggests that HSV antibody effectively depresses CMI, but where cultures are harvested at 5 days, and not at 7 days, the opposite occurs, and there is enhancement of LT (Figure 6.9). It therefore seems that autologous serum contains a factor, probably HSV antibody, which in fact either potentiates LT or shortens the period during which maximum transformation can be obtained.

The evidence concerning the systemic immunological events which accompany and follow herpes simplex keratitis are conflicting, but it would appear that the following conclusions are justified:

(*a*) there is a specific cell-mediated immune response following or accompanying primary infections, associated with the production of lympho-

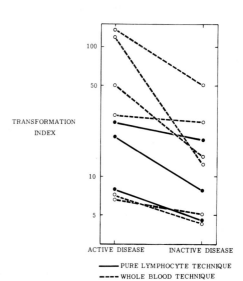

TRANSFORMATION
INDEX

ACTIVE DISEASE   INACTIVE DISEASE

——— PURE LYMPHOCYTE TECHNIQUE
---- WHOLE BLOOD TECHNIQUE

Figure 6.8. Lymphocyte transformation to herpes simplex antigen in patients with active and inactive epithelial disease. (Courtesy, Editor of the *British Journal of Ophthalmology.*)

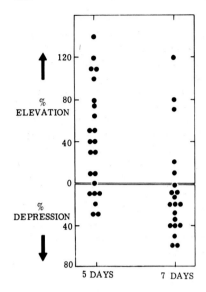

Figure 6.9. Comparison of the influence of autologous serum and lymphocyte transformation at days five and seven, using herpes simplex antigen. There is an enhancement of lymphocyte transformation at the fifth day, in contrast to seven-day cultures where there is depression of LT.

kines, including interferon, which act in some way to prevent the further spread of virus.

(*b*) recurrent ulcerative disease is accompanied by a similar systemic response, but to a lesser extent.

(*c*) the evidence seems to suggest that the production of lymphokines is transitory, and that once the disease has been overcome, the ability of lymphocytes to produce a lymphokine on specific stimulation seems to disappear.

(*d*) there has been little work on the systemic responses in patients with stromal disease, but the evidence suggests that there is minimal systemic immunological change in patients with stromal disease of varying degrees of severity.

(*e*) where there is acquired cell-mediated immunodeficiency, both epithelial and stromal disease may occur with increased severity.

Lysozyme tear levels in patients with herpes simplex virus eye infection have been reported by Eylan *et al.* (1977). The concentration of enzyme in patients during an acute attack of epithelial disease was lower than that of the other eye, and reduced below levels found in healthy control subjects. During convalescence, levels of lysozyme increased but not to normal levels, and the authors considered that reduced levels may be an indicator of a tendency toward further recurrences.

Histopathology of Human Corneal Tissue

Studies of human tissues taken from patients receiving corneal grafts indicate that in spite of the presence of severe stromal disease, which may be either active or quiescent, it has proved difficult to find evidence of virus or its antigen within the tissues. Metcalf and Kaufman (1976) have pointed out that the herpes simplex virus is capable of causing cell-mediated immune responses, and suggests that such responses are seen in stromal disease where virus antigen is fixed either within the keratocyte, or between the collagen fibrils of the stroma. Both in animals models of stromal disease and in human tissues, viral antigen can be demonstrated in the keratocytes, although Metcalf *et al.* (1976) were unable to demonstrate mature infectious virus particles in the same tissues using EM and viral culture. A major infiltrating cell type was the lymphocyte, many of which were found in intimate contact with the keratocytes which were in varying degrees of degeneration. When viral particles invade a living cell, either productive infection involving viral replication and cell destruction, or abortive infection in which viral replication is blocked, may occur (Kelleher *et al.*, 1975; Green, 1970). In the case of abortive infection, the formation of viral antigens on the cell surface would be anticipated and it is likely that these cells would then be recognised as non-self and would eventually be destroyed by the action of antibody-mediated lymphocytotoxicity, or K-cells. However if this is the entire process, it becomes difficult to understand why the stromal disease may be so persistent, unless either further keratocytes are generated which become infected, or virus reaches the stroma by axoplasmic flow from the posterior root ganglion.

In a report concerning the findings made following examination of a corneal disc taken from a 6-year-old girl, Meyers-Elliott *et al.* (1980*b*) reported the presence of viral antigens in the tissues. A central disciform keratitis was surrounded by a circumferential opaque ring, histologically resembling the immune ring first described by Wessely. Along a line of altered keratocytes and ground substance, an infiltration of inflammatory cells was found. Herpes virus particles were seen by EM in the corneal stroma, but these particles had abnormal, non-infective forms such as empty capsids and incomplete virions. By immunoelectron microscopy with a peroxidase-labelled antiherpes antibody reagent, herpes virus antigens were localised in the keratocytes and in the corneal stroma. The major localisation of the virus antigens was in association with the herpes virions and surrounding vacuoles in the keratocyte nucleus and in the corneal stroma in the area of degenerating keratocytes. The report of Meyer-Elliott *et al.* (1980) is interesting because it distinguishes between structurally complete enveloped virus particles indicative of mature replicating infectious virus, which were rarely found, and particles which were incomplete, without cores, which would be considered to be non-infectious but nonetheless antigenic. Such incomplete particles were located within the keratocytes and the stroma. Peroxidase-labelled antibody stained viral capsids within the keratocyte, together with HSV antigens on the nuclear membrane of the keratocyte. Most of the cells within the tissue were PMNs but there was little evidence that these cells were found in juxtaposition with herpes virions and antigen.

Dawson *et al.* (1968) had previously reported the presence of HSV particles using EM in 5 of 19 corneal specimens from patients with herpetic keratitis, undergoing keratoplasty. In two specimens taken from one patient who received two grafts consecutively, virus was found both in the original specimen and in the failed grafts. A positive virus culture for HSV was achieved in only 1 of the 19 corneal specimens. Using prior organ culture of corneal tissue followed by fragmentation of the tissue, HSV was isolated from the corneal buttons taken from a patient with chronic stromal keratitis (Shimeld *et al.*, 1981; Figure 6.10).

The corneal stroma is not a fertile milieu for viral proliferation and it is difficult to explain why the disease is often chronic, and why it goes through periods of recrudescence and remission when it might be anticipated that inflammatory responses occurring in the stroma would control virus proliferation, which, at the same time, does not seem to lead to either mature virus, or eventual clearing of antigen from the site. Clinical disease as seen in Western communities is rarely untreated, which fact should be considered in understanding the processes which occur in the production of stromal disease. The use of topical corticosteroid is just one factor which may serve to reduce the inflammatory events which check the virus within the stroma, but may also enhance the spread of viral antigen by a variety of mechanisms. The factors determining the severity of stromal disease are shown in Table 6.2.

TABLE 6.2

FACTORS DETERMINING THE SEVERITY OF STROMAL DISEASE

Whether primary or recurrent disease;
the magnitude of the non-adaptive and adaptive phase of the
    inflammatory/immune response, and the delay before the
    appearance of the specific phase;
the virulence of the HSV strain;
the frequency of recurrences;
the severity of recurrences;
the stage at which antiviral treatment is introduced;
patient compliance;
the influence of topical corticosteroid;
the influence of systemic immunodeficiency.

Sudden cessation of topical steroid can result in exacerbation of stromal inflammatory disease, whereas a gradual tapering down may often avoid this. One explanation of this rebound is that during a period of treatment virus might be proliferating within the keratocyte, which eventually becomes disrupted and allows the escape of viral particles into the stroma, where they may become trapped, or whence they may diffuse to other sites within the stroma. The rebound phenomenon in itself implies that there may be an increase in antigenic loading during treatment which invites an enhanced inflammatory response on curtailment of the treatment, although how a comparatively small number of keratocytes can provoke marked inflammatory response is unclear. At the same time, once keratocytes have degenerated there is little known about their rate of replacement, or whether this does indeed occur. The possibility that virus enters the corneal stroma through nerves within the stroma has received little attention, and such mechanisms may go some way to explaining recurrent stromal disease which occurs in the absence of epithelial disease. Stromal disease of a disciform type has been

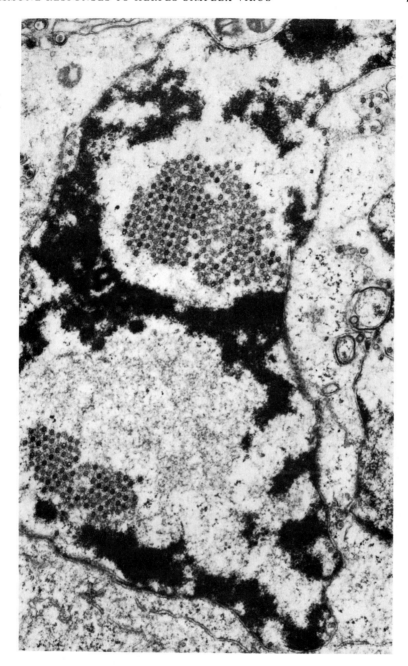

Figure 6.10. Virus particles in vero cells typical of herpes simplex virus type 1, cultured from the corneal disc of a patient with a six-year history of persistent stromal keratitis. (17 000.) (Courtesy, Miss Penny Stirling.)

encountered with a negative history of epithelial disease and an absence of positive serology or cell-mediated immune response. On treatment of such patients with topical steroid there has been eventual ulceration from which HSV has been cultured. Clinical evidence of this type of stromal disease occurring both in the absence of positive serology and preceding epithelial disease suggests that in rare circumstances virus can be introduced into the stroma in the absence of a positive systemic immune response, where it may lay sequestered from the immune system but nevertheless allow proliferation to occur with ascent of live virus up the nerve axon to latently infect the posterior root ganglion. Thus the virus, which may be acquired as HSV 2 infection during birth in the presence of maternal antibody, may remain sequestered in the corneal stroma and/or in the posterior root ganglion of the sensory nerve. It is possible that recurrent disease may occur in the stroma without the appearance of epithelial disease. With the small quantity of virus involved, it seems unlikely that in such circumstances there would be systemic evidence of humoral or cell-mediated responses. Hence it is theoretically possible for stromal HSV to occur in seronegative individuals.

The information that has been presented shows that there are a number of conflicting findings which make it difficult to understand the mechanisms controlling epithelial disease and its recurrence, and the production of stromal disease. It is possible to make the following speculative hypothesis:

1. In primary disease of the skin surrounding the eye, and of the cornea itself, it is possible that proliferating virus may spread from a cutaneous lesion and subsequently involve the cornea and conjunctiva. Thereafter virus would spread into the stroma, endothelium and anterior uvea. The inhibition of virus spread would depend to some extent on adaptive immune responses. Thus it has been shown that epithelial disease starts to heal once adaptive immune responses have been activated. A delay in adaptive response would increase the likelihood of penetration into the stroma.

2. Virus at the same time enters the sensory neuron and eventually reaches the posterior root ganglion (Figure 6.11). It may spread to the central nervous system, and evidently is able to pass across the synapses and enter the sensory neurons of other dermatomes (Tullo et al., 1983). Latency is set up in the ganglia of the other dermatomes. It is likely that the concentration of latent virus, or the number of neurons involved by latent virus, would be less in other dermatomes.

3. The amount of virus which enters a sensory neuron is probably determined by the time interval between initial infection and the adaptive immune response which, if delayed, would be associated with greater viral proliferation. Thus a good early response would serve to limit the primary disease and reduce the concentration of latent virus in the sensory ganglion, and also the amount of virus that is able to penetrate into the eye. The events which occur following primary disease of the cornea and which serve to control the proliferation of the virus occur in the tarsal plates, the ciliary body area, and the stroma.

4. Once latency has been established, then recurrent disease may occur. It is not known precisely how the virus reaches the corneal epithelium, although the probabilities are that it does so via the sensory neuron, if only

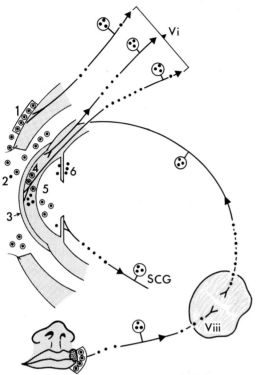

Figure 6.11. Primary herpes simplex infection may occur in the region of the lids (1), and virus may enter the tears (2) and invade the corneal epithelium (3). It may spread via the sensory neuron to become latent in the posterior root ganglion. Virus may penetrate the deeper tissues (4, 5, 6). Labial primary herpes can theoretically spread to set up sites of latent infection in posterior root ganglia which do not necessarily subserve the site of primary disease. Thus labial or oropharyngeal herpes may provide a potential for latency which can cause viral recurrences at other sites, for example the cornea.

because the concentration of nerve terminals is extremely high (Figures 6.11 and 6.12). It would appear that the chances of recurrence occurring are determined by the concentration of neurons containing latent virus. It is conceivable that recurrence may occur in the cornea by a "back door" spread from another dermatome, and this would seem likely as many cases of recurrent epithelial disease are not preceded by primary disease at a clinical level (Tullo et al., 1982). At the same time, auto-inoculation from another site is not very likely, in view of the considerable protection afforded by previous infection elsewhere. The mechanism by which recurrent stromal disease occurs is unclear. The number of sensory neuron endings within the stroma is conceivably much less than that in the epithelium. The time scale of stromal disease also suggests that it may not be due to recurrent leakage of virus because the natural history is prolonged and does not appear to be influenced by the usual trigger factors that caused epithelial recurrence.

5. The responses which occur in recurrent disease are more efficient than those following primary disease, in that the adaptive immune responses already exist and it is probable that they are stimulated rapidly by the presence of viral antigen. In particular the presence of a reservoir of immunoglobulin both in the tears and in the stroma must influence spread of virus in the epithelium and from the epithelium into the stroma in a beneficial way.

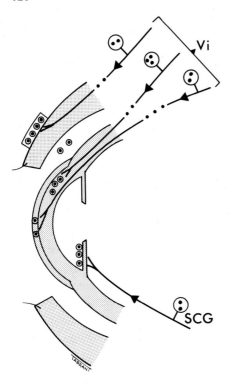

Figure 6.12. Scheme demonstrating routes of entry of virus into the tissues of the eye. Shedding may occur into the conjunctival sac, and the nerve endings supplying the epithelium probably introduce virus to this layer. Whether nerve endings in the stroma act in the same way is unclear. It is possible that virus which exists in a latent form in the superior cervical ganglion may be able to enter the anterior uvea and cause recurrent uveitis.

6. It is conceivable that many cases of serious stromal disease result from an imbalance in the immune mechanisms which serve to control spread of virus. One of the most common causes of this imbalance is the mistaken use of topical corticosteroid. On the other hand there are other factors which influence the spread of virus between layers, including virus sub-type, individual susceptibility and immunodeficiency, whether congenital or acquired.

REFERENCES

ALLISON, A. C. (1972). Immune responses in persistent virus infections. *J. Clin. Path.*, **25**, Supplement (Royal College of Pathologists), **6**, 121.

AL-SAADI, S. and CLEMENTS, G. B. (1983). Recovery of latent HSV-2 from different strains of mice. *International Herpesvirus Workshop, Oxford*, p. 174.

ALTMANN, D. M. and BLYTH, W. A. (1983). Suppressor cells for delayed type hypersensitivity to HSV-1 induced by lipopolysaccharide: nature of suppressor cell and effect on pathogenesis of HSV. *International Herpesvirus Workshop, Oxford*, p. 91.

ANDREWES, C. H. (1930). Tissue-culture in the study of immunity to herpes. *J. Path. Bact.*, **33**, 301–12.

BLACK, F. L. and MELNICK, J. L. (1955). Micro-epidemiology of poliomyelitis and herpes-B infections. Spread of viruses within tissue cultures. *J. Immun.*, **74**, 236–242.

BRIER, A. M., WOHLENBERG, C., ROSENTHAL, J., MAGE, M. and NOTKINS, A. L. (1971). Inhibition or enhancement of immunological injury of virus infected cells. *Proc. Nat. Acad. Sci. (Wash.)*, **68**, 3073–7.

BUDDINGH, J., SCHRUM, D. I., LANIER, J. C. and GUIDRY, D. J. (1953). Studies of the natural history of herpes simplex infections. *Pediatrics*, **11**, 595–609.

BURNET, F. M. and WILLIAMS, S. W. (1939). Herpes simplex: new points of view. *Med. J. Aust.*, **1**, 637–642.

CARTER, C. and EASTY, D. L. (1981). Experimental ulcerative herpetic keratitis. 1. Systemic immune responses and resistance to corneal infection. *Brit. J. Ophthal.*, **65**, 77–81.

CENTIFANTO, Y. M., LITTLE, J. M. and KAUFMAN, H. E. (1970). The relationship between virus chemotherapy, secretory antibody formation and recurrent herpetic disease. *Ann. N.Y. Acad. Sci.*, **173**, 649–656.

CHRISTIAN, R. T. and LUDOVICI, P. P. (1971). Cell-to-cell transmission of herpes simplex virus in primary human amnion cells. *Proc. Soc. Exp. Biol. (N.Y.)*, **138**, 1109–15.

CUNNINGHAM, A. L. and MERIGAN, T. C. (1983). A role for interferon-γ in the pathogenesis of recurrent herpes labialis. *International Herpesvirus Workshop, Oxford*, p. 206.

DAWSON, C. R., TOGNI, B. and THYGESON, P. (1966). Herpes simplex virus particles in the nerves of rabbit corneas after epithelial inoculation. *Nature*, **211**, 316–7.

DAWSON, C. R., TOGNI, B. and MOORE, T. E. (1968). Structural changes in chronic herpetic keratitis studied by light and electron microscopy. *Arch. Ophthal.*, **79**, 740–7.

DAWSON, C. R., WEINSTEIN, A., BRIONES, J. D. and SCHACHTER, J. (1978). Herpes simplex superinfection of trigeminal and autonomic ganglions in immune rabbits. In: *Immunology and Immunopathology of the Eye*. Ed. Silverstein and O'Connor. New York: Masson.

EASTY, D. L., CARTER, C. and FUNK, A. (1981). Systemic immunity in herpetic keratitis. *Brit. J. Ophthal.*, **65**, 82–8.

EASTY, D. L., MAINI, R. N. and JONES, B. R. (1973). Cellular immunity in herpes simplex keratitis. *Trans. Ophthal. Soc. U.K.*, **93**, 171–80.

ENNIS, F. A. (1973). Host defence mechanisms against herpes simplex virus 1. Control of infection by sensitised spleen cells and antibody. *Infection and Immunity*, **7**, 898–904.

ENNIS, F. A. and WELLS, M. I. (1974). Immune control of herpes simplex virus. *Cancer Res.*, **34**, 1140–5.

EY, R. C., HUGHES, W. F., HOLMES, A. W. and DEINHARDT, F. (1963). The effect of IDU on experimental and clinical herpes simplex infections. *Trans. Amer. Ophthal. Soc.*, **61**, 100.

EYLAN, E., RONEN, D., ROMANO, A. and SMETANA, D. (1977). Lysozyme tear level in patients with herpes simplex virus eye infection. *Invest. Ophthal. & Vis. Sci.*, **16**, 850–3.

FIREMAN, P., FRIDAY, G. and KUMATE, J. (1969). Effect of measles vaccine on immunologic responsiveness. *Pediatrics*, **43**, 264–72.

FUJIBAYASHI, T., HOOKS, J. J. and NOTKINS, A. L. (1975). Production of interferon by immune lymphocytes exposed to HSV-antibody Hb complexes. *J. Immun.*, **115**, 1191–3.

GANGE, R. W., DE BATS, A. D., PARK, J. R., BRADSTREET, C. M. P. and RHODES, E. L. (1975). Cellular immunity and circulating antibody to herpes simplex virus in subjects with recurrent herpes simplex lesions and controls as measured by the mixed leucocyte migration inhibition test and complement fixation. *Brit. J. Dermat.*, **93**, 539–44.

GERMUTH, F. G., MAUMENEE, A. E., SENJERFIT, L. B. and POLLACK, F. (1962).

Immunohistological studies on antigen-antibody reaction in the avascular cornea. 1 Reactions in rabbits actively sensitised to foreign protein. *J. Exp. Med.*, **115**, 919–28.

GLASGOW, L. A. (1970). Cellular immunity in host resistance to viral infections. *Arch. Intern. Med. (Chicago)*, **126**, 125–34.

GLORIOSO, J., REES, U., KUMEL, G., KIRCHNER, H. and KRAMMER, P. H. (1983). Limiting dilution analysis of the specificity of cytotoxic T lymphocytes for herpes simplex virus glycoprotein determinants. *International Herpesvirus Workshop, Oxford*, p. 83.

GRABNER, G. and JARISCH, R. (1979). Leucocyte migration inhibitory factor in primary and recurrent ocular infections by herpes simplex virus. *Albrecht v. Graefes Arch. Klin. Exp. Ophthal.*, **211**, 85–93.

GREEN, M. (1970). Oncogenic viruses. In: *Annual Review of Biochemistry*, p. 701. Eds. Snell, E. E., Boyer, P. D., Meister, A. and Simsheimer, R. L. Palo Alto: Annual Reviews, Inc.

GREWAL, A. S., ROUSE, B. T. and BABIUK, L. A. (1977). Mechanisms of resistance to Herpesviruses: comparison of the effectiveness of different cell types in mediating antibody-dependent cell-mediated cytotoxicity. *Infection & Immunity*, **15**, 698–703.

HAAHR, S., RASMUSSEN, L. and MERIGAN, T. C. (1976). Lymphocyte transformation and interferon production in human mononuclear cell microculture for assay of cellular immunity to herpes simplex virus. *Infection & Immunity*, **14**, 47–54.

HALL, C. B. and KANTOR, F. S. (1972). Depression of established delayed hypersensitivity by mumps virus. *J. Immun.*, **108**, 81–5.

HALL, L., MACKNESON, R. G. and ORMSBY, H. L. (1955). Studies of immunity in experimental herpetic keratitis in rabbits. *Amer. J. Ophthal.*, **39**, 226–233.

HENSON, D., HELMSEN, R., BECKER, K. E., STRAND, A. J., SULLIVAN, M. and HARRIS, D. (1974). Ultrastructural localisation of herpes simplex virus antigens on rabbit corneal cells using sheep antihuman IgG antihorse ferritin hybrid antibodies. *Invest. Ophthal.*, **13**, 819–27.

HIRSCH, M. S., ZISMAN, B. and ALLISON, A. C. (1970). Macrophages and age dependent resistance to herpes simplex virus in mice. *J. Immun.*, **104**, 1160–5.

HOGGAN, M. D., ROIZMAN, B. and ROANE, P. R. (1961). Further studies of variants of herpes simplex virus that produce syncytia or pock-like lesions in cell culture. *Amer. J. Hyg.*, **73**, 114–22.

HOLLENBERG, M. J., WILKIE, J. S., HUDSON, J. B. and LEWIS, B. J. (1976). Lesions produced by human herpesviruses 1 and 2. Morphologic features in rabbit corneal epithelium. *Arch. Ophthal.*, **94**, 127–34.

HOLZEL, A., FELDMAN, G. V., TOBIN, J. O. and HARPER, J. (1953). Herpes simplex; a study of complement-fixing antibodies at different ages. *Acta Paediat.*, **42**, 206-14.

IRVINE, A. R., and KIMURA, S. J. (1967). Experimental stromal herpes simplex keratitis in rabbits. *Trans. Amer. Ophthal. Soc.*, **65**, 189–210.

JAYASURIYA, A. K., COBBOLD, S. and NASH, A. A. (1983). *In vivo* relevance of Ly^2 cells in immunity to herpes simplex virus. *International Herpesvirus Workshop, Oxford*, p. 90.

JONES, B. R. and AL HUSSAINI, M. K. (1963). Therapeutic considerations in ocular vaccinia. *Trans. Ophthal. Soc. U.K.*, **83**, 613–31.

KAUFMAN, H. E. (1960). The diagnosis of corneal herpes simplex infection by fluorescent antibody staining. *Arch. Ophthal.*, **64**, 382–84.

KELLEHER, J. J., VARAMI, J. and NELSON, W. W. (1975). Establishment of a non-productive herpes simplex virus infection in rabbit kidney cells. *Infection & Immunity*, **12**, 128–33.

KLEIN, R. J. (1983). The effect of infection with Acyclovir-resistant HSV mutant on subsequent reinfection with pathogenic HSV strains. *International Herpesvirus Workshop, Oxford*, p. 176.

KLEINERMAN, E. S., SNYDERMAN, C. and DANIELS, C. A. (1974). Depression of human monocyte chemotaxis by H.S. and influenza viruses. *J. Immun.*, **113**, 1562–7.

KNOBLICH, A., KAMPE, P., HÄRLE-GRUPP, V. and FALKE, D. (1983). Aspects of regulation of antibody formation against HSV-1 and 2 in the mouse. *International Herpesvirus Workshop, Oxford*, p. 81.

LAUSCH, R. H., SWYERS, J. S. and KAUFMAN, H. E. (1967). Delayed hypersensitivity to herpes simplex virus in the guinea-pig. *J. Immun.*, **96**, 981–87.

LERNER, A. M., SHIPPEY, J. S. and CRANE, L. R. (1974). Serological responses to herpes simplex virus in rabbits: complement-requiring neutralising, conventional neutralising, and passive hemagglutinating antibodies. *J. Infect. Dis.*, **129**, 623–36.

LEWIS, M. E., LEUNG, W.-C., JEFFREY, V. M. and WARREN, K. G. (1983). Detection of multiple strains of HSV-1 within individual human hosts. *International Herpesvirus Workshop, Oxford*, p. 171.

LODMELL, D. L., NIWA, A., HAYASHI, K. and NOTKINS, A. L. (1973). Prevention of cell-to-cell spread of herpes simplex virus by leukocytes. *J. Exper. Med.*, **137**, 706–20.

McCULLEY, J. P., SLANSKY, H. H., PAVAN-LANGSTON, D. and DOHLMAN, C. H. (1970). Collagenolytic activity in experimental herpes simplex keratitis. *Arch. Ophthal.*, **84**, 516–9.

MALONEY, E. D. and KAUFMAN, H. E. (1965). Dissemination of corneal herpes simplex. *Invest. Ophthal.*, **4**, 872–5.

MARKHAM, R. H. C., CARTER, C., SCOBIE, E. M., METCALF, C. and EASTY, D. L. (1977). Double-blind clinical trial of adenine arabinoside and idoxuridine in herpetic corneal ulcers. *Trans. Ophthal. Soc. U.K.*, **97**, 333–40.

METCALF, A. F., HAMILTON, P. S. and REICHERT, R. W. (1979). Herpetic keratitis in athymic (nude) mice. *Infect. Immun.*, **26**, 1164–71.

METCALF, J. F. and HELMSEN, R. (1977). Immunoelectron microscopic localisation of herpes simplex virus antigens in rabbit cornea with antihuman IgG-antiferritin hybrid antibodies. *Invest. Ophthal. & Vis. Sci.*, **16**, 779–86.

METCALF, J. F. and KAUFMAN, H. E. (1976). Herpetic stromal keratitis: evidence for cell-mediated immunopathogenesis. *Amer. J. Ophthal.*, **82**, 827–34.

METCALF, J. F., McNEILL, J. I. and KAUFMAN, H. E. (1976). Experimental disciform oedema and necrotising keratitis in the rabbit. *Invest. Ophthal.*, **15**, 979–85.

MEYERS, R. L. and CHITJIAN, P. A. (1976). Immunology of herpesvirus infections; immunity to herpes simplex virus in eye infections. *Survey Ophthal.*, **21**, 194–204.

MEYERS, R. L. and PETTIT, T. H. (1974). Chemotaxis of polymorphonuclear leukocytes in corneal inflammation: tissue injury in herpes simplex virus infection. *Invest. Ophthal.*, **13**, 187–97.

MEYERS, R. L. and PETTIT, T. H. (1973). Corneal immune response to herpes simplex virus antigens. *J. Immun.*, **110**, 1575–90.

MEYERS-ELLIOTT, R. H. and CHITJIAN, P. A. (1978). Role of T- and B-lymphocytes in acute herpes simplex virus keratitis. In: *Immunology and Immunopathology of the Eye*. Eds. Silverstein and O'Connor. New York: Masson.

MEYERS-ELLIOTT, R. H. and CHITJIAN, P. A. (1980a). Induction of cell-mediated immunity in herpes simplex virus keratitis: kinetics of lymphocyte transformation and the effect of antiviral antibody. *Invest. Ophthal. & Vis. Sci.*, **19**, 920–929.

MEYERS-ELLIOTT, R. H. and CHITJIAN, P. A. (1980b). Immunopathogenesis of corneal inflammation in herpes simplex virus stromal keratitis; role of polymorphonuclear leukocyte. *Invest. Ophthal. & Vis. Sci.*, **20**, 86–99.

MEYERS-ELLIOTT, R. H., PETTIT, T. H. and MAXWELL, W. A. (1980). Viral antigens in the immune ring of herpes simplex stromal keratitis. *Arch. Ophthal.*, **98**, 897–904.

MOLLER-LARSEN, A., HAAHR, S. and BLACK, F. T. (1978). Cellular and humoral immune responses to herpes simplex virus during and after primary gingivostomatitis. *Infection & Immunity*, **22**, 445–51.

MONTGOMERIE, J. Z., BECROFT, D. M. O., CROXSON, M. C., DOAK, P. B. and NORTH, J. D. K. (1969). Herpes simplex virus infection after renal transplantation. *Lancet*, **2**, 867–70.

MUNK, K., KIRCHNER, H., REISER, H. and BRAUN, R. (1983). Infection of human T lymphocytes with herpes simplex virus: restriction to a specific T cell subset and evidence for receptor structures on the cell surface. *International Herpesvirus Workshop, Oxford*, p. 82.

NAGY, R. M., McFALL, R. C. and SERY, T. W. (1980). Cell-mediated immunity in herpes corneal stromal disease. *Invest. Ophthal. & Vis. Sci.*, **19**, 271.

NAGY, R. M., McFALL, R. C., SERY, T. W., NAGLE, B. T. and McGREEVY, L. M. (1978). Scanning electron microscopic study of herpes simplex virus experimental disciform keratitis. *Brit. J. Ophthal.*, **62**, 838–42.

NAHMIAS, A. J. and DOWDLE, W. R. (1968). Antigenic and biologic differences in *Herpesvirus hominis*. *Prog. Med. Virol.*, **10**, 110–159.

NAHMIAS, A. J., DOWDLE, W. R., KRAMER, J. H., LUCE, L. F. and MANSOUR, S. C. (1969). Antibodies to *Herpesvirus hominis* types 1 and 2 in the rabbit. *J. Immun.*, **102**, 956–62.

NOTKINS, A. L. (1974). Immune mechanisms by which spread of viral infections is stopped. *Cell. Immun.*, **11**, 478–83.

OAKES, J. E. (1975*a*). Invasion of central nervous system by herpes simplex virus type 1 after subcutaneous inoculation of immunosuppressed mice. *J. Infect. Dis.*, **131**, 51–7.

OAKES, J. E. (1975*b*). Role for cell-mediated immunity in the resistance of mice to subcutaneous herpes simplex infection. *Infection & Immunity*, **12**, 166–72.

OH, J. O. (1970). Endothelial lesion of rabbit cornea produced by herpes simplex virus. *Invest. Ophthal.*, **9**, 196–205.

OH, J. O., MOSCHINI, G. B., OKUMOTO, M. and STEVENS, T. (1972). Ocular pathogeniety of types 1 and 2 *Herpesvirus hominis* in rabbits. *Infection and Immunity*, **5**, 412.

OKUMOTO, M. JAWETZ, F. and SONNE, M. (1959). Studies on herpes simplex virus. *IX*. Corneal responses to repeated inoculation with herpes simplex virus: rabbits. *Amer. J. Ophthal.*, **47**, 61–66.

OPENSHAW, H. and SEKIZAWA, T. (1983). HSV-1 latency and reactivation in nervous tissue. In: *International Herpesvirus Workshop, Oxford*, p. 175.

O'REILLY, R. J., CHIBBARO, A., ANGER, E. and LOPEZ, C. (1977). Cell-mediated immune responses in patients with recurring herpes simplex infections. II. Infection associated with deficiency of lymphokine production in patients with recurrent herpes labialis or herpes progenitalis. *J. Immun.*, **118**, 1095–1102.

PAVAN, P. R. and ENNIS, F. A. (1977). The elimination of herpes simplex plaques by antibody and the emergence of resistant strains. *J. Immun.*, **118**, 2167–75.

PAVAN-LANGSTON, D. and NESBURN, A. B. (1968). The chronology of primary herpes simplex infection in the eye and adnexal glands. *Arch. Ophthal.*, **80**, 238–64.

PETTIT, T. H., KIMURA, S. J. and PETERS, H. (1964). The fluorescent antibody technique in diagnosis of herpes simplex keratitis. *Arch. Ophthal.*, **72**, 86–98.

PFIZENMAIER, K., JUNG, H., STARZINSKI-POWITZ, A., RÖLLINGHOFF, M. and WAGNER, H. (1977). The role of T cells in anti-herpes simplex virus immunity. I. Introduction of antigen-specific cytotoxic T lymphocytes. *J. Immun.*, **119**, 939–944.

PLAEGER-MARSHALL, S. and Smith, J. W. (1978). Experimental infection of sub-populations of human peripheral blood leukocytes by HSV. *Proc. Soc. Exp. Biol. (N.Y.)*, **158**, 263–8.

POLLIKOFF, R., CANNAVALE, P. and DIXON, P. (1972). Herpes simplex virus infection in rabbit eye. *Arch. Ophthal.*, **88**, 52–7.

RAGER-ZISMAN, B. and ALLISON, A. C. (1976). Mechanism of immunologic resistance to herpes simplex virus 1 (HSV-1) infection. *J. Immun.*, **116**, 35–40.

RAND, K. H., RASMUSSEN, L. E., POLLARD, R. B., ARVEN, A. and MERIGAN, T. C. (1976). Cellular immunity and herpes infections in cardiac transplant patients. *New Engl. J. Med.*, **296**, 1372–7.

RASMUSSEN, L. E., JORDAN, G. W., STEVENS, D. A. and MERIGAN, T. C. (1974). Lymphocyte interferon production and transformation after herpes simplex infections in humans. *J. Immun.*, **112**, 728–36.

ROCKLIN, R. E. (1975). Inhibition of cell migration as a correlate of cell-mediated immunity. In: *Laboratory Diagnosis of Immunologic Disorders*, p. 111. Ed. G. Vyaset Al. New York: Grune & Stratton.

ROSENBERG, G. L., FARBER, P. A. and NOTKINS, A. L. (1972). *In vitro* stimulation of sensitised lymphocytes by herpes simplex virus and vaccinia virus. *Proc. Nat. Acad. Sci. (Wash.)*, **69**, 756–60.

ROSENBERG, G. L. and NOTKINS, A. L. (1974). Induction of cellular immunity to herpes simplex virus: relationship to the humoral immune response. *J. Immun.*, **112**, 1019–25.

ROSENBERG, G. L., SNYDERMAN, R. and NOTKINS, A. L. (1974). Production of chemotactic factor and lymphotoxin by human leukocytes stimulated with herpes simplex virus. *Infection & Immunity*, **10**, 111–15.

RUSSELL, A. S. (1973). Cell-mediated immunity to herpes simplex virus in man. *Amer. J. Clin. Path.*, **60**, 826–30.

RUSSELL, A. S. and MILLER, C. (1978). A possible role for polymorphonuclear leucocytes in the defence against recrudescent herpes simplex virus infection in man. *Immunology*, **34**, 371–8.

RUSSELL, A. S., PERCY, J. S. and KOVITHAVONGS, T. (1975). Cell mediated immunity to herpes simplex in humans: lymphocyte cytotoxicity measured by ^{51}Cr release from infected cells. *Infection & Immunity*, **11**, 355–9.

SCOTT, T. F. M. (1957). Epidemiology of herpetic infections. *Amer. J. Ophthal.*, **43**, 134–147.

SERY, T. W. and NAGY, R. M. (1977). Cellular reaction in experimental herpetic disciform keratitis. *Amer. J. Ophthal.*, **84**, 675–80.

SERY, T. W., NAGY, R. M. and NAZARIO, H. (1972). Experimental disciform keratitis. II. Local corneal hypersensitivity to a highly virulent strain of herpes simplex. *Ophthal. Res.*, **4**, 99.

SERY, T. W., PINKES, B. H. and NAGY, R. M. (1962). Immune corneal rings: I. Evaluation of reactions to equine albumen. *Invest. Ophthal.*, **1**, 672–85.

SERY, T. W., RICHMAN, M. W. and NAGY, R. M. (1966). Experimental disciform keratitis. I. Immune response of the cornea to herpes simplex virus. *J. Allergy*, **38**, 338–51.

SHABO, A. L., PETRICCIANI, J. C. and KIRSCHSTEIN, R. L. (1973). Identification of herpes simplex and vaccinia viruses in corneal cell cultures with immunoperoxidase: a light and electron microscopic study. *Invest. Ophthal.*, **12**, 839–47.

SHILLITOE, E. J., WILTON, J. M. A. and LEHNER, T. (1977). Sequential changes in T and B lymphocyte responses to herpes simplex virus in man. *Scand. J. Immun.*, **7**, 357–66.

SHIMELD, C., TULLO, A. B., EASTY, D. L. and THOMSITT, J. (1982). Isolation of herpes simplex virus from cornea in chronic stromal keratitis. *Brit. J. Ophthal.*, **66**, 643–647.

SKINNER, G. R. B., MUSHI, E. Z. and WHITNEY, J. E. (1975/76). Immune inhibition of virus release from herpes simplex virus infected cells. *Intervirology*, **6**, 296–308.

SMITH, I. W., PEUTHERER, J. F. and McCALLUM, F. O. (1967). The incidence of herpesvirus hominis antibody in the population. *J. Hyg. (Lond.)*, **65**, 395–408.

SPENCER, W. H. and HAYES, T. L. (1970). Scanning and transmission electron microscopic observations of the topographic anatomy of dendritic lesions in the rabbit cornea. *Invest. Ophthal.*, **9**, 183–95.

STEELE, R. W., VINCENT, M. M., HENSEN, S. A., FUCILLO, D. A., CHAPA, I. A. and CANALES, L. (1975). Cellular immune responses to herpes simplex virus type 1 in recurrent herpes labialis: *in vitro* blastogenesis and cytotoxicity to infected cell virus. *J. Infect. Dis.*, **131**, 528–34.

STEVENS, T. R. and OH, J. O. (1973). Comparison of types 1 and 2 *Herpesvirus hominis* infection of rabbit eyes. II. Histologic and virologic studies. *Arch. Ophthal.*, **90**, 477–80.

SWYERS, J. S., LAUSCH, R. H. and KAUFMAN, H. E. (1967). Corneal hypersensitivity to herpes simplex. *Br. J. Ophthal.*, **51**, 843–6.

TANAKA, N. and KIMURA, S. (1967). Localisation of herpes simplex antigen and virus in the corneal stroma of experimental herpetic keratitis. *Arch. Ophthal.*, **78**, 66–73.

THONG, Y. H., VINCENT, M. M., HENSEN, S. A., FUCILLO, D. A., ROLA-RIESZCZYNSKI, M. and BELLANTI, J. A. (1975). Depressed specific cell-mediated immunity to herpes simplex virus type 1 in patients with recurrent herpes labialis. *Infection & Immunity*, **12**, 76–80.

TULLO, A. B., SHIMELD, C., BLYTH, W. H., HILL, T. J. and EASTY, D. L. (1982). Latent infection following ocular herpes simplex in non-immune and immune mice. *J. Gen. Virol.*, **63**, 95–101.

TULLO, A. B., SHIMELD, C., HILL, T. J., BLYTH, W. H. and EASTY, D. L. (1983). Ocular herpes simplex in non-immune and immune mice. *Arch. Ophthal.*, **101**, 961–964.

UCHIDA, Y. and KIMURA, S. J. (1965). Fluorescent antibody localisation of herpes simplex virus in the conjunctiva. *Arch Ophthal.*, **73**, 413–9.

VESIKARI, T. and BUINOVICI-KLEIN, E. (1975). Lymphocyte responses to rubella antigen and phytohemagglutinin after administration of R.A. 27/3 strain of live attenuated rubella virus. *Infection & Immunity*, **11**, 748–53.

WANDER, A. H., CENTIFANTO, Y. M. and KAUFMAN, H. E. (1980). Strain specificity of clinical isolates of herpes simplex virus. *Arch. Ophthal.*, **98**, 1458–61.

WESTMORELAND, B. (1978). HSV-1 and human lymphocytes: virus expression and the response to infection of adult and foetal cells. *J. Gen. Virol.*, **40**, 559–75.

WHEELER, C. E. (1960). Further studies on the effect of neutralising antibody upon the course of herpes simplex infections in tissue culture. *J. Immun.*, **84**, 394–403.

WHEELER, C. E. (1964). Biologic comparison of a syncytial and a small giant cell-forming strain of herpes simplex. *J. Immun.*, **93**, 749–756.

WILLIAMS, L. E., NESBURN, A. B. and KAUFMAN, H. E. (1965). Experimental induction of disciform keratitis. *Arch. Ophthal.*, **73**, 112–4.

WILTON, J. M. A., IVANYI, L. and LEHNER, T. (1972). Cell-mediated immunity in herpes-virus hominis infections. *Brit. Med. J.*, **1**, 723.

CHAPTER SEVEN

Clinical Aspects of Ocular Herpes Simplex Virus Infection

THE first descriptions of disease caused by the herpes group of viruses go back into antiquity, and have been well summarised by Kaplan (1973), Juel-Jensen and MacCallum (1972) and Thygeson (1976). Aphthous ulcerations in children was described by Celsus in 1516, and Cooke in 1676 wrote the earliest account in English of the manifestations of herpes simplex disease. In 1817 Bateman recognised six types of clinical herpes, including herpes zoster and herpes labialis. Somewhat later Pringe (1890) recognised herpes zoster and simplex, designating the latter herpes catarrhalis and dividing it into two types, herpes facialis and herpes genitalis. Astruc in 1736, however, is believed to have been the first to provide a clinical description of genital herpes, now known to be caused by herpes simplex virus 2. Thygeson (1976) has well summarised the history of the frequent experiments with the virus.

Human inoculation experiments were first carried out by Vidal (1873), and Steiner in 1875 was able to distinguish the difference between HSV infection and pox virus infection on cytological grounds. Grüter (1920) established that the virus could be transmitted to rabbits. Horner in 1871 was reputedly the first to describe herpes corneae febrilis, and the term dendritic keratitis was coined by Hansen Grut in 1885 (MacNab, 1907). In 1912 Grüter inoculated the corneas of rabbits with material taken from subjects with herpetic keratitis, a finding which was confirmed by Kraupa (1920) and Lowenstein (1919); the latter was able to demonstrate that material taken from cutaneous lesions at various sites, including the genital tract, could produce a specific keratitis in rabbits. Dour and Vöchting (1920) showed that in certain experiments, brain damage occurred following inoculation of the cornea, from which they concluded that the virus had invaded the central nervous system and induced an encephalitis. Early workers recognised the frequency and severity of dendritic keratitis in malaria and atopic dermatitis, with wide dissemination often occurring in children (Thygeson, 1976). Elliott in 1920 referred to the deep keratitis seen in patients with malaria, which was often central and disciform in character. The reasons for the severity of herpetic keratitis occurring in association with malaria are related to the high fever, and the immunosuppression induced by malaria (Thygeson, 1976).

Although HSV 2 was not identified until 1961 (Schneweis and Brandis), genital disease was first described in 1736. The reasons for the long delay appear to have been the variation among strains of herpes simplex viruses which are now being recognised at the molecular level (Pereira *et al.*, 1976). Such variations have long been appreciated clinically because of the differences which occur in the disease processes induced in rabbits, particularly in regard to the potential to cause an encephalitis (Nahmias and Dowdle, 1968). The clinical and epidemiological significance of the distinction between the types became evident some years later when it was demonstrated that human genital isolates were predominantly, but not exclusively, HSV 2, whereas non-genital isolates were HSV 1.

HERPES SIMPLEX KERATITIS

Epidemiology

Infection with herpes simplex virus is the single most frequent cause of corneal opacities in developed countries. Ocular infection can be a source of considerable suffering to the patient, and because of the many different manifestations of the disease it may often leave the clinician in a dilemma as to the best form of treatment to initiate. The incidence is more difficult to estimate in the developing countries, but in a limited estimate made in Tunisia, the incidence was found to be 14 per million (Whitcher *et al.*, 1976). The authors report that dendritic and geographic ulcers were complicated by deep stromal keratitis in 31 per cent, which is similar to the incidence in Europe and the United States of America. Sixty patients with ulcerative herpes simplex of the eye out of a total of 7,113 new patients were seen in a Bristol eye casualty clinic over a period of six months (Vernon, personal communication).

Norn (1970*a*) assessed the incidence over a period of 7 years, when 157 patients with one or more attacks of herpetic keratitis were seen, against a background of 50,220 out-patients. The number of patients with dendritic ulcers occurred at a rate of 1:196 of the total number of patients attending with ophthalmic diseases. The approximate estimate was that there are probably some 500 patients presenting yearly with dendritic ulcers per million population. Age and sex incidence indicated that below the age of 16 years the sexes were equally affected, while above this age a greater number of males than females were affected. The maximum incidence occurred between the ages of 40 and 50 years. Most cases were unilateral, bilateral disease occurring in 1–2 per cent of affected patients. Primary keratitis according to Norn (1970*b*) was in the region of about 5 per cent of new cases. Associated recurrent herpes of the lips was reported to occur in 50 per cent of this group of patients. Recurrence was found in 61 per cent of 109 cases. Out of the complete series the average number of attacks was 3·4. The time interval between a first and second attack averaged 5·7 years, ranging from less than 1 year up to 47 years. The interval between the first attack and the recurrence was considered to be unrelated to the age of the patient. Visual acuities recorded in 107 of the patients treated with antiviral, steroid or cauterisation therapy or combinations of these therapies showed that about 46 per cent of the group retained a visual acuity of 6/6 or better, while 17 per cent had a reduction of visual acuity to 6/18 or less. Steroid therapy had a significant influence in reducing the visual acuity. Corneal opacities of various types was seen in 85 per cent. Blood-vessel invasion was found in half the affected eyes. The size of the opacity together with the vascularisation was aggravated by treatment with steroid, relapses, and possibly treatment with IDU.

In a study of 152 patients with ulcerative herpetic keratitis over a five-year period, with respect to recurrence of epithelial disease, the development of stromal disease, and the utilisation of topical corticosteroid, Wilhelmus *et al.* (1981*a*) reported a recurrence rate of 40 per cent with over half occurring during the first six months. This contrasted with other studies in which the rate of recurrence had varied between 35 per cent and 71 per cent over a two- to seven-year follow-up. Recrudescences tended to occur in the first two weeks in 46 per cent of patients with mechanical debridement. Important factors associated with ulcer recurrence were a history of previous herpetic ulcer and the sex of the patient; patients with prior ulceration, and males, were more likely to develop recurrence. Fifty-three per cent of patients with at least one previous ulcer developed a third recurrent ulcer, compared with 28 per cent of those with no prior history of ocular herpes. Fifty per cent of male patients developed recurrences compared with 22 per cent of females.

The recurrence of stromal inflammation occurred in 25 per cent of a population studied by Wilhelmus *et al.* (1981*b*). Two-thirds occurred in the form of a disciform keratitis, and the other third occurred as non-disciform stromal infiltrates. Disciform keratitis occurred in the first month following resolution of the original ulcer, with the remainder occurring progressively less frequently over a five-year period. Only 11 per cent of cases of stromal keratitis occurred during the first month post-treatment, but 78 per cent had occurred by the end of the first year of follow-up. The different morphological appearances and timings of presentation implied that the two types of stromal involvement were produced by different immunological mechanisms. Topical corticosteroid therapy was associated with a higher incidence of stromal disease.

A classification of herpes simplex eye disease is shown in Table 7.1 and corneal ulceration in Table 7.2.

CLINICAL MANIFESTATIONS OF HERPETIC KERATITIS

Primary Disease

Primary herpes simplex virus disease is the first infection in a host who has no immunity against the virus. It may present in various forms and affect a number of different patient groups (Table 7.3). The incubation period ranges from 2 to 12 days, and the infection occurs in both sexes and all races. It is a common infection and may occur in 50 to 60 per cent in people living in good

TABLE 7.1

CLASSIFICATION OF HERPES SIMPLEX EYE DISEASE

Primary	Cutaneous (lids and lid margins)
	Conjunctival (follicular conjunctivitis)
	Corneal (true primary of the cornea without lid involvement probably rare; generally occurs shortly following cutaneous eruption of lids)
Secondary	Possibly rare (protection induced by primary or recurrent disease elsewhere prevents reinfection by auto-inoculation, and also partially protects against reinfection by another virus strain)
Recurrent epithelial keratitis	Common form of herpetic keratitis; rarely follows primary corneal disease, but more often follows a primary focus elsewhere with internal neurogenic spread and subsequent presentation
Recurrent stromal disease	Associated with epithelial disease
	Associated with cutaneous disease
Prolonged stromal disease	
Chronic kerato-uveitis	
Recurrent uveitis	
Bilateral disease	Keratitis
	Uveitis
	Bilateral disease in association with immunosuppression
	Bilateral disease in association with atopic disease

hygienic conditions, but may reach a level of 100 per cent in those in less good hygienic surroundings.

Primary infection usually occurs early in life after maternal antibodies have declined and there is no longer useful protection, attack rates being maximal between 1–5 years and between 16 and 25 years. The antibody titres show an overall occurrence rate of 97 per cent by the age of 60 years (Smith *et al.*, 1967). However with the passing of time and with the improvement in environmental and hygienic conditions it is to be expected that the frequency of subjects with positive antibody titres will wane.

In 50 per cent of cases, the primary infection is not recognised and is merely associated with the appearance of antibodies. The recognisable infections may be minimal with few symptoms, but on occasions may be severe and produce a significant clinical disease. The site of entry is thought to be the place where the disease becomes manifest; herpes simplex virus 1 may produce a gingivostomatitis, infection of the upper respiratory tract, such as pharyngitis, tonsillitis and rhinitis, ocular infections or cutaneous infections (Ostler, 1976). HSV 2 generally produces genital and neonatal disease. The first sign of primary infection is oedema which is followed by the appearance of vesicles in the skin, or by ulceration in moist situations. The regional lymph nodes may often be enlarged in primary infections. Primary gingivostomatitis is one of the most frequent modes of infection, the symptoms being sore throat, chills and fever and myalgia. On the first or second days, vesicles appear on the soft palate, gums or tongue and buccal mucosa (Figure 7.1 and Plate I*a*). It is of some importance that the virus may be isolated from the oral lesions for up to

TABLE 7.2

CLASSIFICATION OF ULCERATION OF THE CORNEA ASSOCIATED WITH THE HERPES SIMPLEX VIRUS

Primary disease	Punctate epithelial keratitis Necrotic plaque epitheliopathy Areolar dendritic figure Classical dendritic figure
Recurrent dendritic figure	Single or multiple dendritic figures
Ulcerative disease in patients treated with topical steroid	(a) Geographic ulcer. (b) Dendritic figure
Ulcerative disease associated with active stromal keratitis	(a) Geographic if treated with topical steroid without antiviral cover (b) Dendritic figure
Recurrent ulcerative lesions in patients with increased risk due to immunosuppression and immunodeficiency	Dendritic figures, occurring with increased frequency
Fine, localised punctate epithelial keratitis	(a) Persistent, overlying site of the dendrite (b) Recurrent, sterile, possibly related to use of topical steroid (c) Recurrent or persistent conglomerate superficial erosion
Fine punctate epithelial keratitis extending onto conjunctiva	Resulting from the prolonged use of topical antivirals; may be associated with vortex patterns in Bowman's membrane or the superficial stroma
Trophic corneal ulcer	Persistent ulcer often with rolled edge; if prolonged, may be associated with overproduction of collagenase with subsequent corneal thinning or threatened perforation
Recurrent abrasion	Following cautery, debridement techniques.
Ulcerative disease in organ-transplanted patient	(a) Dendritic figure } appear on host and extend onto (b) Geographic figure } donor tissue

several weeks after the infection and therefore such disease would continue to act as a reservoir from which the disease might spread to other patients.

Primary disease occurs with the typical skin eruption which nevertheless may not always be easy to detect. The eruption may consist of a large number of vesicles which can be situated around the eyes and involved the skin of the lids and periorbital skin (Figure 7.2). On the other hand, the lesion may be a single, isolated one which is situated along the lid margin such that it evades detection, if not specifically thought of and searched for with the microscope. Follicular conjunctivitis may be associated with the eruption involving the upper and lower tarsal plates together with a punctate epithelial keratitis.

The cornea becomes involved in about 30 per cent of these patients. The initial punctate keratitis may clear without progressing to the more diffuse disease which may sometimes occur. Occasionally, islands of necrotic cells may coalesce to form white elevated plaques which eventually desquamate and spread to form a large dendritic figure (Plate I*b*). The affected epithelial cells, their nuclei laden with replicating virus, balloon just prior to releasing newly formed virus that will infect adjacent cells, and it is at this time that virus can be isolated in quantity. According to clinical observation, primary

TABLE 7.3

CLASSIFICATION OF PRIMARY ULCERATIVE HERPES SIMPLEX KERATITIS

	Type or disease	Immunological status
Neonatal	Ulcerative and stromal	Occurs in the presence of maternal antibody
Infantile	Follicular conjunctivitis, skin vesicles and dendritic figure	Immunity absent at initiation
Childhood	As in infantile, but rare	As in infancy
Adolescence and young adulthood	Isolated vesicle hidden from view, follicular conjunctivitis, punctate epithelial keratitis, dendritic figure	Persists until local and systemic immune responses are turned on
Mature adulthood	Primary disease rare	Increasing chance of systemic immunity due to prior cutaneous infection, or subclinical infection
Immunosuppressed subjects	Rare but severe; associated with systemic manifestations e.g. encephalitis	Systemic and local immune reactions delayed
Immunodeficient patients	Primary disease of increased severity with associated stromal disease	Usually occurs in patients with depleted cell-mediated immunity
Atopic subjects	Primary disease severe (e.g. Kaposi's varicelliform eruption)	No specific deficiency in protective immunity located.

ocular herpetic keratitis is not always followed by recurrent ulcerative disease, and deep stromal involvement is by no means common. The lesions of the skin or lid margin become vesicular, crusted and dessicated and eventually heal without scarring. The conjunctivitis may persist for two to three weeks. A reactive iritis may occasionally occur with cells in the anterior chamber, and a slight flare detectable with a narrow beam on the slit-lamp microscope. However, although severe iritis is rare in primary disease, it may occur with a greater degree of severity in the newborn.

Eye infections with herpes simplex virus in neonates have been reviewed by Nahmias *et al.* (1976). Of 297 newborns with HSV type 1 or 2 infections, about 20 per cent demonstrated ocular involvement including conjunctivitis, keratitis, chorioretinitis, optic neuritis and cataracts. In a case described in depth by these authors there was bilateral corneal opacification with vascular ingrowth and ulceration on the left side. The ocular disease was accompanied by a diffuse vesicular skin eruption from which HSV was cultured. The diagnosis should be suspected if there is a history of genital herpes in the mother, particularly if it occurs during pregnancy. It was considered that the infection had occurred some three weeks before birth, but the authors state that it is not possible to know whether the infection is acquired by a transplacental route or via an ascending infection. Although such an infection can be designated as primary, it is somewhat different from primary disease in later life, as

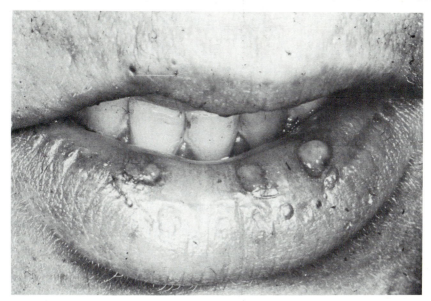

Figure 7.1.   Herpes simplex vesicles affecting the lower lip in a patient with herpetic stomatitis. (Courtesy of Dr. Robin Davies.)

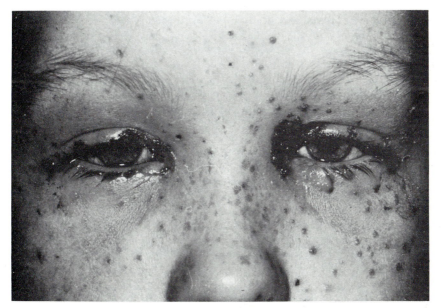

Figure 7.2.   Peri-orbital skin eruption in primary herpes simplex virus infection.

presumably the infection occurs in the presence of passively transmitted maternal antibodies which might play a role in determining the clinical presentation of the disease and its eventual outcome.

Recurrent Follicular Conjunctivitis

An acute herpetic follicular conjunctivitis or keratoconjunctivitis resembling adenovirus ocular infection can present and can be a trap for the unwary. There is a moderate to severe follicular and papillary reaction in the tarsal plates with epithelial and sometimes subepithelial punctate keratitis associated with little sign of systemic disease, this appearance, occurring in the absence of a facial or corneal lesion, being closely similar to adenoviral infections caused by types 8 and 19. It is important that such cases of acute follicular conjunctivitis should arouse suspicion of HSV infection, and the diagnosis must be supported by appropriate laboratory tests. Darouger et al. (1978) have stressed the importance of reaching an accurate diagnosis and avoiding the use of topical corticosteroid. The majority of patients are aged between 20 and 35 years, with males and females equally affected. It is possible that typical herpetic lesions of the lids and cornea will follow in a portion of these patients.

Recurrent Ulcerative Herpetic Keratitis

Recurrent disease is often related to a trigger which is pyrexial in nature, but there are a number of other factors, not least of which is trauma. In childhood, both sexes are involved equally, but in adult life males predominate. Gundersen (1936) reported a male:female ratio of 2.4:1, while Laibson and Leopold (1964) reported a ratio of 3:1. Bilateral disease is uncommon and is usually associated with immunodeficiency or severe atopic disease (Easty et al., 1975).

The clinical picture of recurrent epithelial disease is variable, but whereas in primary diseases both the cornea and the conjunctiva can be simultaneously affected, it is unusual for the conjunctiva to be involved in the presence of active epithelial disease (Table 7.4). Corneal ulcers present with a painful eye and the appearance of fine granular spots in the epithelium. Epithelial bedewing, vesicles, cracks and fissures may occur in association, which produce differing appearances such as superficial punctate keratitis, stellate areolar keratitis, or superficial striate keratitis where the punctate opacities arrange themselves into a criss-cross pattern. The common manifestation is the branching ulcer known as a dendritic ulcer or figure, which stains with fluorescein or rose bengal drops (Plate Ic). Surrounding the invaded area the epithelium becomes loosely attached to the basement membrane, and it can easily be removed. In primary ulcerative herpetic keratitis the underlying stroma does not seem to be involved to the same extent as in recurrent disease, where a subepithelial keratitis is often present.

The dendritic figure is of an irregular zig-zag shape with side-branchings forming a complicated arborescent figure. The ulcer is surrounded by a vertical edge where the cells are opaque and contain invading virus. Staining with fluorescein demarcates the ulcer for a short period, following which the dye spreads into the unhealthy surrounding epithelium. It may also seep into the stroma and disguise important clinical signs such as the degree of cellular

PLATE I

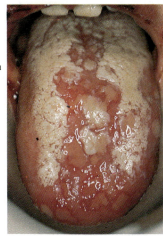

(a) Vesicles on the tongue of a patient with severe primary herpetic stomatitis. (Courtesy, Dr Robin Davies.)

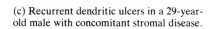

(b) Large primary dendritic ulcer in a 20-year-old patient with primary disease.

(c) Recurrent dendritic ulcers in a 29-year-old male with concomitant stromal disease.

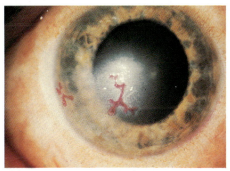

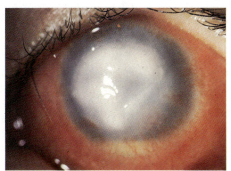

(d) Diffuse corneal abscess in a patient with a history of herpetic keratitis.

TABLE 7.4

FEATURES OF ULCERATIVE HERPETIC KERATITIS OF VARYING TYPES

	Primary disease	Recurrent disease
Immune status	Absent at time of infection	Immunity present
Frequency in population	Uncommon	Common
Trigger	Absent	Fever, sunburn, stress, menstruation, depressed CMI
Frequency of recurrence	Recurrence infrequent	Frequency of recurrences vary: depends on trigger and possibly on immune status
Clinical disease		
Cutaneous manifestations	Diffuse periorbital vesicles; Large isolated vesicles; Single vesicle (small and evasive)	Recurrent dendrite occasionally but not always preceded by cutaneous disease
Conjunctival manifestation	Follicular conjunctivitis	Occasional cause of follicular conjunctivitis in absence of corneal disease. Conjunctival reaction; follicular/papillary or minimal specific change
Corneal manifestation Epithelial	Punctate epithelial keratitis Plaques of necrotic epithelial cells Desquamation and coalescence to produce large dendrite	Dendritic figure Single Multiple
Stromal disease	Rare	Stromal disease of varying grades of severity in approximately 30% of patients.

infiltration in the stroma, the amount of oedema, and the presence of a proteinaceous flare and cells in the anterior chamber. Rose bengal drops, on the other hand, remain isolated in the ulcerated area, and do not disguise clinical signs by diffusion into the surrounding tissue.

The dendritic ulcer heals in 5–12 days in the untreated state. Epithelial deficits may remain for longer periods and can cause concern to the clinician, but may represent inability of the epithelium to regenerate rather than continuing virus replication; on the other hand such persistent lesions can be the result of the use of topical antiviral therapy which can inhibit the rate of epithelial regeneration (Table 7.2) or to the development of resistant strains of virus.

Resolution of a dendritic figure may occur in the absence of treatment. Thygeson (1976) was convinced early in his career that the natural history of recurrent ulcerative herpetic keratitis was essentially benign, and that the disease was usually over-treated by procedures that temporarily or permanently increased the opacity in Bowman's membrane beneath the original lesion. Such observations are supported by the early placebo-controlled clinical trials of antiviral agents, one of which was thought to be aureomycin (Thygeson and Hogan, 1950). Following treatment with a product that is now known to have no antiviral properties, ulcerative disease cleared in 60 per cent of patients within 7 days. That the aureomycin was acting as a placebo was later shown by Geller and Thygeson (1951).

The recurrence of epithelial deficits following the apparently successful treatment of a dendritic ulcer may sometimes leave the clinician in a dilemma, as it is not always clear whether the deficit is due to the presence of virus which is replicating or due to the secondary effects of over-zealous treatment regimes. The prolonged use of antiviral agents or of cautery/debridement techniques can lead to either persistent staining areas, or to later reappearance of epithelial deficits, so that it is not clear what the true aetiology is. Clarification can be obtained by a careful history directed particularly towards the presence of recurrence elsewhere or the recent occurrence of a trigger factor.

Epithelial Trophic Ulcers (Metaherpetic)

After the resolution of a typical epithelial lesion, breakdown of the epithelium may recur with the formation of a chronic ovoid ulcer with a grey, thickened border formed by heaped cells which are seemingly unable to move across damaged basement membrane (Figure 7.3). It is important to recognise that trophic ulcers are not due to active proliferation of virus but rather to basement-membrane damage from the prior disease process. The treatment regime is therefore aimed at assisting epithelium to regenerate, rather than being against the virus.

Trophic ulcers which persist, failing to heal after a time-interval of some

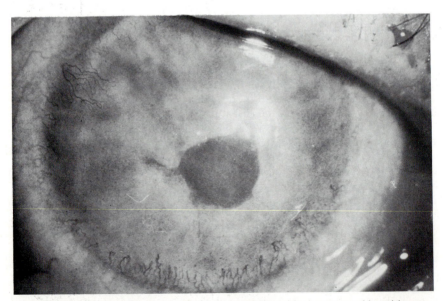

Figure 7.3   A trophic ulcer persisting in association with severe stromal keratitis.

weeks, may become complicated by secondary bacterial invasion or by stromal melting induced by the local production of collagenase.

Stromal Herpes Simplex Keratitis

In approximately 30 per cent of all patients who have experienced ulcerative herpetic keratitis, the virus or its antigens may spread into the corneal stroma. The factors which determine the spread of virus into the corneal stroma are complex, and involve the balance between the attempts of the immune system to dispose of the virus, and the tendency of both the virus and the immune reactions which are directed against it to cause tissue damage. It must be recalled that in most animal models of epithelial disease, there has been good laboratory evidence of penetration of virus antigen into the stroma, which in many patients must be cleared. Some of the factors which influence this spread are shown in Table 7.5, but it is probably the use of topical corticosteroid which has been an important cause of this unfortunate complication in the past. The manifestations of deep stromal keratitis show considerable variety

TABLE 7.5

FACTORS INFLUENCING THE SEVERITY OF HERPES SIMPLEX KERATITIS

Source of virus	Labial Oral Mucocutaneous ⎫ Cutaneous ⎬ HSV 1 Genital ⎭ HSV 2
Mode of transmission	Transfer from exogenous source (kissing, physical contact such as during various sports; venereal routes)
Distribution of virus in the CNS	Virus probably spreads during a first attack, via the brain stem, from the primary dermatome to create latency in ganglia subserving other dermatomes
Amount of virus introduced onto the corneal surface	Dependent upon the amount of virus present in the reservoir of infection and the precise mechanism of transfer
State of the corneal epithelial barrier at the time of inoculation	Interruption to barrier caused by trauma at the time of inoculation, or present prior to inoculation
Frequency and severity of recurrent attacks	Determined by frequency of triggers; local trauma, associated eye disease, e.g. immediate allergic responses to external allergens systemic: fever, immunosuppression, menstruation, psychological stress external: exposure to UV light
The host response	Primary infections; time taken for immune response to occur Recurrent disease; efficacy of immune response
Associated diseases	Immunodeficiency; immunosuppression; atopic disease; local external eye disease
Age and sex ratio	Trend towards severe stromal disease in the elderly; Males:females, 7:3 approximately

in appearance, but it is possible to distinguish a number of patterns which can help in leading the clinician towards a suitable treatment policy. It is particularly important in management to document the corneal changes with accuracy, so that the influence of treatment can be monitored in order to recognize improvement or deterioration at each examination.

Stromal herpetic keratitis may be defined as an inflammatory reaction occurring in the presence of, or following, a dendritic figure, to a degree greater than that to be expected or than that caused by herpes simplex virus proliferation in the epithelium. Thus for the purist there is an inevitable stromal reaction directed against any epithelial disease process, manifest at a microscopic level by the preliminary appearance of polymorphonuclear leuco-cytes at an early stage. Careful scrutiny of underlying stroma can allow the detection of such cells during epithelial disease. Figures 7.4 and 7.5 demon-strate schematically some ways in which the cornea reacts to the herpes simplex virus.

Stromal disease may follow primary herpetic keratitis immediately in the form of superficial stromal opacities generally underlying the sites of the previous epithelial disease. A somewhat delayed stromal focus of inflammation may occur well after the primary disease has apparently healed (Figure 7.6). Stromal inflammation following ulcerative disease depends upon the frequency of recurrence and its treatment. Whatever the factors are which contribute to the entry of virus into the stroma and its resultant severity, a number of syndromes may be recognised.

Ghost of Dendritic Figure

Following the healing of a dendritic figure a superficial stromal opacity may remain which outlines the area covered by the previous ulcer. The opacity may itself be dendritiform, or appear as a series of superficial stromal punctate opacities.

Stromal disease may be said to be present if stromal inflammation persists beyond the time taken for the epithelial disease to completely resolve. The reactions induced in the stroma by the virus are similar to inflammatory responses induced in other tissues, but are unique in that they can be witnessed in detail *in vivo* with the binocular microscope. Cellular infiltration, inflam-matory oedema, oedema due to endothelial decompensation, vascular ingrowth, and tissue damage which may result in permanent scarring may be seen. Uveitis may occur in association with keratitis, and keratitic precipitates may form which are largely composed of plasma cells of lymphocytes (Inomata and Smelser, 1970). There is a certain amount of clinical evidence for involvement of the endothelium (Vannas and Ahonen, 1981).

In Figures 7.4 and 7.5 can be seen a classification of stromal keratitis which serves to highlight the various syndromes which may be encountered, although it is emphasised that no one case of stromal keratitis is exactly the same as another, and that each case encountered will have unique characteristics and clinical problems. It is convenient to think of the disease as being a balance between dissemination or spread of the virus or antigen in varying concentra-tions, countered by the host response which would be expected also to vary.

Figure 7.4. Schematic representation of the varieties of herpetic keratitis:

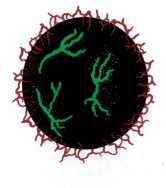

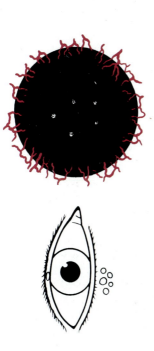

(a) Punctate epithelial keratitis with isolated vesicles

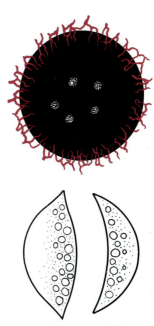

(b) Necrotic epithelial plaques with follicular conjunctivitis and a pre-auricular gland palpable

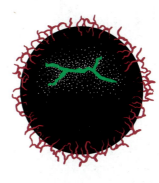

(c) Multiple dendritic ulcers which eventually coalesce

(d) Recurrent dendritic ulcer

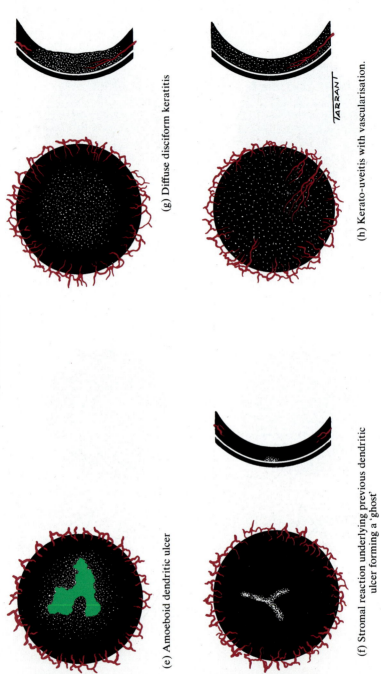

Figure 7.4. (*continued*)

(e) Amoeboid dendritic ulcer

(f) Stromal reaction underlying previous dendritic
ulcer forming a 'ghost'

(g) Diffuse disciform keratitis

(h) Kerato-uveitis with vascularisation.

Figure 7.5. Schematic representation of various syndromes in herpes simplex keratitis.

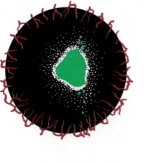

(c) Trophic ulceration

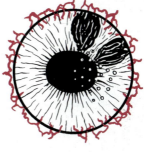

(d) Anterior uveitis and iris atrophy

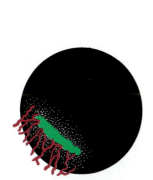

(a) Marginal keratitis

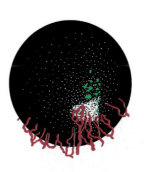

(b) Dense infiltration and vascularisation

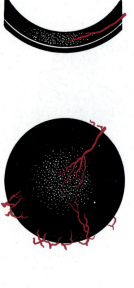

(g) Deep stromal scarring and vascularisation

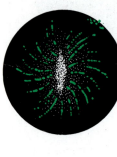

TARRANT

(h) Antiviral toxicity.

Figure 7.5. (*continued*)

(e) Geographic ulceration
due to topical
corticosteroid

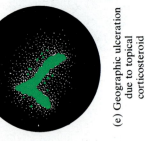

(f) Geographic ulceration
following penetrating
keratoplasty

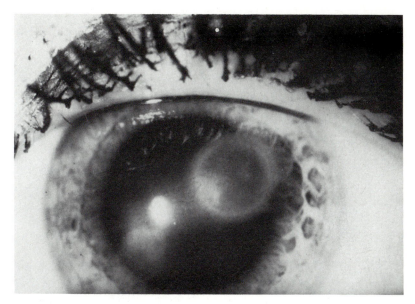

Figure 7.6.   Stromal keratitis forming an immune ring in a patient with a history of primary ulcerative herpetic keratitis three months previously.

The amount of antigenic material available for absorption or spread into the stroma will depend upon a number of factors, not least of which is the host immune response which serves to inhibit virus proliferation in the epithelium.

Superficial Punctate Keratitis

Punctate opacities may appear to be dispersed further afield than an initial dendrite, producing a superficial punctate keratitis.

Disciform Keratitis

Occasionally a keratitis may occur following a history of a dendritic figure previously, where a localised, often central, opacity appears in the cornea with stromal oedema and mild infiltration, and inflammatory cells visible with the slit-lamp (Figure 7.7). The stromal swelling is rarely accompanied by vascularisation, but can be associated with the formation of keratic precipitates and a mild anterior uveitis. In such lesions the prognosis is good, the condition often resolving with the use of topical anti-inflammatory therapy in minimal dosages.

Immune Ring Formation

The formation of an immune ring due to inflammatory cells in the stroma is a not uncommon happening at some stage of stromal disease (Figure 7.6). On occasions it may occur in isolation, or it can accompany stromal disease of various types and be one manifestation of virus spread. It is thought to be due to the formation of immune complexes and may be part of a disciform keratitis.

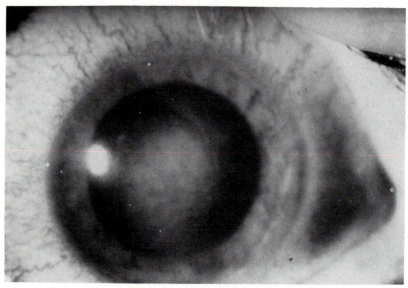

Figure 7.7.   Central disciform keratitis due to the herpes simplex virus in a male patient.

It can be seen developing in the stroma towards the end of a dendritic figure during the phase of healing as a circular halo around the ulcerated area, or it may occur later, somewhat in the manner of disciform keratitis, where its appearance may be delayed well after the resolution of the ulcerative disease. It has generally been our experience that the appearance of an immune ring at the time of ulceration indicates the subsequent onset of severe and persistent stromal disease.

Limbal Keratitis

Keratitis occurring close to the limbus can be associated with persistent disease, deep and superficial vascularisation, recurrent epithelial deficits, and often with the formation of dense collections of inflammatory cells (Figure 7.5). There can occasionally be a localised area of episcleral or scleral hyperaemia which, rarely, can lead to thinning at the limbus with the appearance of pigmented ciliary body.

Kerato-uveitis

The occurrence of a diffuse keratitis affecting the greater part of the stroma may be accompanied by an anterior uveitis which adds considerably to the problems which can be met in the management of stromal disease. The keratitis is diffuse and may involve the whole cornea, and be associated with vascular ingrowth, inflammatory oedema, endothelial decompensation, and large keratic precipitates (Figure 7.8). The opacification of the stroma prevents detailed observation of the anterior chamber; the inflammatory response can be such that a hypopyon can occur which may be missed unless particular care

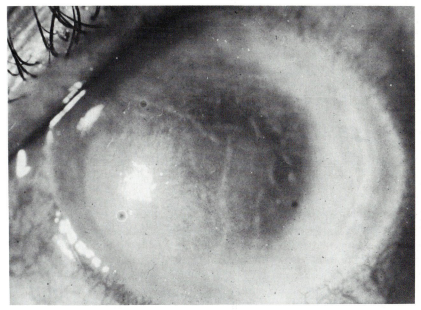

Figure 7.8.   Severe diffuse stromal keratitis and uveitis.

is taken to observe it. Uveitis can result in the formation of posterior synechiae, iris atrophy, secondary cataract and elevation of the intra-ocular pressure.

Active Stromal Keratitis in the presence of Dendritic Ulceration

When stromal disease of various descriptive types occurs in the presence of proliferative viral disease in the epithelium, the ocular syndrome becomes the more difficult to manage, and it is from this point of view that it should be regarded as a specific entity (Plate I*c*).

Corneal Abscess Following Herpes Simplex Keratitis

Severe corneal abscesses may occur rarely, following the inexpert use of topical corticosteroid, when the stroma becomes densely infiltrated with inflammatory cells. Abscesses may be diffuse (Plate I*d*), or localised (Plate II*a*), and may exist in the presence of live virus proliferating in the epithelium, or be situated in the deeper stroma without a surface deficit. It is in this group of patients that care must be taken to exclude the presence of other invasive organisms by careful investigation with smears and bacterial and mycotic culture.

Stromal Thinning, Descemetocele or Perforation

Stromal thinning can be associated with persistent epithelial deficits of a trophic type, and can lead to actual or threatened perforation. These changes are not necessarily associated with cellular infiltration in the stroma, and may occur in the patient with a localised keratitis which can be of only a moderate degree of severity from a clinical point of view (Figure 7.9).

Permanent Stromal Scarring

Stromal inflammation may lead to the formation of a scar which, situated in the centre of the cornea, may overlie the visual axis and cause distortion and loss of vision. The scarring may be situated at various levels within the stroma, or may on the other hand involve the whole thickness. Where blood vessels have penetrated the stroma it is rare for them to disappear, and a single arteriole may supply a central plexus of capillaries from which a number of venous channels drain towards the limbus (Figure 7.10). Faceting of the corneal surface may result in prolonged disease which may serve to reduce the visual acuity or cause visual distortion.

Herpes Simplex Uveitis

Oh (1976) studied the dynamics of HSV uveitis induced as a primary and secondary event in laboratory animals. The study showed that live HSV could be isolated from eyes with primary herpetic uveitis during the acute stage of the disease, but virus could not be isolated in secondary uveitis at any stage of the disease, even as early as 5 hours after intravitreal injection of live HSV. The failure to isolate infectious HSV from eyes with secondary uveitis was thought to be due to the neutralising effect on the virus of high titres of specific antibody in the eye. The antibody persisted in the rabbit eyes for more than 10 months after their recovery from the primary infection.

The role of immune mediated reactions in the pathogenesis of primary and secondary HSV uveitis was also studied by Oh (1979). Primary uveitis was induced by the intracameral injection of live HSV in normal rabbits, and secondary uveitis was induced by re-injection into eyes which had recovered from a primary infection. Primary uveitis reached a peak on the fourth day post-injection, whereas secondary uveitis was most severe on the first day post-injection. Infectious virus was required to induce primary disease, but either live or inactivated virus was able to produce secondary disease. In primary uveitis immunosuppressive agents did not effect either the uveal inflammation or virus replication during the early stages of the disease, but it nevertheless attenuated the uveitis while enhancing virus growth in the late stage of the disease. It was concluded that primary herpetic uveitis is mediated first by infection of uveal tissue by live virus, and later by immune-mediated mechanisms, these mechanisms probably operating to induce secondary uveitis. Immunity was thought to play a considerable part in both primary and secondary herpetic uveitis.

Herpes simplex uveitis in humans may accompany an attack of severe epithelial ulcerative disease, and more commonly is associated with stromal keratitis. On occasions it may present a recurrent problem without corneal manifestations although these are often apparent in the past history. It is particularly in patients where the cornea shows no involvement that care should be taken in deciding on treatment; it is imperative in such cases that topical corticosteroid therapy should be covered by an antiviral agent which possesses good penetrating properties so that the anterior uvea is reached.

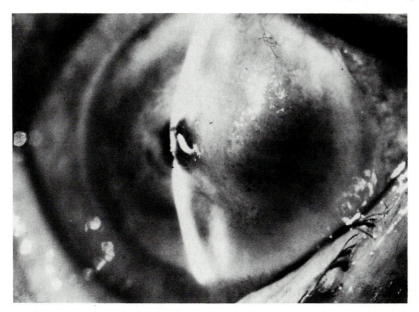

Figure 7.9.   Diffuse keratitis with a descemetocele and threatened perforation.

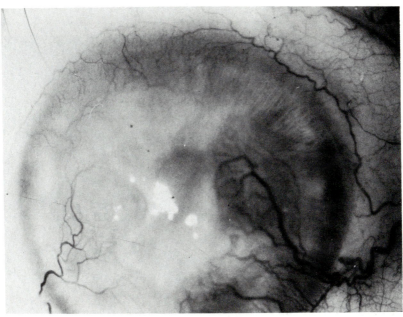

Figure 7.10.   Diffuse scarring and vascularisation in a 55-year-old male, following severe kerato-uveitis.

Uveitis is characterised by the sudden onset of photophobia and soreness, accompanied by severe blurring of vision on occasions. Cells and flare are present in the anterior chamber, and posterior synechiae may form at the pupil margin (Figure 7.11). In a significant proportion of patients secondary glaucoma may occur, adding considerably to the difficulties encountered in clinical management. Herpes simplex uveitis is one of the more common causes of spontaneous hyphaemia. In adults the anterior uvea is characteristically involved, but in the newborn and in immunologically compromised hosts chorioretinitis may occur (Minkler *et al.*, 1976). In neonatal ocular herpes, where there may be an associated encephalitis, the posterior uvea is quite often involved. In adults when the disease accompanies stromal disease, the latter is often severe and prolonged and shows poor response to treatment. It may also occur in the absence of preceding stromal disease; presumably latency is established in the superior cervical sympathetic ganglion, whence virus may enter the uvea by axoplasmic flow.

The isolation of herpes simplex virus has provided the same difficulties as in the case of identification of the virus in preparations taken from patients or animals with stromal keratitis. Using fluorescein-tagged antibodies, Patterson *et al.* (1968) found evidence of herpes simplex antigens in cells aspirated from the anterior chamber, but confirmation that the antigens were infectious was not obtained. Witmer and Iwamato (1968) were able to demonstrate particles with the morphological characteristics of herpes virus in the iris of a 71-year-old male who had undergone iridectomy during operative treatment of painful secondary glaucoma.

There has been some disparity in the reported results of investigation into

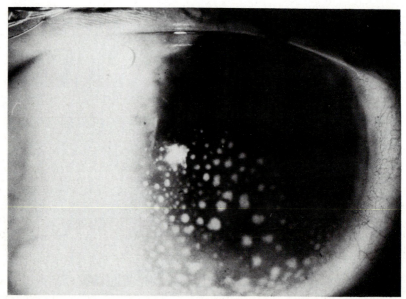

Figure 7.11.   Keratic precipitates in a patient with herpes simplex virus uveitis.

the presence of viable virus in aqueous humour taken from patients with uveitis. Some investigators have not been able to isolate virus (Hogan *et al.*, 1964; Kimura, 1962), while other workers have been able to isolate viable agent; Cavara (1955) isolated virus from aqueous humour in 7 out of 13 patients; Hewson (1957), Pavan-Langston and Brockhurst (1969), and Bock *et al.* (1972) have reported an isolation of virus from one of their series of cases.

Sundmacher and Neumann-Haefelin (1979) assessed the aqueous humour for virus in 33 patients with uveitis. Eight cultures taken from seven patients were positive for herpes simplex virus. It was considered that there are criteria which indicate that there is live HSV in the anterior chamber. HSV-positive patients exhibited secondary glaucoma, and the presence of glaucoma was in itself highly predictive in assessing the chances of positive virus isolation. A focal, serous HSV-positive iritis healed with treatment with topical cortico-steroid and mydriatic. In particular there were diffuse and large keratic precipitates covering most of the endothelium.

The diagnosis of herpetic uveitis is usually made because of the presence of active epithelial or stromal disease, but on the occasions where there is no evidence of this the uveitis may present a trap for the unwary physician. Such patients may show sectorial iris atrophy (Figure 7.5) which although similar to the sectorial atrophy which may be seen following herpes zoster uveitis, differs from this in that the deficits, which may be visualised in the pigment epithelium of the iris with a co-axial beam of the slit lamp, are ovoid with their long axis radial, rather than triangular (Marsh *et al.*, 1974). Fluorescein studies show that the atrophy of the iris occurring in the uveitis which accompanies herpes zoster ophthalmicus is due to a local ischaemia, whereas that which is due to the HSV does not present findings suggesting an ischaemic process.

Elevation of the intra-ocular pressure occurs in 28 per cent of patients with herpetic kerato-uveitis, and 10 per cent of these patients develop glaucoma (Falcon and Williams, 1978).

Herpes Encephalitis

Although the first few months of life present a period of relative insuscep-tibility to HSV infection, there are exceptions. Rarely, shortly before birth, during parturition or immediately after birth, a susceptible infant can be infected through its mother, father or from its attendants. In some 80 per cent of cases, such a fetus or newborn develops a severe generalised disease, with multi-organ involvement and a mortality of over 80 per cent. Involvement of the brain is often a dominant sign, but in neonatal herpes this encephalitis is part of a pathological process which also involves the lungs, liver adrenal glands, the skin and the eye. Encephalitis, as a manifestation of HSV infection of the neonate, is a different disease from herpes encephalitis in later childhood or adult life (Longson, 1979).

There are a number of possible outcomes of HSV infection of the central nervous system (Table 7.6). In the first case that was reported by Smith *et al.* (1941), there was an associated necrosis of the brain which was focal in type. The usual site for such necrosis is in the cerebral hemisphere, particularly in

TABLE 7.6

EFFECTS OF HSV INFECTIONS ON THE
HUMAN CENTRAL NERVOUS SYSTEM

1 Latent infection
2 Minor or subclinical disease (? psychiatric disorders—chronic
   nervous system disease)
3 Herpes meningitis with encephalitis (prognosis good)
4 Mild diffuse encephalitis (with good prognosis)
5 Severe diffuse encephalitis (poor prognosis)
6 Acute necrotising encephalitis, focal, with poor prognosis
7 Brain-stem encephalitis, with poor prognosis

(From Longson, 1979)

the temporal or frontal lobes, where the focus can mimic a space-occupying lesion.

Estimated total death rates are considered to occur in the region of 25 per year in the United Kingdom (Longson, 1979). The incidence of herpes simplex encephalitis lies in the region of about 50 patients per year, which is about 1 per million population per year.

The natural history of herpes encephalitis has long been a matter of dispute, many authorities assuming it to be a manifestation of a primary infection, while others hold the view that it is the result of virus reactivation. Longson (1979) has observed that the disease is rarely accompanied by any of the lesions otherwise associated with primary HSV infections elsewhere, there being little evidence of dermatrophic and mucotrophic manifestations, which are curiously suppressed. Other evidence may be cited suggesting that the disease is not primary, such as the presence of a different age distribution between those suffering from primary infections compared to those suffering from encephalitis. The contrast is compatible with the hypothesis that herpes encephalitis is the result of a reactivation of an infection originally acquired months, years or decades before. Electroencephalography at the time of primary herpetic acute gingivostomatitis often reveals abnormalities, which may be non-specific changes related to the pyrexia associated with the illness, but could also signal the arrival of HSV in the brain prior to the establishment of latent infection in that organ. Many patients with herpes encephalitis have well documented histories of previous recurrent herpes labialis. It is likely that many patients with encephalitis have had gingivostomatitis at an earlier time, which is probably one of the most convincing pieces of evidence in favour of the reactivation hypothesis. Ocular disease is sometimes seen in patients with herpes encephalitis, though this is rare. Savir et al. (1980) have described retinal vasculitis occurring in adults with encephalitis. With the increasing sophistication of techniques for the identification and isolation of the herpes simplex virus from tissues, it is to be anticipated that the virus will be found in retinal disease (Openshaw, 1983). There is now good laboratory evidence for the spread of virus to the retina from the opposite eye following intra-ocular inoculation (Howe et al., 1979; Tullo et al., 1982).

Herpes Simplex Virus Type 2 Disease

The two types of herpes simplex virus have distinctive antigenic and biological properties. Infections with the type 1 strain usually affect the oral cavity or the skin, these manifesting as oral ulcers, gingivostomatitis and herpes labialis, with rarely an encephalitis. Type 2 is the genital strain which is associated with vulvovaginitis, cervicitis and cervical cancer, with the various lesions of herpes simplex occurring in the newborn, such as keratoconjunctivitis and chorioretinitis (Tuffli and Nahmias, 1969). Its occurrence in adults has been less commonly reported, but nevertheless it does occasionally cause disease (Oh et al., 1976), which appears to be transmitted from genital sites. Hanna et al. (1976) reviewed 171 isolates during the period 1950 to 1975, and found that 161 could be readily typed by indirect immunofluorescence. Of 81 typable isolates from mouth, eye or skin above the waist, 84 per cent were HSV 1 and 13 per cent were HSV 2 and 1 could not be typed. The clinical findings in 5 patients with ocular disease due to HSV 2 indicate that the disease is severe; in one patient there was a dendritic figure with a pseudomembrane, with deep stromal infiltrates and iritis. In a second case there was a keratoconjunctivitis with a geographic ulcer.

A comparison between the lesions induced by HSV 1 and 2 in the rabbit has been made by Oh and Stevens (1973). It was reported that type 2 strains were much slower to produce lesions, but the lesions were more severe and of longer duration; an extensive deep keratitis was regularly produced and led to corneal scarring and pannus. The differences between the clinical appearances of the two types of disease was clear. It was considered that type 2 virus was able to penetrate the epithelial barrier more easily than type 1 virus, but no explanation could be given for this. Histopathological and virological studies (Stevens and Oh; 1973) indicated that there was epithelial loss followed by rapid regeneration in type 1 disease, while in contrast there was persistent epithelial loss and marked epithelial hyperplasia in type 2 disease. The stromal infiltration with inflammatory cells was more severe and deeper in type 2 infection, as was the inflammatory infiltration of the corneal endothelium, iris and choroid. Virus could be isolated from the rabbit cornea up to day 31 in type 2 infection, but could not be cultured in type 1 infections beyond day 15 or 16. However, the virus was recovered in low titres from corneas at the end of four weeks, which suggests that the stromal disease was not necessarily due to the presence of proliferating virus alone. Specific differences between the appearances of epithelial diseases have been described using light and electron microscopic techniques. Scanning EM confirmed that the edges of the type 2 epithelial lesions are raised.

Herpetic Keratitis in Children

A series of 21 paediatric patients with ocular herpes simplex infections were divided into two groups (Poirer, 1980), those with documented recurrences and those with clinical primary herpes. Stromal keratitis and visual loss were not marked in the group with primary disease.

Herpetic Keratitis and Atopic Disease

Herpes simplex keratitis can occur with increased severity in patients with atopic disease, and who are subject to hypersensitivity reactions involving various target organs. The term allergy indicates that a patient has a changing reactivity as a result of an antigenic stimulus. In order to define more clearly a group of patients who were at risk of developing severe allergic reactions, Coca and Cook (1923) introduced the term 'atopy', meaning 'strange disease', which was defined as a 'type of hypersensitivity peculiar to man, subject to hereditary influence, presenting the characteristic immediate wealing type reaction, having circulating antibody reagin, and manifesting peculiar clinical syndromes such as asthma and hay fever'. Reaginic antibody, which is now known as IgE, is often elevated in atopic disease. Allergic disease in general occurs in the population in 1 in 10 individuals, where it commonly takes the form of allergic rhinitis. In certain patients with an increased level of hypersensitivity, eczema and asthma as well as allergic rhinitis may occur in varying combinations. The diseases of the eye which can be associated are as unusual as the other manifestations of atopy and include mild, moderate or severe allergic conjunctivitis (vernal disease), lid eczema, severe blepharitis, allergic keratitis, keratoconus, corneal infections (particularly with the herpes simplex virus), and cataract (Easty *et al.*, 1975). In patients with keratitis following herpetic infections it has proved difficult to achieve successful corneal transplantation, and it is important to tissue-match using the HL-A antigen in patients who are at risk of developing such complications (Easty *et al.*, 1979).

The impression that herpes simplex keratitis can be more severe in patients with severe atopy is supported by the well-known association of eczema with severe reactions following vaccination, and wide dissemination of virus can occur following infection with HSV, where the typical cutaneous lesion may be umbilicated, with facial lesions which become ulcerative (Figures 7.12 and 7.13). The increased risk of this unfortunate group of patients is not understood but insight into the difficulties which are to be expected in those with atopic disease and herpetic keratitis is of aid in the clinical management of the patient.

Herpetic keratitis can be particularly severe in subjects with atopy, and may be of varying degrees of severity (Table 7.7). It is possible to recognise a number of syndromes where the disease may be either primary or secondary. In primary disease, the cutaneous eruption may be particularly severe and diffuse, and may affect the skin of the face and body, or be localised in certain patients to the periorbital region. Ocular herpes can be associated during the primary stage, and it is in these patients that the dendrite may be bilateral and extensive (Figure 7.14). The dendritic ulcer can heal without leading to recurrence or to stromal disease. Patients with primary disease in association with atopy are predominantly male, and children and young adults are most often affected.

Recurrent epithelial disease may occur in adult patients, who may have associated disease of the tarsal plates in the form of vernal disease, or of the lid margins in the form of chronic staphylococcal blepharitis. The frequent recurrences are eventually associated with stromal opacification (Figure 7.15).

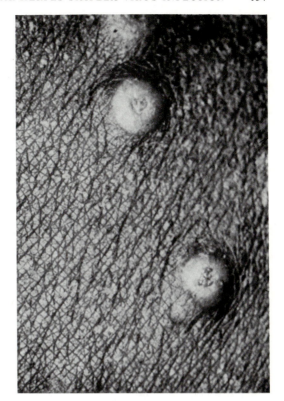

Figure 7.12. Umbilicated cutaneous lesions due to disseminated herpes simplex virus infection in a two-year-old child.

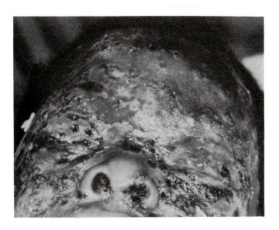

Figure 7.13. The facial appearance in a two-year-old child with disseminated herpes simplex virus infection. The child was severely atopic.

TABLE 7.7

HERPES SIMPLEX INFECTION IN ATOPIC INDIVIDUALS

PRIMARY	mild
	moderate
	severe (diffuse facial, rarely generalised)
	epithelial disease plus follicular conjunctivitis
RECURRENT	unilateral ⎱ (sometimes triggered by exacerbation of
	bilateral ⎰ local conjunctival allergic responses)
STROMAL	unilateral
	bilateral
	superficial
	deep
	perforating
	associated with secondary infections (bacterial or mycotic)

The presence of allergic disease of the external eye in association with herpetic disease creates severe problems in management in view of the fact that vernal disease may necessitate the use of topical corticosteroid, which would carry serious risks if there should be a recurrence of herpetic disease during their use. It is our clinical impression that recurrences are sometimes triggered by reactivation of the vernal disease, which increases the difficulties in the management of these unfortunate patients.

Stromal disease may be severe, and can take a number of forms. Figure 7.16 shows the appearance seen in a patient with vernal disease, keratoconus and recurrent stromal disease with frequent ulceration and secondary infection. In Figure 7.17 the appearance of the cornea in a patient with severe atopic disease is shown. There is hyperkeratosis and diffuse opacification. In the opposite

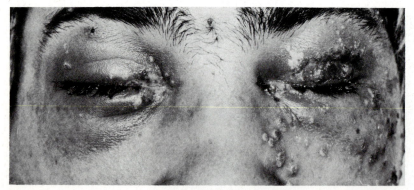

Figure 7.14.   Severe primary cutaneous herpes simplex virus infection in a 19-year-old youth with severe asthma and eczema. He suffered bilateral corneal disease.

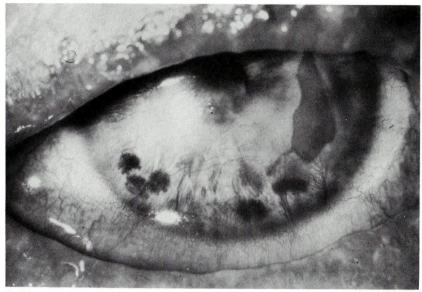

Figure 7.15.   Severe epithelial ulceration due to herpes simplex virus infection, together with stromal opacification in a patient with severe atopy and vernal disease.

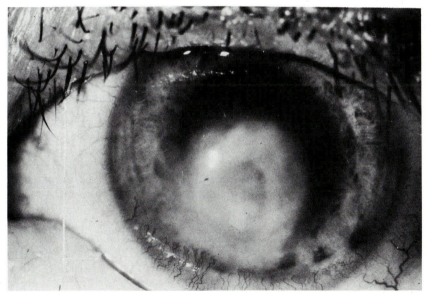

Figure 7.16.   Herpes simplex keratitis which eventually caused a perforation in a patient with keratoconus and severe atopy.

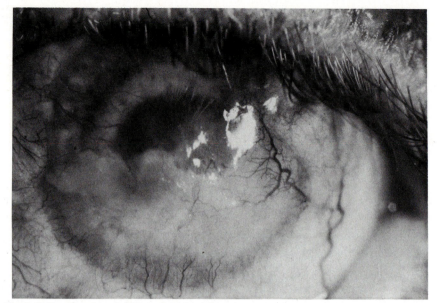

Figure 7.17. Severe and diffuse corneal opacification and epithelial keratinisation in an atopic patient. There was severe infection with *Candida albicans* in the other eye.

eye there was secondary infection with *Candida albicans*. Patients with severe atopy and corneal herpes are poor risks for keratoplasty, and surgical treatment should be contemplated only when all other forms of therapy have been tried.

This association between atopy and herpetic keratitis has been recently re-emphasised by Bloch-Michel and his colleagues (1981). Roussus and Denis (1981) found that the frequency of allergic disease in patients with ocular herpes was 37 per cent in the group with herpetic keratitis, and 17 per cent in controls.

Bilateral Disease

Bilateral disease may occur as keratitis on one side and uveitis on the other without preceding evidence of stromal keratitis. It is difficult to explain a disease of this type, and in particular the means by which the virus enters a uveal tract when there is no history of external disease. As understanding increases concerning the neurotropism of the herpes simplex virus and the mechanisms of its spread between dermatomes and along other neurological pathways such as the optic chiasma (as has been found in laboratory animals (Howe *et al.*, 1979; Tullo *et al.*, 1982)), it can be speculated that bilateral eye disease in humans may also occur as a result of spread via the nervous system along a number of possible routes. It has also, rarely, been experienced that severe unilateral disease can be associated with central retinal venous occlusion in the opposite eye. The probability of this association is extremely low, and it therefore may be speculated that one condition is related to the other.

Thirty patients with bilateral herpetic keratitis were identified in a population of approximately one thousand patients with corneal disease due to human herpes virus. Immediately preceding the initial episode of keratitis, four of the patients had had systemic illnesses, which were malaria, pulmonary tuberculosis, lumbar herpes zoster and gastric carcinoma. Atopy was present in 40 per cent of the patients. The initial episode of keratitis occurred simultaneously in 17 of the group, and on different occasions in 13 patients (43 per cent). Four of the atopic patients developed secondary microbial keratitis. One patient had bilateral suppurative keratitis due to *Staphylococcus aureus*. Of the remaining three, one was due to *Staphylococcus aureus*, one to *Pseudomonas aeruginosa* and one to *Candida albicans* (Wilhelmus *et al*. 1981*b*).

The Pathogenesis of Human Ocular HSV Infection

The presence of the virus in epithelial disease can be determined by direct examination of the specimens, or by isolation techniques. The histology of the vesicle occurring in the skin and the dendritic figure has received extensive study in experimental animals and in patients. The basic pathology is one of epithelial hyperplasia, with cell fusion and subsequent necrosis, the extent of which depends on the site of the lesion (Juel-Jenson and MacCallum, 1972). In a typical skin lesion, there is ballooning of the cells, between which a serous exudate forms containing exfoliated epithelial cells, leucocytes and possibly some giant cells, together with a deposit of fibrin. Lesions of the oral, nasal and genital mucosa show early ulceration in contrast to lesions in the skin. It is uncommon to witness herpetic ulceration of the bulbar or palpebral conjunctiva, the disease generally being confined to the cornea, although in primary infections and occasionally in recurrent disease a follicular reaction may occur in the tarsal conjunctiva, extending into the fornices.

The first complete virus particles are formed in the nucleus of the corneal epithelial cell; the nucleoli enlarge and disappear, but at the same time small masses of nucleoprotein coalesce until the nucleus is filled with inclusion material which is thought to contain early virus particles (Figure 7.18). Later, the inclusion shrinks from the nuclear membrane, becoming eosinophilic with H and E staining when it becomes known as Cowdrey type A inclusion. Replication of the virus within the nucleus is thought to affect the chromosomes and mitosis is arrested in metaphase, which, it is suggested, is responsible for the formation of giant cells. The virus may also act on the cell membranes themselves or the adjacent infected and non-infected cells, so that fusion between cells occurs when the cytoplasmic membranes disappear.

In corneal disease the pathological changes occur in the cells which are host to proliferating virus, but also inflammatory changes occur in the surrounding tissues. In epithelial disease changes in the cell have been described by Duke-Elder (1965). Eosinophilic inclusions occur which are probably a non-specific degeneration; subsequent nuclear swelling attains the diameter of a normal cell, balloon degeneration occurs and the inclusion bodies become cytoplasmic. A diffuse necrosis follows with the formation of bullae. The eventual appearance of multinucleated giant cells is of some diagnostic value, although these also occur in zoster and vaccinia.

Stromal involvement occurs in primary or recurrent disease with the appearance of acute and chronic inflammatory cells, with large collections of

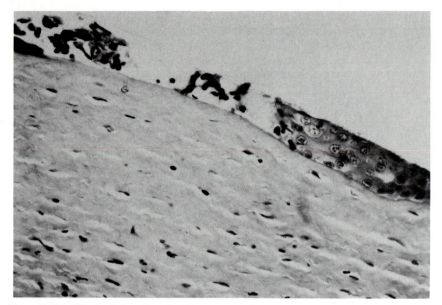

Figure 7.18.   Histological section of rabbit cornea shortly after inoculation with HSV. A synctium
of cells is seen. PMNs are present in the epithelium.

cells occurring at the corneal limbus and in the tarsal plates of laboratory
animals (Table 7.8). In stromal disease without ulceration there is lamellar
separation by oedema, with dense collections of acute and chronic inflammatory cells which vary according to whether adaptive immune responses have
occurred (Figure 7.19a, b). The endothelium may be involved, with loss of
cells and the formation of keratic precipitates.

Although the infective agent can be isolated from 75 per cent of large
dendritic ulcers (Coleman et al., 1969) it is interesting that it can be cultured
less frequently from geographic ulcers. It has proved difficult in the past to
recover the virus from tissue taken during transplantation of corneal tissue
from patients with stromal keratitis of various types.

Virus has been located in corneal stroma, which is a mesodermal layer,
using electron-microscopical techniques (Dawson et al., 1968a; Dawson et al.,
1968b). Particles were found resembling herpes virus in the stromal layers in
5 of 19 specimens obtained from patients with stromal disease. Virus particles
were found in the superficial stroma, mid-stroma, and the deep stroma, and
were not apparently related to the site of previous epithelial disease. The
presence of virus particles in cell nuclei suggests that the keratocyte is capable
of supporting viral replication (Figure 7.20). The presence of enveloped
particles outside the cell membrane of stromal cells which also contain nuclear
particles is evidence that the final step in the formation of fully mature virus
particles can take place (Holmes and Watson, 1963). In spite of the presence
of virus particles in the stroma it has generally proved impossible to isolate the
virus in tissue culture (Dawson et al., 1968b), and it has been suggested that

TABLE 7.8

REACTIONS INDUCED IN THE CORNEAL STROMA BY THE HSV

(a) Cellular infiltration
    (i) polymorphonuclear
    (ii) lymphocytic
    (iii) macrophage
(b) Inflammatory oedema
(c) Oedema due to endothelial pump malfunction
(d) Vascular ingrowth
    (i) conjunctival (isolated or multiple vessels)
    (ii) deep stromal (peripheral or central; single or multiple)
(e) Permanent tissue damage
    (i) epithelial (trophic ulceration)
    (ii) stromal damage with loss of lattice structure
    (iii) transformation of keratocytes into fibroblasts and formation of scar tissue
    (iv) permanent damage in the form of scarring
    (v) permanent damage in the form of faceting of the surface
    (vi) permanent endothelial damage with stromal oedema
(f) Lipid degeneration
(g) Keratic precipitates

the reasons for this are that virus particles are trapped between the tightly packed lamellae of the cornea, and that the outer envelope in many of the particles is absent (Holmes and Watson, 1963). However, Figure 7.21 demonstrates the appearance of stromal disease prior to keratoplasty. Live virus was cultured from the recipient button using preliminary corneal organ culture (Shimeld et al., 1982). Electron-microscopy examination can identify virus in stromal cells in organ cultured corneal buttons (Figure 7.22a, b).

It is because of the large size of intact virus particles that they may not diffuse easily out of the cornea, and may become trapped between the corneal lamellae; such fixed particles could thereby produce an inflammatory response. Evidence of the presence of actively proliferating virus has been reported by Collin and Abelson (1976), where the presence of virus particles was established with electron-microscopy in corneal stroma, retrocorneal fibrous membrane and vitreous, and confirmation of this was made by culture of the virus from the vitreous. The presence of live virus capable of proliferation in the stroma and elsewhere in the eye is of importance in the often difficult decision concerning the use of topical steroids in the treatment of prolonged stromal inflammatory disease.

Factors Influencing the Severity of Herpes Simplex Keratitis

The factors which influence the severity of herpes simplex keratitis are biological, immunological, therapeutic and environmental. There are a number of ways in which the severity of epithelial disease may be influenced. It is probable that the severity of stromal disease is related to the quantity of virus or antigen which penetrates into the stroma and beyond.

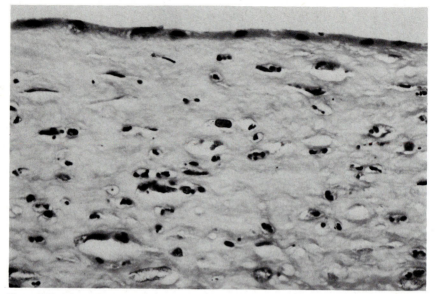

Figure 7.19 (*a*). The stromal reaction following primary inoculation of HSV in rabbits. The epithelium is reduced to a single layer. The majority of cells in the stroma are PMN.

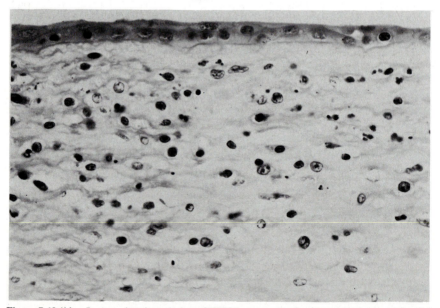

Figure 7.19 (*b*). In secondary inoculation of HSV the stromal cells are mostly mononuclear; they are also seen in the epithelium. (Courtesy, Miss Clare Carter.)

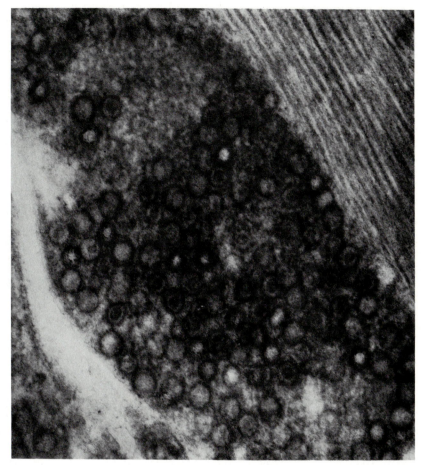

Figure 7.20. Herpes simplex viral particles packed in the cytoplasm of a keratocyte in tissue taken from a patient with a failed lamellar keratoplasty (EM x 76 650). (Courtesy, Dr. Ramesh Tripathi and Professor Barrie Jones.)

Frequency

The frequency of recurrence of epithelial disease must in part be decided by the frequency of the trigger for reactivation in a particular patient. Carroll *et al.* (1967) reported a 26 per cent rate of clinical recurrence within two years following the first attack, the rate rising to a level of 43 per cent following a second recurrence. It is of some interest that patients with frequent recurrences of ulcerative disease do not necessarily go on to develop severe stromal disease. Thus many patients who have experienced recurrent ulcers over a number of years may be left with little visual deficit (Thygeson, 1976).

The factors which stimulate recurrence are often highly stereotyped in their nature, although varying widely in their apparent nature (Baringer, 1976).

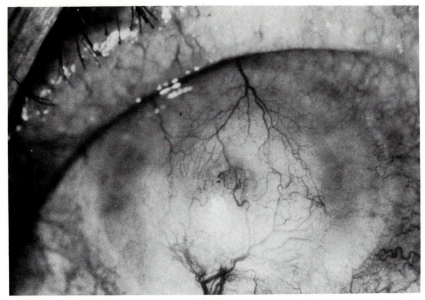

Figure 7.21. Herpetic keratitis in a 30-year-old patient with a six-year history of stromal inflammation. Viable virus was cultured from the disc removed at keratoplasty.

Fever is a common cause and this was highlighted when cutaneous herpes occurred in a large percentage of patients subjected to fever therapy (Warren *et al.*, 1940). Less consistent has been the association of herpes recurrence with sunlight, emotional or physiological stress, or menstruation.

Type of Herpes Simplex Virus

The majority of isolates taken from patients with ocular disease have been reported to be HSV 1 (Nahmias and Dowdle 1968). On the other hand Hanna *et al.* (1976) reported that 7 out of 54 isolates (13 per cent) could be identified as HSV 2. When the clinical records of these patients were reviewed, it seems that the eye disease had been unusually severe, and one case was an immunosuppressed patient who had undergone a renal transplant.

Transmission and Dosage

Type 1 HSV is transmitted primarily from labial herpes by kissing, from an exogenous source, or possibly via an autogenous route where the agent is transmitted by hand from a focus elsewhere; commonly this would be expected to occur following type 1 infection, but it is theoretically possible that a type 2 focus could be a source of self-infection of the eye. The severity of the ensuing disease must depend upon the amount of live virus which has been transmitted, and which is allowed to enter the tissues. Where there is a primary infection the degree of viral proliferation permitted before immune responses occur, which would curtail the infection, depends upon the dynamics of the prime immune reaction; thus a delay in such a response would be expected to allow increased proliferation of virus with increased risks of penetration of the corneal stroma, or of penetration of the axon of the sensory neuron and the consequent establishment of a latent infection. When transmission of virus is accompanied by trauma, which is also thought to be a trigger factor, virus penetration into the stroma can be severe, presumably due to the loss of the mechanical barrier afforded by the tight junctions between the cells of the epithelium.

The precise method by which the virus is introduced on to the corneal surface controls the magnitude of the amount of virus introduced, and hence may determine the severity of the lesion; thus a large inoculum of virus would be introduced into the conjunctival sac where there is direct contact between a cutaneous lesion containing proliferating virus, whereas a smaller number of viral particles would be expected to be transferred via an intermediate carrier such as the patient's hand. The feasibility of the introduction of the virus from a latent reservoir set up during the original primary attack at another site must be considered to be a real possibility (Figure 7.23).

The Host Response

The response of the host following primary infection and recurrent disease is discussed elsewhere. These responses may be affected by a number of systemic disturbances of the immune system (Table 7.9). These syndromes may be congenital or acquired, and although diseases such as the Wiskott-Aldrich syndrome may be associated with severe infections with the herpes simplex virus, the more common influences on the immune processes, directed against proliferation of the virus, are acquired. It is therefore valuable to take careful note of the patient's previous history of disease, and at the same time to be alert to the possible disease processes which may be active at the time of the presentation of active keratitis.

In children, acquired causes of immunodeficiency include certain of the haemopoietic disorders, severe burns, exudative enteropathy, the nephrotic syndrome, sarcoidosis, splenectomy, uraemia, severe virus infection and malnutrition. On occasions more than one of these causes of transient immunoincompetence may occur together in the same patient and co-operate to reduce the immune processes which will protect the host from infection, or respond to established disease. These factors go some way to explain the high incidence of herpes simplex virus found in corneal ulcers associated with measles keratitis in 34 children in Nigeria (Sandford-Smith and Whittle, 1979; Plate IV*b*). The incidence of positive isolates amounted to 47 per cent of the group. The morphology of many of the ulcers was typical of herpetic ulcers occurring in an immunosuppressed patient, which was confirmed by culture and immunofluorescence studies.

In addition to the immunodeficiency syndromes of childhood, it is to be remembered that a number of diseases occur in childhood, adolescence and adulthood which are associated with a reduced defence against infective disease, and it is in such patients that herpes simplex keratitis can occur, although to the clinician the association may not be apparent unless a complete history is recorded and a systemic examination and investigation made. In patients in whom the disease is severe, with frequent recurrences which do not

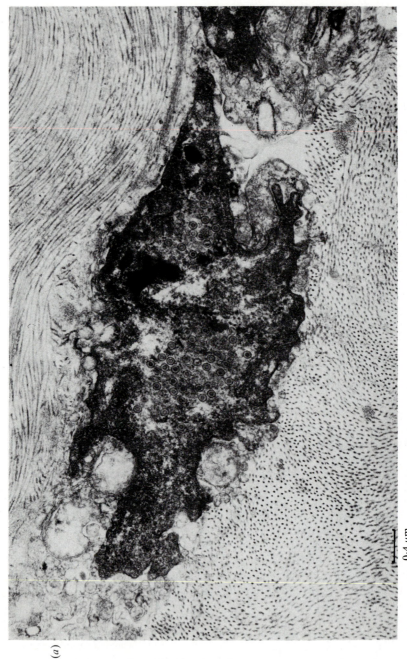

(a)

0·4 μm

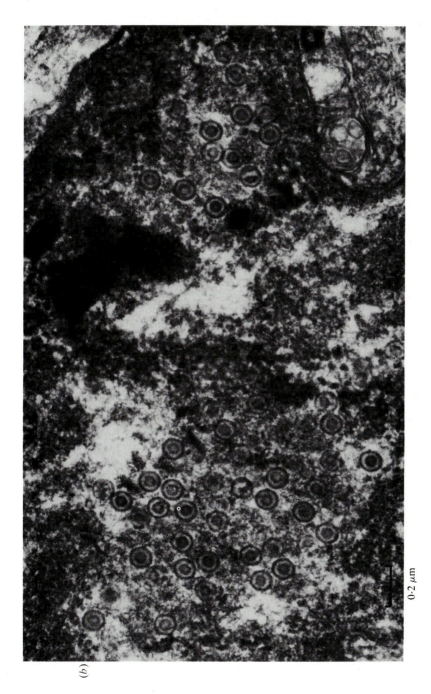

0·2 μm

(b)

Figure 7.22 a and b.   Herpes simplex virus particles in a stromal cell apparent after 5–10 days on organ culture of a corneal button.

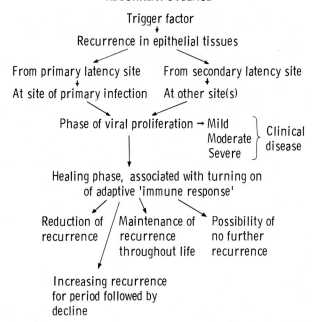

Figure 7.23. A modified scheme to demonstrate the possible disease patterns following recurrent herpes simplex virus disease. It would be expected that the most severe recurrence would occur at the site of primary disease.

seem to be related to an identifiable trigger, such further investigation can be helpful.

Good (1975) has summarised the situations where perturbation of immune function may exist, and has suggested that increasing understanding of the congenital immunodeficiency syndromes may help in the understanding of how serious infections are incurred in adult patients. Significant and severe depressions of immune function are encountered during the ageing process in man and animals, with what has been thought to be an involution of the thymus and thymus-dependent system. Many malignancies, particularly of the cells of the immune apparatus, but also other tumours including carcinomas and sarcomas in their widely disseminated state, may be accompanied by depression of cell-mediated and humoral immunities. Further, oncogenic viruses and chemical carcinogens frequently have immunosuppressive properties. Serious virus disease may depress immunological function, as can certain bacterial infections such as leprosy and tuberculosis, both of which, on the other hand, may sometimes *stimulate* immunological function. In the same way, immune function may be suppressed in fungus or protozoan infection. Other causes of acquired immunodeficiency include alcoholic beverages, cigarette smoke or environmental pollutants. Malnutrition can profoundly depress humoral and cellular immunities, and many of the most powerful anticancer drugs or other agents that are used in modern medicine can act as

TABLE 7.9

IMMUNE DEFICIENCY DISEASES IN CHILDHOOD

1. Immunodeficiency of immaturity
    (a) Transient hypogammaglobulinaemia of infancy
    (b) Immunodeficiency of the newborn
2. Antibody immunodeficiency
3. Selective IgA deficiency
4. Immunodeficiencies with thymic hypoplasia
    (a) Thymic hypoplasia (Di George syndrome)
    (b) Severe combined immunodeficiency
        (Swiss-type agammaglobulinaemia)
    (c) Autosomal recessive immunodeficiency with lymphopenia
    (d) Immunodeficiency with generalised haemopoietic hypoplasia
5. Other cellular immunodeficiencies
    (a) Immunodeficiency with ataxia-telangiectasia
    (b) Immunodeficiency with thrombocytopenia and eczema
        (Wiskott-Aldrich syndrome)
6. Disorders of the phagocytic system
7. Disorders of the complement system
8. Acquired and transient immunodeficiencies
    (a) Haemopoietic disorders
    (b) Associated with burns
    (c) With exudative enteropathy
    (d) With nephrotic syndrome
    (e) With sarcoidosis
    (f) With virus infection
    (g) With malnutrition

immunosuppressants, or can interfere with biological amplification or effector mechanism in relation to immune defence mechanisms. Organ transplantation requires carefully controlled depression of immunological function, with the use of corticosteroids and other immunosuppressive agents.

In relation to the occurrence of herpetic keratitis it is clear that these factors contribute to the severity of the disease, its recurrence rate, and the spread of the virus into the stroma. It has been our clinical impression that the severity can be influenced by increasing age, and stromal disease can be particularly chronic and unresponsive to treatment in patients who take an excessive amount of alcohol. The immunosuppression occurring in association with disseminated carcinomatosis was accompanied by a severe dendritic ulcer and followed by prolonged stromal disease in a patient of 70 years, and in three patients who had undergone renal transplantation there was severe ulcerative and stromal disease, accompanied by perforation in one and serious and unremitting stromal disease in another (Figure 7.24; Easty, 1977; Howcroft and Breslin, 1981). The increasing use of immunosuppressive regimes in the treatment of autoimmune disease is liable to be accompanied by a risk of ocular involvement.

Influences of Topical Medication

The influence of topical medications on the severity of ulcerative and stromal herpetic keratitis is an indication for constant vigilance by clinicians

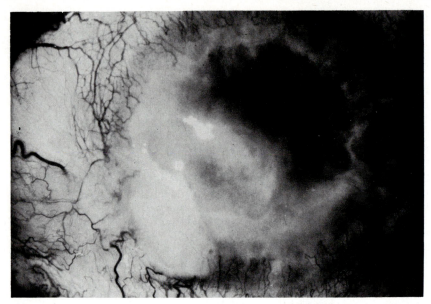

Figure 7.24.   Recurrent epithelial and stromal keratitis in a renal transplant patient. There is a plaque of hyperkeratinisation due to prolonged use of topical antiviral in the lower nasal corneal periphery.

involved in the management of the disease. In spite of the emphasis against the use of topical steroid medication in patients with ulcerative disease, these patients are still referred to casualty departments in the United Kingdom while undergoing treatment with topical steroid. In a recent survey it was found that 20 per cent of patients entered into a trial of a new antiviral were being treated with topical steroid to the affected eye. However, it is not only primary treatment prescribed by a non-trained practitioner that leads to the development of serious keratitis; self-medication by a patient without appropriate advice, and the fact that in certain countries steroid medication can be obtained without prescription can also do so. At the same time there is some controversy amongst ophthalmologists concerning the best form of management in stromal disease, and it may be that the use of such medication at all may be in part responsible for the slow development of more serious disease. Thygeson (1976) has discussed the corticosteroid disaster in relation to herpetic keratitis, and points out that the short-term benefits of obtaining resolution of symptoms and signs in stromal disease do not outweigh the long-term dangers. At the same time he equally considers that the dendritic figure is a self-limiting lesion and will resolve without the help of any form of medication, without adverse effect on the corneal stroma. It is widespread experience that those patients with kerato-uveitis have often been treated in error with topical steroid at the onset of the disease, and it is in such subjects that management has often proved to be extremely difficult. With the increase in understanding of the dosages of topical steroid which can be used locally to reduce inflammatory responses, the avoidance of steroids where epithelial disease exists, and the employment of a minimal dose which will nevertheless induce a therapeutic effect, it is becoming apparent that the severe management problems which were encountered in the 1960s are now declining.

The use of topical corticosteroid in the treatment of an active dendritic ulcer causes local immunosuppression so that the virus appears to proliferate, inducing the formation of an extensive area of ulceration which no longer bears the dendritic appearance, but becomes map-like, geographic or amoeboid (Figure 7.25). Although it may not necessarily appear to be affecting the stroma at the stage of ulceration, it appears likely that significant amounts of virus or its antigenic subunits spread into the stroma, but the effects of the penetration of the tissue may become manifest somewhat later. Thus there may be a latent period between the period of enhanced ulcerative disease and the onset of stromal keratitis.

The difficulties associated with the use of topical steroids in the treatment of stromal disease must depend upon the fact that they are performing two essentially different tasks which are nevertheless closely related, the clinical intention being to reduce the hypersensitivity element of the stromal disease, but at the same time not suppress the immune responses which are being directed against virus which may be propagating in the keratocytes of the stroma. It would seem unlikely that the two responses can be separated, but clinical experience indicates that the use of dilute preparations of topical

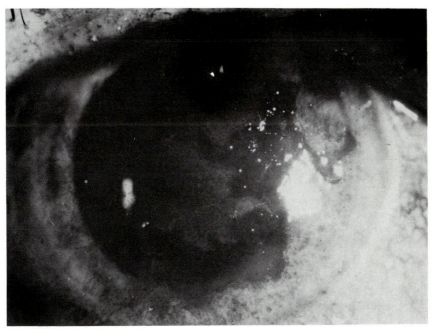

Figure 7.25.   Geographic ulcer due to herpes simplex virus infection following corticosteroid therapy.

steroid provides suppression of inflammation without causing increased viral proliferation in the stromal cells.

Sudden curtailment of topical steroid, without tapering off over a period of several weeks using increasing dilutions, can result in a rebound of activity which can be more serious than the original stromal disease—a situation which may be particularly difficult to manage in the patient who has undergone a penetrating keratoplasty following HSV infection.

The use of topical corticosteroid in the treatment of prolonged stromal disease should be accompanied by the use of antiviral cover to avoid the chance of exacerbating an epithelial recurrence should there be live virus in either the conjunctival sac or corneal epithelium. Even the careful tapering off of topical corticosteroid can be associated with the appearance of the corneal and conjunctival changes which are thought to be due to the use of topical antiviral drugs such as idoxuridine. The use of anti-inflammatory reagents goes some way to suppressing such toxic phenomena which only appear on reducing the dosage below a certain threshold level.

The toxicity which can be induced by the antiviral group of drugs may in itself occasionally provide considerable difficulties in management of herpetic keratitis, as can a cutaneous hypersensitivity reaction to the drops. Thus, in addition to the tendency to cause superficial punctate keratopathy and vortex patterns in the epithelium, it has been considered that there is an increased incidence of so-called ghost opacities beneath the dendrite (Thygeson, 1976), together with an immunosuppressive effect which can cause the onset of stromal infection by secondary opportunistic agents, an effect which was first described by Gunderson (1964); *Staphylococcus aureus* was then the offending agent, while on other occasions the offender has been *Streptococcus viridans*.

In summary, there are many influences which can determine the clinical severity of both epithelial and stromal keratitis following infections with the herpes simplex virus. It remains a strong clinical impression that one of the major problems in the management of HSK is the injudicious use of topical corticosteroid and the clinical decision whether to treat or not to treat with topical medication remains at the centre of the debate concerning management of an all-too-common eye disease. The emergence of therapeutic agents capable of passage through the corneal epithelium to neutralise virus in the stroma and the anterior part of the uvea has now allowed topical corticosteroids to be used with less anxiety in the management of the afflicted patient.

REFERENCES

BARINGER, J. R. (1976). The biology of herpes simplex virus infection in humans. *Survey Ophthal.*, **21**, 171–174.

BLOCH-MICHEL, E., VAMVOUKOS, D., CAMPINCHI, R. and NIESSEN, F. (1981). Atopy and herpetic keratitis. In: *Herpetic Eye Diseases*. Ed. Sundmacher. Munich: J. F. Bergman Verlag.

BOCK, J., FANTA, D., SÖLTZ-SZOTS, J. et al. (1972). Isolierung von Herpes simplex virus aus dem kammerwasser eines an rezidivierender Iridocyclitis erkranten Auges. Albrecht von Graefes Arch. Klin. Ophthal., 185, 349–353.

CARROLL, J. M., MARITOLA, E. L. and LAIBSON, P. R. (1967). The recurrence of herpetic keratitis following idoxuridine therapy. Amer. J. Ophthal., 63, 103–7.

CAVARA, V. (1955). The role of viruses in the aetology of uveitis. Acta XVII. Concilium Opthalmologicum (1954), Vol. 2. Toronto: University of Toronto Press.

COCA, A. F. and COOK, R. A. (1923). On the classification of the phenomena of hypersensitiveness. J. Immunol., 8, 163–182.

COLEMAN, V. R., THYGESON, P., DAWSON, C. R. et al. (1969). Isolation of virus from herpetic keratitis: influence of idoxuridine in isolation rates. Arch. Ophthal., 81, 22–24.

COLLIN, H. B. and ABELSON, M. B. (1976). Herpes simplex virus in human cornea, retrocorneal fibrous membrane and vitreous. Arch. Ophthal., 94, 1726–1729.

DAROUGER, S., HUNTER, P. A., VISWALINGHAM, M., GIBSON, J. A. and JONES, B. R. (1978). Acute follicular conjunctivitis and keratoconjunctivitis due to herpes simplex virus in London. Brit. J. Ophthal., 62, 843–9.

DAWSON, S., TOGNI, B., and MOORE, T. E. (1968b). Structural changes in chronic herpetic keratitis studies by light and electron microscopy. Arch. Ophthal., 79, 740–748.

DAWSON, S., TOGNI, B., MOORE, T. E. and COLEMAN, V. (1968a). Herpes virus infection of human mesodermal tissue (corneal) detected by electron microscopy. Nature, 217, 460–467.

DOUR, R. and VÖCHTING, K. (1920). Etudes sur le virus de l'herpes febrile, Rev. Gen. Ophthal. (Paris), 34, 409–421.

DUKE-ELDER, S. (1965). Diseases of the outer eye. In: System of Ophthalmology, Vol. III, Pt. 1. London: Henry Kimpton.

EASTY, D. L. (1977). Manifestations of immunodeficiency diseases in ophthalmology. Trans. Ophthal. Soc. U.K., 97, 8–17.

EASTY, D. L., BIRKINSHAW, M., MERRITT, T., MERRETT, J. and MADDEN, P. (1979). Immunology of vernal disease. In: The Mast Cell, pp. 493–502. Eds. Pepys and Edwards. London: Pitman Medical.

EASTY, D. L., ENTWHISTLE, C., FUNK, A. and WHICHER, J. (1975). Herpes simplex keratitis and keratoconus in the atopic patient. Trans. Ophthal. Soc. U.K., 95, 267–76.

FALCON, M. G. and WILLIAMS, H. P. (1978). Herpes simplex kerato-uveitis and glaucoma. Trans. Ophthal. Soc. U.K., 98, 101–104.

GELLER, H. O. and THYGESON, P. (1951). Aureomycin, chloromycetin and terramycin in experimental herpes simplex virus infections. Amer. J. Ophthal., 34 165–174.

GOOD, R. A. (1975). Immunodeficiencies of man and the new immunobiology. In: Immunodeficiency in Man and Animals. Ed. D. Beresna. Sunderland, Mass.: Sinauer Associates Inc.

GRÜTER, W. (1920). Experimentalle und Klinische untersuchungen uber den sogenannten Herpes corneae. Ber. Dtsch. Ophthal. Ges. 42, 162.

GUNDERSEN, T. (1936). Herpes corneae with special reference to its treatment with strong solutions of iodine. Arch. Ophthal., 15, 225–249.

GUNDERSEN, T. (1964). In discussion of Ey, R. C., Hughes, W. F., Holmes, A. W. and Deinhardt, F.: The effect of IDU on experimental and clinical herpes simplex infections. Trans. Amer. Ophthal. Soc., 61, 109.

HANNA, L., OSTLER, H. B. and KESHISHYAN H. (1976). Observed relationship between herpatic lesions and antigenic type of Herpesvirus hominis. Survey Ophthal., 21, 110–114.

HEWSON, G. E. (1957). Iritis due to herpes virus. Irish J. Med. Sci., 372–373.

HOGAN, M. J., KIMURA, S. J. and THYGESON, P. (1964). Pathology of herpes simplex kerato-iritis. *Amer. J. Ophthal.*, **57**, 551–564.

HOLMES, I. H. and WATSON, D. H. (1963). An electron microscope study of the attachment and penetration of herpes virus in BHK 21 cells. *Virology*, **21**, 112–123.

HOWCROFT, M. J. and BRESLIN, C. W. (1981). Herpes simplex keratitis in renal transplant recipients. *Can. Med. Assoc. J.*, **124**, 292–4.

HOWE, J. W., NARANG, H. K. and CODD, A. A. (1979). Herpes simplex virus uveitis and optic neuropathy. *Trans. Ophthal. Soc. U.K.*, **99**, 111–16.

INOMATA, H. and SMELSER, G. K. (1970). Fine structural alterations of corneal endothelium during experimental uveitis. *Invest. Ophthal.*, **9**, 272–85.

JUEL-JENSEN, E. E. and MACCALLUM, F. O. (1972). *Herpes Simplex and Varicella Zoster.* London: W. Heinemann Medical Books.

KAPLAN, A. S. (1973). *The Herpes Viruses.* New York and London: Academic Press.

KIMURA, S. J. (1962). Herpes simplex uveitis: a clinical and experimental study. *Trans. Amer. Ophthal. Soc.*, **60**, 440–470.

KRAUPA, E. (1920). Zu grüters äteiologischen Untersuchungen über den fieberhaften Herpes. *Münch. Med. Wschr.*, **67**, 1236.

LAIBSON, P. R. and LEOPOLD, I. N. (1964). An evaluation of double-blind IDU therapy in 100 cases of herpetic keratitis. *Trans. Amer. Acad. Ophthal. Otolaryng.*, **58**, 22–34.

LONGSON, M. (1979). Herpes encephalitis. In: *Virus Diseases.* Ed. R. B. Heath. London: Pitman Medical.

LOWENSTEIN, A. (1919). Ätiologie Untersuchungen über den fieberhaften Herpes. *Münch. Med. Wschr.*, **66**, 769–70.

MACNAB, A. (1907). *Ulceration of the Cornea.* p. 162. London: Baillière Tindall & Cox.

MARSH, R. J., EASTY, D. L. and JONES, B. R. (1974). Iritis and iris atrophy in herpes zoster ophthalmicus. *Am. J. Ophthal.*, **78**, 255–61.

MINCKLER, D. S., McLEAN, E. B., SHAW, C. M. and HENDRICKSON, A. (1976). Herpesvirus hominis encephalitis and retinitis. *Arch. Ophthal.*, **94**, 89–95.

NAHMIAS, A. J. and DOWDLE, W. R. (1968). Antigenic and biologic differences in Herpesvirus hominis. *Prog. Med. Virol.*, **10**, 110–159.

NAHMIAS, A. J. VISINTINE, A. M., CALDWELL, D. R. and WILSON, L. A. (1976). Eye infections with herpes simplex viruses in neonates. *Survey Ophthal.*, **21**, 100–105.

NORN, M. S. (1970*a*). Dendritic herpetic keratitis: 1. Incidence, seasonal variations, recurrence rate, visual impairment, therapy. *Acta Ophthal.*, **48**, 91–107.

NORN, M. S. (1970*b*). Dendritic (herpetic) keratitis: 2. Follow up examination of corneal opacity. *Acta Ophthal.*, **48**, 214.

OH, J. O. (1976). Primary and secondary herpes simplex uveitis in rabbits. *Survey Ophthal.*, **21**, 178–184.

OH, J. O. (1979). The role of immunity in the pathogenesis of herpes simplex uveitis. In: *International Symposium on Immunology and Immunopathology of the Eye.* Eds. A. M. Silverstein, and R. O'Connor, New York: Masson.

OH, J. O., KIMURA, S. J., OSTLER, H., DAWSON, C. R. and SMOLIN, G. (1976). Oculogenital transmission of type 2 herpes simplex virus in adults. *Survey Ophthal.*, **21**, 106–109.

OH, J. O. and STEVENS, T. R. (1973). Comparison of Types 1 and 2 Herpesvirus hominis infection of rabbit eyes. I. Clinical manifestations. *Arch. Ophthal.*, **90**, 473–476.

OPENSHAW, H. (1983). Latency of herpes simplex virus in ocular tissue of man. *Infection and Immunity*, **39**, 960–962.

OSTLER, H. B. (1976). Herpes simplex: The primary infection. *Survey Ophthal.*, **21**, 91–99.

PATTERSON, A., SOMMERVILLE, R. G. and JONES, B. R. (1969). Herpetic keratouveitis with herpes virus antigen in the anterior chamber. *Trans. Ophthal. Soc. U.K.*, **88**, 243–249.

PAVAN-LANGSTON, D. and BROCKHURST, R. J. (1969). Herpes simplex pan-uveitis. A clinical report. *Arch. Ophthal.*, **81**, 783–787.

PEREIRA, L., CASSAI, E. and HONESS, R. W. (1976). Variability in the structural polypeptides of herpes simplex virus 1 strains: potential application in molecular epidemiology. *Infection & Immunity*, **13**, 211–20.

POIRER, R. H. (1980). Herpetic ocular lesions in childhood. *Arch. Ophthal.*, **98**, 704–6.

PRINGE, J. J. (1890). Herpes. In: *A Dictionary of Practical Medicine*, p. 344. Ed. J. K. Fowler. London: J. & A. Churchill.

ROUSSUS, J. and DENIS, J. (1981). Interference between ocular herpes and allergic diseases. An epidemiological approach. In: *Herpetic Eye Diseases*. Ed. R. Sundmacher. Munich: J. F. Bergmann Verlag.

SANDFORD-SMITH, J. H. and WHITTLE, H. C. (1979). Corneal ulceration following measles in Nigerian children. *Brit. J. Ophthal.*, **63**, 720–724.

SAVIR, H., GROSSWASSER, Z. and MENDELSON, L. (1980). Herpes virus hominis encephalomyelitis and retinal vasculitis in adults. *Ann. Ophthal.*, **12**, 1369–71.

SCHNEWEIS, K. E. and BRANDIS, H. (1961). Serologische untersuchungen zur typendifferenzierurig der Herpesvirus hominis. *Z. Immunitetsforsch.*, **124**, 24.

SHIMELD, C., TULLO, A. B., EASTY, D. L. and TOMSITT, J. (1982). Isolation of herpes simplex virus from cornea in chronic stromal keratitis. *Brit. J. Ophthal.*, **66**, 643–647.

SMITH, I. W., PEUTHERER, J. F. and MacCALLUM, F. O. (1967). The incidence of Herpesvirus hominis antibody in the population. *J. Hyg.*, **65**, 395–408.

SMITH, M., LENNETTE, E. H. and REAMES, H. R. (1941). Isolation of virus of herpes simplex and demonstration of intranuclear inclusions in case of acute encephalitis. *Amer. J. Path.*, **17**, 55–68.

STEVENS, T. R. and OH, J. O. (1973). Comparison of Types 1 and 2 Herpesvirus hominis infection of rabbit eyes. II. Histopathologic and virologic studies. *Arch. Ophthal.*, **90**, 477–480.

SUNDMACHER, R. and NEUMANN-HAEFELIN, D. (1979). Herpes simplex virus—positive and negative keratouveitis. In: International Symposium on *Immunology and Immunopathology of the Eye*, p. 255. Eds. A. M. Silverstein and R. O'Connor. New York: Masson.

THYGESON, P. (1976). Historical observations on herpetic keratitis. *Survey Ophthal.*, **21**, 82–90.

THYGESON, P. and HOGAN, M. J. (1950). Aureomycin in the treatment of herpes simplex corneae. *Amer. J. Ophthal.*, **33**, 958–960.

TUFFLI, G. A. and NAHMIAS, A. J. (1969). Neonatal herpetic infection. *Amer. J. Dis. Child.*, **118**, 909–914.

TULLO, A. H., SHIMELD, C., HILL, T. J., BLYTH, W. and EASTY, D. L. Virus spread to the retina of the opposite eye following primary herpetic uveitis in mice. (*In preparation*).

VANNAS, A. and AHONEN, R. (1981). Herpetic endothelial keratitis. A case report. *Acta Ophthal. (Kbh.)*, **59**, 296–301.

VIDAL, J. B. (1873). Inoculabilite des pustules d'ecthyma. *Ann. Dermat. Syph. (Paris)*, **4**, 350.

WARREN, S. L., CARPENTER, C. M. and BOAK, R. A. (1940). Symptomatic herpes, a sequelae of artificially induced fever. *J. Exp. Med.*, **71**, 155–168.

WHITCHER, J. P., DAWSON, C. R. and HOSHIWARA, I. (1976). Herpes simplex keratitis in a developing country. *Arch. Ophthal.*, **94**, 587–592.

WILHELMUS, K. R., COSTER, D. J., FALCON, M. G. and JONES, M. C. (1981a).

Longitudinal analysis of ulcerative herpetic keratitis. In: *Herpes Eye Diseases*, p. 375. Ed. R. Sundmacher. Munich: J. F. Bergmann Verlag.

WILHELMUS, K. R., FALCON, M. G. and JONES, B. R. (1981*b*). Bilateral herpetic keratitis. *Brit. J. Ophthal.*, **65**, 385–7.

WITMER, R. and IWAMATO, T. (1968). Electron microscopic observations of herpes-like particles in the iris. *Arch. Ophthal.*, **79**, 331–337.

CHAPTER EIGHT

The Management of Herpes Simplex Keratitis

The Management of HSK

The ideals in the therapy of HSV infections, although not yet all attained, help in the approach to the management of the affected patient. Today, much is understood concerning the treatment of epithelial disease with the use of topical antiviral drugs. However, these drugs have limitations; it is not certain how they are able to penetrate the corneal epithelium to enter the stroma, and when they do, whether they are able to reduce the rate of viral proliferation which is thought to occur in the stromal cells. At the same time, they have little influence on the recurrence rate of the disease. Whether the total inactivation of the virus in the posterior root ganglion can be achieved has yet to be seen, but it can be anticipated that this objective will be difficult to attain because it is suspected that the virus within the ganglion becomes part of the DNA of the genome when not undergoing active proliferation.

The ultimate aim in the care of the patient is the prevention of visual loss in those in whom the disease has become apparent. The objective is therefore to prevent active virus or viral antigen entering the stroma where it is thought to be capable of invading the keratocytes, or lying dormant between the lamellae of the collagen fibrils, whence it is incapable of escaping or being removed. In order to prevent this spread, antiviral therapy should be introduced early in the disease, and where the trigger factor is known there seems to be little contra-indication to the use of prophylactic therapy prior to, or at an early stage of, ulcerative disease.

A further objective, not yet attained, is the development of an anti-inflammatory agent which does not increase the rate of viral proliferation. Although the use of topical steroid in experienced hands can be valuable in the clearing of stromal opacities, patients develop more serious disease as a result, and are not always helped.

In the following chapter the therapeutic armamentarium available in the treatment of HSK will be reviewed, and the problems which may be encountered in their use will be described. There are many manifestations of the disease where the best form of treatment is not clear, and these will be discussed. The management of patients with herpetic keratitis who require keratoplasty will also be described, together with the difficulties which can be encountered in their postoperative care.

Cautery Debridement

Simple debridement by gently removing all loose epithelium around a dendrite or a geographic ulcer may be performed with a sterile cotton-wool applicator. This may be followed by the instillation of local antibiotic, and a pad should be applied for 24 hours, following which the condition of the eye should be reviewed. The use of carbolic acid, ether or iodine carefully applied to the edge of the lesion with the tip of an orange stick, although effective, has been considered to induce damage to the basement membrane, Bowman's membrane, or the superficial stroma. Debridement has been compared with idoxuridine (IDU) in clinical trials, and there is some evidence that the rate of healing can be more rapid using such techniques. Thus, Wellings *et al.* (1972) state that IDU-treated ulcers heal more slowly than those treated by debridement. Mackenzie (1964) and Ibraham (1967) and Whitcher *et al.* (1976), found that debridement or 'cauterisation' was superior to IDU. At the same time, the efficacy of patching was demonstrated well before the advent of IDU (Gunderson, 1936; El Korashy, 1942). In spite of the apparently beneficial effects of debridement, the question of recurrence rates following such techniques has recently been raised, and it is considered that there is a recurrence of at least 50 per cent within 14 days (Coster *et al.*, 1977). The latter have pointed out that debridement techniques aim at removing the diseased epithelial cells at the wound edge which harbours replicating virus, thereby reducing the quantity of virus in the locality. In addition to the cells nurturing replicating virus, the wound edge also contains degenerate epithelial cells, occasional inflammatory cells, and free virus. Removal of the tissue which is considered to be a potent inducer of inflammation results in the rapid diminution of this response.

Debridement using other methods includes sharp dissection with the blade of a scalpel; it is precise and convenient, but there is a risk of injury to Bowman's membrane. An erosion may form which may take some time to heal and at the same time act as an entry portal for free virus into the stroma. Coster *et al.* (1977) consider that the use of chemicals undoubtedly causes damage to the stroma, is inconvenient to perform and causes discomfort to the patient. Zinc sulphate, carbolic acid and trichloroacetic acid all have similar disadvantages in that considerable experience and an element of skill is required to prevent the induction of a disease process, involving either the epithelium or the stroma, which is more serious than the initial lesion.

In a similar way to cautery techniques, the use of cryotherapy is beset with difficulties (Amoils and Maier, 1973; Fulhorst *et al.*, 1972) in that it lacks precision and appears to have a lasting influence on the stroma and corneal endothelium, although the mechanism for this is not clear. There is little histopathological evidence that corneal freezing damages the stroma or the endothelium. However, there is no doubt that the stromal disease in patients following cryotherapy of dendritic figures is more severe than that which follows other methods of treatment, and from the clinician's point of view, the technique is not efficacious. It seems likely that the severe stromal disease which follows is due to the increased amount of viral agent penetrating the stroma.

Photodynamic Inactivation

Herpes simplex virus particles are rendered non-infective by the visible-light spectrum after a period of exposure to certain heterotricyclic dyes. Known as photodynamic inactivation, the technique has been fully investigated *in vitro* where it has application in the production of vaccines and maintenance of viral cultures free of other viral contaminants. There were encouraging reports in the management of recurrent cutaneous herpes, which were followed by similar findings in herpetic keratitis in rabbits (Lahav *et al.*, 1975; Allen and Szjnader, 1976).

Photodynamic inactivation is a sensitised photo-auto-oxidation reaction in which the first step is the binding of a photo-active dye to specific sites on viral DNA, the sites probably being the base guanine in the case of herpes virus. Dyes which may have such reactions include toluidine blue, neutral red, proflavine, and members of the thiazine, phenazine and acridine series. The result of the process of inactivation brought about is thought to be a break in single-stranded DNA induced when the virus is replicating.

O'Day *et al.* (1975) treated a group of patients with ulcerative herpetic keratitis who had IDU toxicity or resistance. Using a group of patients treated with IDU as a control group, photodynamic inactivation with proflavine dye in a 0·1 per cent solution showed a significant therapeutic effect. However, hazards were associated with the technique. The first was a keratitis similar to an ultraviolet-light burn of the cornea, with photophobia, conjunctival injection and epithelial punctate keratopathy. A second complication reported by O'Day and his associates was the appearance of iritis which became more severe following photo-inactivation.

Clearly, further investigation concerning concentration of the photosensitising dye, the time of exposure and light intensity are required before such methods can be considered for investigation in human disease. Using proflavine dye, blue light peaking at 450 nm is more effective than white fluorescent light or incandescent light in the photodynamic inactivation of herpes simplex keratitis in rabbits.

THE ANTIVIRALS

The Early Studies

The discovery of the topical antiviral drugs was a vital stage in the development of therapy of herpetic keratitis. Kaufman first reported that idoxuridine (IDU; Figure 8.1) was active against herpetic keratitis first in rabbits and then in man (Kaufman, 1962). Idoxuridine was synthesised by Prusoff (1959), and Herrmann (1961) reported that IDU, when tested in the

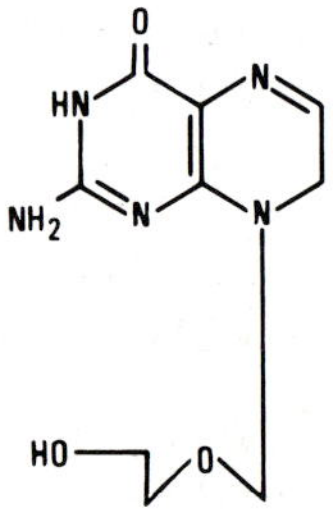

Figure 8.1. The structural formulae of the antiviral compounds compared:
1. Thymidine
2. Idoxuridine
3. Trifluorothymidine
4. Adenine arabinoside
5. Acyclovir

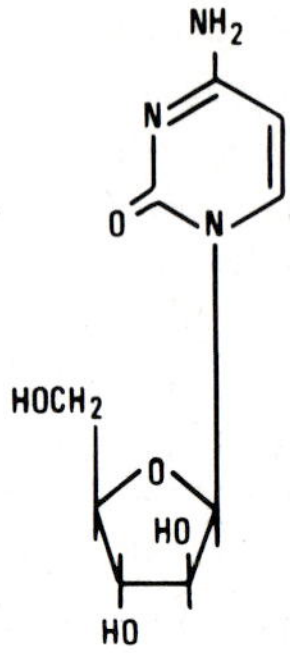

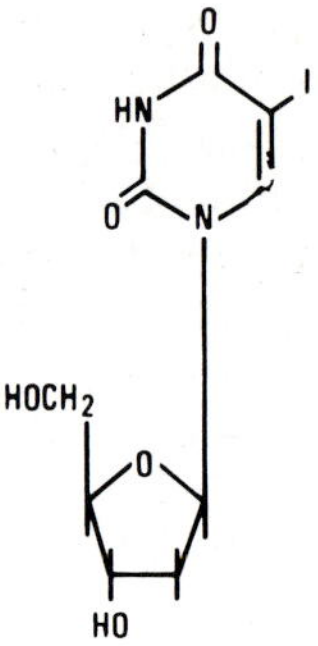

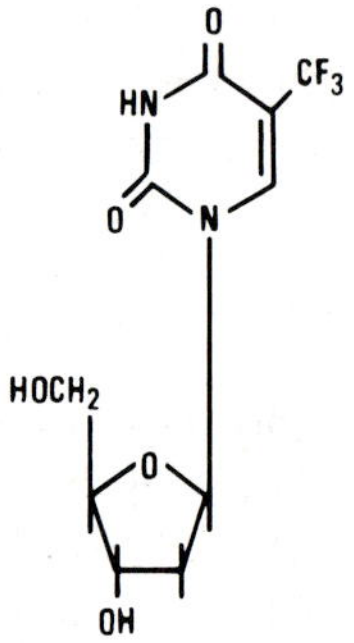

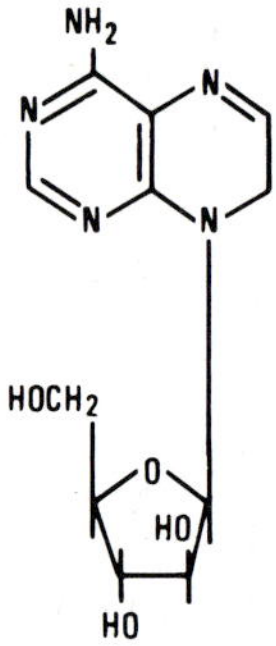

agar-diffusion plaque inhibition test, was found to inhibit plaque formation of vaccinia and herpes simplex virus. Rapp and Vanderslice (1964) showed that IDU was active against varicella zoster virus *in vitro*. Kaufman (1962) reported that herpetic lesions could be successfully treated both in rabbit eyes and in humans without significant toxicity to the host. It was initially considered that IDU had negligible toxicity when applied locally to the skin, but this has not been borne out in prolonged application to the external eye. However, following investigations of systemic introduction it was considered that the toxicity rating was low. Calabresi *et al.* (1961) reported that only large dosages, when given intravenously to cancer patients, induced leucopenia, stomatitis and alopecia. The value of systemic therapy was investigated in mice by

Sidwell *et al.* (1968), following intraperitoneal injection, where it combated vaccinial encephalitis, but Sloan *et al.* (1969) found that it was inactive in herpes simplex encephalitis in mice, possibly because therapeutic levels were not obtained.

Following the reports by Kaufman that topically applied IDU was effective in herpes simplex keratitis, the therapeutic efficacy was investigated in cutaneous herpes, but the therapeutic effect was limited because of poor penetration of the water-soluble drug into the tissues (Hall-Smith, Corrigan and Gilkes, 1962; Burnett and Katz, 1963; Juel-Jensen and MacCallum, 1964; Kibrick and Katz, 1970). When administered as an injection (Juel-Jensen and MacCallum, 1965) the drug had a significant advantage over placebo. The insolubility of IDU remained a problem until investigations were made using dimethyl sulphoxide (DMSO) as a vehicle known to increase the penetration of various dyes and steroids through the skin (Kligman, 1965). A 5 per cent solution of IDU applied three times daily to cold sores of recent onset showed that the drug was effective in a controlled trial (MacCallum and Juel-Jensen, 1966). There was a difference in healing of two days between the two groups. DMSO alone seemed to confer some benefit however, and it remains possible that the entry of specific antibody into the virus-infected cell was facilitated by this reagent.

A number of groups have reported that IDU is effective in the treatment of herpes simplex keratitis. Placebo-controlled trials have been reported by Patterson *et al.* (1963), Laibson and Leopold (1965) and Hart *et al.* (1965) who demonstrated that the drug was favourable in comparison to a placebo. However, Markham *et al.* (1977) were not able to show statistically significant superiority of IDU over placebo in ulcerative disease, although the results of the trial were highly suggestive. Difficulties were also experienced by a number of workers in earlier trials; Burns (1963) found IDU better than placebo but not strikingly so, 60 per cent of his placebo treated cases being improved. Luntz and MacCallum (1963) and Jepson (1964) could not demonstrate a significant difference between IDU and placebo. Placebo-controlled trials of antiviral drugs in ulcerative disease require 50 subjects per group to achieve statistical significance (Markham *et al.* 1977).

There are a number of factors which may make comparison between different cases and different controlled series difficult, such as the time lapse between infection and treatment, initial size of the ulcer, virulence of virus, resistance to antivirals, local and systemic immunity, patient difficulty in instilling therapy, or observer variation.

In spite of such difficulties, it is hard to explain why placebo-controlled trials do not show clear-cut results, in view of the dramatic responses to IDU found in the original animal studies by Kaufman *et al.* (1962) and Corwin *et al.* (1963), where the therapeutic effects were pronounced. Antiviral effects were investigated in rabbits by Markham *et al.* (1977), and it was found that the differences between animals where one eye was treated with placebo and the other with an antiviral (IDU or Vira A) was greater in primary infections than in secondary infections. It was considered that previous experience of herpetic infection was able to protect the cornea against re-infection, so that in such animals the difference between placebo and antiviral treated eyes was

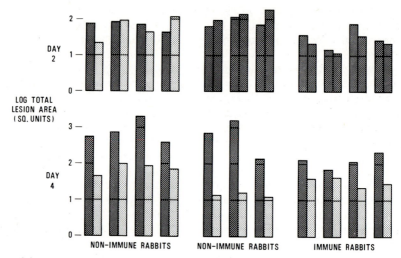

Figure 8.2. Comparison of placebo with the antiviral adenine arabinoside in groups of non-immune and immune rabbits. The contrast between placebo- and antiviral-treated eyes is less in the immune rabbits as compared with the non-immune rabbits.

considerably reduced (Figure 8.2). This would to some extent explain the difficulties which have been encountered in the conduct of clinical trials with convincing statistical results in patients who also are probably protected by previous infections. The dendritic ulcer would be expected to be a useful clinical disease in which a therapeutic effect might be measured but experience has not been able to demonstrate this with any conviction, and the same is true of other diseases caused by the herpes simplex virus, such as in the case of cutaneous herpes (Burnett and Katz, 1963; Juel-Jensen and MacCallum, 1964 and 1972). In the case of ulcers which have been treated with topical steroid a statistically significant effect can be obtained. Recently, Coster *et al.* (1979) have reported the superior therapeutic efficacy of trifluorothymidine (F_3T) over adenine arabinoside in a steroid-treated group of patients.

The Recent Antivirals

The structural formulae of the other antiherpes compounds are presented in Figure 8.1. They act by inhibition of one or more stages in the synthesis of viral DNA. Idoxuridine inhibits thymidine kinase, thymidine monophosphate kinase and DNA polymerase (Delamore and Prusoff, 1962) and is incorporated into DNA. Cytarabine inhibits deoxycytidine kinase, thymidylate synthetase and DNA polymerase, and is incorporated into DNA and into RNA to a lesser extent. Trifluorothymidine inhibits thymidine kinase, and thymidylate synthetase and is incorporated into DNA. The mechanism of adenine arabinoside is known in less detail. It acts by inhibition of DNA polymerase and is also incorporated into DNA. These compounds in addition to inhibiting virus proliferation also inhibit mechanisms in the host cell, but there is a quantitative difference which allows the antiviral effect to be evident at lower than toxic levels. Acyclovir has relatively little effect on host cell systems and its inhibitory activity is directed against the replication of virus DNA. It is converted to the monophosphate by thymidine kinase produced by herpes virus and further to the triphosphate which inhibits virus DNA polymerase. Formation of triphosphate is reduced in uninfected cells and the inhibitory activity against the DNA polymerase of the cell is low. There is some evidence that acyclovir is incorporated into the viral DNA.

Cheng (1981) has summarised the molecular basis and pharmacological considerations in selective antiherpetic agents. There are a number of thymidine-kinase-dependent agents which exert their selective antiherpes virus effect by being able to act as 'selective alternative substrates' of virus thymidine kinase. There are many possible agents, but acycloguanosine is presently available. Uninfected cells are not affected by these agents since their thymidine kinase cannot efficiently utilise the compounds as substrate. However, the selective antiviral effect of the group of agents relies on the ability of the herpes virus to induce a thymidine kinase which can recognise them as substrates in infected cells. Different types of herpes virus have different abilities to induce thymidine kinase. Field (1981) has reported the clinical implications of resistant mutants of herpes simplex virus. Thus the virus has been shown to readily develop resistance to acyclovir *in vitro*. This mutation is associated with the virus losing its ability to induce thymidine kinase. The herpes virus thymidine-kinase-dependent agents include phosphonoacetate (Gordon *et al.*, 1977), phosphonoformate, adenine arabinoside, and 2-deoxyglucose.

After instillation into the conjunctival sac IDU passes into the corneal epithelium, and to a lesser extent into the iris and lens (Bakhle *et al.*, 1965). On the other hand, F_3T has been shown to pass into the aqueous when given in the form of eye drops (Sugar *et al.*, 1973). Acyclovir has been given experimentally, both intravenously and orally, and has achieved significant bio-availability. It penetrates into the aqueous humour in rabbits as a topical therapy in an ophthalmic ointment, and is absorbed through the skin after topical application in rats and guinea-pigs (De Miranda *et al.*, 1978).

The antiviral activity of these compounds vary over a wide range. Values of ID50 (the 50 per cent infectious dose) against a strain of type 1 herpes are shown in Table 8.1 (Bauer, 1980*a*). Acyclovir is more active than the other compounds available. Trifluorothymidine and acyclovir are equally effective against type 1 and type 2 herpes viruses whereas other compounds are somewhat less effective against type 2 strains. The properties of the antiherpes compounds are demonstrated in Table 8.2 (Bauer, 1980*a*). Acyclovir is active in animal models when given orally (Schaeffer *et al.*, 1978). The only known compounds to cross the blood-brain barrier and probably the blood-ocular barrier are vidarabine and acyclovir. In addition to acyclovir, bromovinyl deoxyuridine (BVDU) is a potent agent found after screening of compounds of the 5 substituted 2-deoxyuridines, because of its ability to inhibit replication of HSV 1 and varicella-zoster virus (VZV) in cell culture at low concentration. Preliminary observations in man indicate that BVDU may be efficaceous in the treatment of herpetic keratitis where virus has become resistant to other antiviral compounds. BVDU appears to be less toxic than IDU in laboratory

TABLE 8.1

RELATIVE POTENCIES AGAINST TYPE I HERPESVIRUS.
(BAUER, 1980a)

Compound	ID50 (μM)	Potency
Vidarabine (Vira A)	16	6
Trifluorothymidine	1·5	67
Idoxuridine	1	100
Cytarabine	0·2	500
Acyclovir	0·1	1000

TABLE 8.2

PROPERTIES OF THE ANTIHERPES COMPOUNDS (BAUER, 1980a)

	Cytarabine	Idoxuridine	Trifluoro-thymidine	Vidarabine	Acyclovir
Solubility	10	0·8	5	0·05	0·14
Stability at pH 7	unstable	stable	unstable	—	stable
Half-life (min)	30–60	—	30	60	120–180
Metabolites	inactive	inactive	inactive	active	active
Activity (oral)	no	no	no	yes	yes
Crosses blood-brain barrier	—	no	—	yes	yes
Enters aqueous	no	yes	yes	yes	yes
Teratogenic	yes	yes	yes	yes	no
Immunosuppressive	yes	yes	—	no	yes

animals. Prompted by the clinical efficacy of BVDU in animal models (i.e. cutaneous herpes infection in athymic nude mice and herpetic keratitis in rats), and its apparent freedom from toxicity when applied topically to the skin or the eye, trials have been initiated on the influence of topical treatment in herpes labialis with 0·1 per cent BVDU ointment, and with drops of the same concentration in patients with herpetic keratitis.

Adenine Arabinoside (vidarabine; Vira-A)

Adenine arabinoside has been investigated in a number of trials where it has generally been compared with idoxuridine (Pavan-Langston and Dohlman, 1972; Markham et al., 1977; Laibson and Krachmer, 1975; Chin, 1978). Other studies were performed investigating the efficacy of trifluorothymidine (F_3T) compared to Vira A (McGill et al., 1974; Coster et al., 1976). In trials where Vira A was compared to IDU, the former proved to be as effective as idoxuridine in the treatment of epithelial keratitis (Pavan-Langston, 1975). Vira A in addition offered some safety advantages over idoxuridine such as less toxicity to corneal wound healing (Langston et al., 1974). Vira-A appears to be more effective than idoxuridine in vaccinial keratitis (Pavan-Langston *et al.*, 1973), and it has been shown to be effective against herpes simplex virus where resistance or intolerance has proved to be a problem in patients.

In a clinical trial of Vira-A and idoxuridine compared with placebo (Markham *et al.*, 1977) the average duration of treatment was similar with the active agents, but was less for the placebo-treated group. Treatment was discontinued in more patients in the placebo group than in the treatment groups because of inefficacy. The most common reason for treatment failure in placebo-treated patients was that epithelial lesions were larger on day 5 or unchanged by day 7. The fact that patients in the placebo group had their treatment discontinued earlier than patients in the other two groups reflected the effectiveness of Vira-A and idoxuridine over the placebo. However, the differences were not significant between idoxuridine and Vira-A during any observation period, although both agents were shown to be more effective than placebo in the parameters of reduction of dose and in the investigator's evaluation.

The importance of the virus in the induction of stromal disease and anterior uveitis have already been stressed. The treatment of herpes simplex uveitis presents the clinician with a dilemma which also haunts him in the treatment of stromal disease, the difficulty being in the determination of how much topical steroid medication can be given without inducing a harmful increase in the rate of viral proliferation. Abel *et al.* (1975) investigated the effect of intravenous Vira-A on herpes simplex kerato-uveitis in humans, which may be refractory to topical antivial therapy. It was concluded that Vira-A possessed all of the characteristics desirable for an antiviral agent because it has a broad spectrum of activity against the DNA family of viruses. In addition it lacks resistance *in vitro*, and is rapidly excreted. It is thought not to cause immunosuppression, and has low toxicity in significantly therapeutic cases. In a controlled series of patients it was found that Vira-A as intravenous infusions (20 mg/kg/day) for 7 days was effective in the treatment of herpetic kerato-uveitis, while being accompanied by only minimal adverse reactions (Kaufman *et al.*, 1970). The adverse reactions included myalgia, nausea and leucopenia. In addition to the efficacy of Vira-A in uveitis, it has been shown to have some beneficial effect in herpes encephalitis, herpes zoster, particularly when disseminated in immunosuppressed hosts (Luly *et al.*, 1975), and in cytomegalic inclusion disease (Baublis *et al.*, 1975).

Vira-A becomes deaminated to hypoxanthine arabinoside, which also has some antiviral activity although to a lesser extent, the antiviral effect being about one fifth of Vira-A. It has latterly been considered that Vira-A, although a safe systemic therapeutic agent, is not truly selective. The possibility remains that host DNA can be altered, and there is therefore concern of possible metagenesis and teratogenesis (Itoi *et al.*, 1975; Gasset *et al.*, 1976).

Trifluorothymidine (F_3T)

Controlled experiments were carried out by Kaufman and Heidelberger (1964) to evaluate the efficacy of F_3T, compared with idoxuridine, cytosine arabinoside and 5-brom-2-deoxyuridine, and it was established in laboratory animals that F_3T was more active than the other therapies when used in equal concentrations. The low solubility of idoxuridine and its poor penetration into the corneal stroma were limiting factors in the effectivity of what was and is a valuable drug (O'Brien and Edelhauser, 1977). Trifluorothymidine is 10 times more soluble in water than idoxuridine, and does not produce toxic effects in rabbit corneas when used topically for prolonged periods of time. Wellings *et al.* (1972) carried out a clinical evaluation of F_3T in the treatment of herpes simplex corneal ulcers where a comparison was made with idoxuridine. It was found that the percentage of treatment failures was significantly lower for F_3T than for idoxuridine, and the mean time taken to heal on F_3T was significantly shorter. Other studies showed that F_3T was a superior alternative to idoxuridine (McGill *et al.*, 1974), but in a similarly designed study, Pavan-Langston (1977) demonstrated that there was no significant difference between F_3T and IDU in healing rate. However, there was a difference in the *chance* of healing, 96 per cent of all F_3T-treated eyes and only 75 per cent of idoxuridine-treated eyes healing completely within 14 days. Other trials have compared F_3T with Vira-A (Coster *et al.*, 1976), when there was no significant difference between the two drugs. Data from a small group of subjects withe amoeboid ulcers suggested that F_3T may be more effective than Vira-A in the treatment of these ulcers. In a clinical trial comparing F_3T and Vira-A, Van Bijsterveld and Post (1980) were not able to show that there was a difference in efficacy between the two drugs, but stressed the importance of the relation of healing time to the time between the onset of symptoms and the introduction of therapy.

Antiviral Toxicity

IDU, Vira-A and F_3T may all produce toxicity to the external eye if used in the long term (Table 8.3). Treatment regimes generally involve the use of an antiviral in epithelial disease for periods of 2 weeks, the drops or ointment being instilled four or five times per day. By the end of this time the epithelium has regenerated, and there is on occasions little evidence of a previous herpetic ulcer. Occasionally, a scar will form beneath the ulcerated area forming a ghost of the previous ulcer. With the passage of time this small opacity clears, leaving faint scarring which has little influence on vision.

TABLE 8.3

TOXIC EFFECTS OF IDOXURIDINE

Follicular conjunctivitis
Bulbar chemosis and hyperaemia
Constriction of puncti of lacrimal canaliculi
Punctate epithelial keratopathy (whorled appearance)
Chronic or persistent epithelial deficits
Confluent opacities in epithelium or Bowman's membrane
Reduced tear secretion ⎫ after prolonged use
Keratinisation of tarsal plates ⎭

Where the synthetic antivirals are used for long periods, the cornea and bulbar and tarsal conjunctiva are seriously affected. The punctate keratitis may be persistent and take some weeks to resolve. There may be conjunctival chemosis and redness and follicular reaction (Figures 8.3 and 8.4). The condition may remain unrecognised because it is thought that it is a manifestation of the virus disease itself, and therefore no decision is made to stop the antiviral treatment. Since acyclovir is not thought to influence cell metabolism there is hope that its toxicity to the cornea and the conjunctiva will become less of a clinical problem. It is worth remembering that the influence of antiviral therapy on cell metabolism has a secondary effect on the immune response within the conjunctival sac. Thus it has been shown experimentally that IDU may worsen infection with *Staph. aureus*, inducing a more severe keratitis and a more prolific growth of micro-organisms (Yamaguchi *et al.*, 1979). This immunosuppressive influence is probably compounded where antiviral therapy is prescribed simultaneously with corticosteroid.

The adverse reactions which result from topical therapy with idoxuridine, adenine arabinoside and trifluorothymidine have been summarised by Falcon *et al.* (1981). In a substantial group of patients, both IDU and F_3T were found to cause the typical toxic changes. Toxicity due to adenine arabinoside was infrequent. There were two principle types of toxic response to F_3T. A marked corneal epitheliopathy with diffuse epithelial oedema occurred in a small number of patients on short-term therapy, whereas in a larger group of patients receiving long-term therapy, punctate lesions in the conjunctiva and corneal

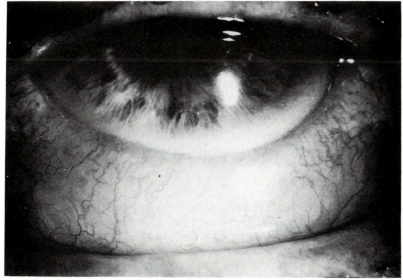

Figure 8.3. Severe conjunctival chemosis and hyperaemia following the prolonged use of antiviral therapy in herpes keratitis.

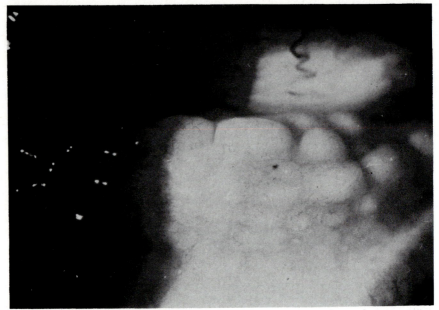

Figure 8.4.   Follicles forming in the lower fornix as a result of antiviral toxicity.

epithelium occurred, together with punctal occlusion. Substitution of adenine arabinoside for F_3T allowed the toxic sites to improve. These studies are supported by the *in vitro* work of Taylor and O'Brien (1981), who tested the cyototoxicity of nucleoside antivirals to epithelial cells of conjunctival origin. The relative toxicity was measured by inhibition of growth in the presence of a number of antiviral compounds. It was found that trifluorothymidine was the most toxic, followed by IDU, Vira A and acyclovir in diminishing order.

Acycloguanosine

Acycloguanosine (acyclovir; zovirax) is the generic name of 9-(2-hydroxy-ethoxymethyl) guanine (Figure 8.1). The antiviral activity *in vitro* of acyclovir against herpes simplex virus was first described by Schaeffer *et al.* (1978) and in greater detail by Collins and Bauer (1979). Standard antiherpes compounds were compared with acyclovir by means of plaque-inhibition tests and the latter was found to be more active than IDU, F_3T, Vira-A and phosphonoacetic acid. Acyclovir was effective against herpes-varicella-zoster virus in plaque-reduction assays (Biron and Elion, 1979). However, varicella-zoster was less sensitive to acyclovir than the herpes simplex virus but it has been considered that the drug's activity is great enough for it to be investigated for its clinical efficacy. The effect of acyclovir in the animal model was explored by Bauer *et al.* (1979); it produces satisfactory cures of cutaneous herpes and has a protective effect in herpetic encephalitis (Bauer, 1980). It was effective when given topically, intravenously, or by mouth. Its spectrum of activity included varicella-zoster, EB virus, and cytomegalovirus and B virus. Early studies indicated that it might prevent the establishment of latency after primary infection. Its mode of action is unique in that it is phosphorylated by the thymidine kinase specified by herpes virus, and in the form of the triphosphate it inhibits herpes virus DNA polymerase. These reactions take place to a limited extent in unaffected cells. This is one of the features which reduces the toxicity of this important drug. Acyclovir was evaluated in experimental herpes simplex keratitis in rabbits and compared with F_3T and preparations of IDU and Vira A in clinical use. The compounds were used in the form of ophthalmic ointments applied five times per day at intervals of 2 hours. The treatment was begun on the third day of infection and continued for 4 days. Complete cure was obtained with acyclovir and IDU while F_3T and Ara A were less effective. Acyclovir was equally effective when given intravenously in the form of the sodium salt, and could be detected in tears in inhibitory concentrations when it was given by mouth. The compound was relatively free from toxicity (Bauer et al., 1979). A further study investigated the influence of acyclovir in rabbits with herpetic ulcers of the cornea (Shiota, et al., 1979. Falcon and Jones, 1979). The therapeutic effect of 3 per cent acyclovir was equal to that of 0·5 per cent IDU. There were no toxic signs using slit-lamp examination following treatment for four days. In a short-term comparison of acyclovir, Vira A and Ara AMP ointments, a potent therapeutic effect was shown at three days when these agents were used as ointments, but the therapeutic effect was not so clear when drops were used as the vehicle.

In order to prove that the acyclovir compound had an effective antiviral action in clinical herpes virus infection in man, whilst exposing the least number of persons to the minimal amount of drug, a placebo-controlled randomised double-blind trial was devised (Jones et al., 1980). Twenty-four men were treated by minimal wiping debridement which was followed by the use of acyclovir or placebo. There were recurrences of microscopic foci of epithelial disease in 12 patients treated with placebo, but none in the group of 12 patients treated with acyclovir. A second double-blind randomised trial was carried out contrasting acyclovir ointment (3 per cent) with idoxuridine ointment (1 per cent). The results showed that there was a trend in favour of acyclovir. This work proved that acyclovir was active in ulcerative herpetic disease of the cornea and that it was at least as effective as 1 per cent IDU. In this trial, 7 out of 38 patients on one batch of acyclovir developed minor punctate staining with rose bengal in the lower third of the bulbar conjunctiva (Collum et al., 1980). McGill and Tormey (1981) showed that acyclovir was equivalent in efficacy to adenine arabinoside in a controlled study. Subsequent clinical trials showed that the use of acyclovir in the treatment of herpetic corneal ulceration in patients was highly effective with low toxicity (Jones et al., 1979; Coster et al., 1980). Subsequently, it was shown that the combination of debridement and acyclovir produced a significantly more rapid healing rate than acyclovir alone (Wilhelmus et al., 1981).

The results of systemic studies in man show that absorption of the drug from the gut is incomplete, but that intravenous administration demonstrates a satisfactory pharmacokinetic profile. There are no adverse effects. Introduction of the drug as a therapeutic agent in patients with severe systemic herpetic infection at a dose of 5 mg per kg 8-hourly for five days confirmed a lack of toxicity (Brigden *et al.*, 1980).

Resistance to the Antivirals

McGill and Ogilvie (1980) have drawn attention to the fact that following treatment with IDU some herpes simplex ulcers failed to heal. Such ulcers usually heal following treatment with another antiviral (Pavan-Langston and Dohlman, 1972; McGill *et al.*, 1975; Nesburn *et al.*, 1977). Similarly, ulcers which have been treated with Vira-A may also show a poor response to therapy, and may heal with trifluorothymidine (McGill *et al.*, 1975). The results of sensitivity tests in virus culture against a number of antiviral agents indicate that there is a 33 per cent failure rate in healing of those ulcers treated with IDU. McGill and Ogilvie (1980) showed that in seven patients with IDU-resistant organisms, the healing time was greater than in a group of patients in whom the virus was sensitive. It is considered that where the patient presents with a persistent ulcer, this may be due to viral drug resistance. It is possible that drug-resistant strains are now in circulation. It is therefore advisable, where ulcers increase in size despite full treatment, remain of a similar size at the end of seven days, or fail to heal by fourteen days, that the virus should be deemed to be clinically resistant to the particular antiviral in use, and a second antiviral should be introduced.

The evidence that antiviral resistance exists is accumulating, and so it is therapeutically advisable that antivirals should be used according to routine; IDU remains the drug of choice, but where antiviral resistance occurs or toxicity ensues, adenine arabinoside or acycloguanosine must be considered.

The introduction of antivirals against the herpes simplex virus in corneal disease has made a major impact in the practice of ophthalmology. The main indications for their therapeutic use against the herpes simplex virus are:

1. In the treatment of primary disease of the cornea.

2. As a prophylactic treatment where primary disease affects the peri-orbital cutaneous tissue, to protect the cornea.

3. In recurrent disease. Where a trigger factor is known, patients with frequent recurrences or disease affecting the visual axis should be provided with an antiviral for immediate introduction into the asymptomatic eye, but with instructions to seek clinical advice at the earliest opportunity if symptoms should occur.

In the above situations it is not recommended that the antivirals should be used for longer than two weeks. If there is a failure of resolution of the dendritic ulcer at the end of fourteen days, then a second antiviral agent should be employed.

4. It is recommended that IDU remains the antiviral of choice for short-term use. Other antivirals should be kept in reserve in case toxicity or viral resistance occur.

5. Where full-strength topical corticosteroid is used, it is advisable that an antiviral umbrella is employed at the same time. Where topical corticosteroid is tapered off, antiviral toxicity may become unmasked.

Where very dilute topical steroids are employed, antiviral cover is probably not necessary.

6. Where corneal grafts have been carried out for herpes simplex keratitis, it is recommended that an antiviral be used in the postoperative phase. This is a controversial point, but it is considered that many grafts fail because of herpes simplex recurrence in the presence of high dosage of topical steroid. Antiviral cover significantly reduces this.

7. In herpes simplex kerato-uveitis, antiviral agents with good intra-ocular penetrating properties, such as trifluorothymidine or acycloguanosine, should be employed when used with topical corticosteroid.

Interferon

Interferon was discovered by Isaacs and Lindenmann in 1957 after investigating the biology of interference. This refers to occasions when cells inoculated with one virus, either alive or inactivated, are then inoculated with the second which is found not to grow because the first virus has induced a state of interference. They used chick membranes infected with influenza virus, and found that a mediator was released into the region which rendered other cells resistant to infection by a different virus. This mediator of interference was a protein and was named interferon. Since then it has been shown that there are families of interferons, differing between species and also within an animal according to the cell that makes it. A number of research groups in various parts of the world are investigating both the biology and chemistry of interferon, and developing large-scale production methods for studying its use in clinical medicine. It was discovered that double-stranded RNA and other similar molecules, such as poly I:C, stimulated interferon production. This gave rise to a concept that an interferon inducer might be superior to interferon itself as a medication, and work on interferon production was therefore limited for a while. It was later found that poly I:C was toxic. In the 1970s in Helsinki, Kantel improved the production of leucocyte interferon (IFN) from leucocytes provided by the Finnish Red Cross. Clinical trials were then done with this material. It was eventually possible, with the larger amounts of interferon that were produced, to show that the common virus infections of man could be prevented or treated. For example, a therapeutic effect was shown in rhinovirus infection and in varicella and zoster infections.

The first efforts to purify interferon began after 1957, and almost exactly twenty years later, success was achieved. DNA for interferon has now been cloned into bacteria and sequenced (Mantei et al., 1980), and the nucleoside sequences in these molecules are now being checked. Human interferon from such sources may provide useful amounts for clinical study in the next few years.

The mechanism of action of interferon has been extensively studied. Cytocidal viruses are neutralised because viral gene expression is inhibited in interferon-treated cells. Other types of virus, such as murine RNA tumour viruses, are inhibited by a different mechanism in a later stage of infection, either during the assembly or release of virus progene particles. Of particular interest for potential in clinical medicine are the inhibitory effects of interferon on the growth of tumour cells, and the effects on the cells of the immune system.

Interferon has been used topically in the eye in a number of virus diseases. Using human leucocyte interferon, McGill *et al.* (1976) demonstrated that there was a linear relationship between inhibition of herpetic lesions formed in an experimental model of herpetic keratitis in rabbits, and the log concentration of topically applied human interferon. Using these models it was possible to identify an appropriate concentration that could be used in clinical trials. Although there had been convincing data from the animal model that interferon would be valuable as a prophylactic agent, there had been no consistent demonstration of an effect in the therapy of established lesions in animals. Using the technique of minimal wiping debridement of the diseased epithelial cells at the border of a dendritic ulcer, when there is recurrence in half the cases during the convalescent period, it was found that when leucocyte interferon drops were compared with placebo, there was a significant inhibition of recurrence or recrudescence of corneal lesions (Jones *et al.*, 1976). Topical human interferon has also been used for the therapy and prophylaxis of dendritic keratitis in patients by Sundmacher and his colleagues (1978 and 1981). Evaluating its effect as a long-term prophylaxis of late dendritic recurrences, no therapeutic effect using interferon eye drops could be established. In addition the therapy of dendritic keratitis alone did not seem to offer a clinically relevant therapeutic effect. It was noted however that a combination of interferon with thermomechanical debridement of the diseased corneal epithelium, or with trifluorothymidine eye drops proved to be more effective than either single therapy. The possible role of interferon in the future therapy of herpetic keratitis is uncertain. Although the animal models predict that interferon would be a useful therapeutic agent, it has not been a simple matter to prove this in the human. It seems likely that this is because interferon is induced by the virus disease within the corneal epithelium, and it is therefore feasible that further interferon introduced topically would thus be without visible clinical effect. However, where there is primary disease, and disease caused by the erroneous use of topical steroid, it might be anticipated that interferon would have a recognisable therapeutic effect.

Immune Gamma Globulin in Ulcerative Disease

Gamma globulin and other antibody-containing preparations have been used in the treatment of herpetic keratitis (Amoils and Maier, 1973; Bonamour and Dugarre, 1959), but the value has never been clearly defined in the animal model of herpetic keratitis. Carter and Easty (1981c) have fully assessed the potential value in experimental animals, using normal gamma globulin, and hyperimmune gamma globulin. A possible potential for human gamma globulin is suggested by its high level of antibody to HSV, its lack of toxicity, and its availability at a comparatively low cost. Using the Jones and Al Hussaini (1963) model for the disease, with appropriate modifications, it was shown that HGG therapy in early disease in normal rabbits was very effective, producing a tenfold rise in the concentration of virus required to infect 50 per cent of inoculated sites. The therapeutic efficacy of HGG depended on its anti-HSV antibody content. Established disease was less responsive to HGG therapy, which was most effective where the initial extent of ulceration was small. Keratitis in animals with previous HSV skin infection showed no significant effect with early HGG therapy. Geographic ulceration induced by corticosteroid treatment was not prevented by concurrent administration of HGG. The findings indicated that HGG is unlikely to be clinically useful as a therapy, but that it may have a potential as a prophylactic agent. In a small, randomised double-blind controlled trial using HSV-negative gamma globulin as a placebo in a series of 12 patients with ulcerative herpetic keratitis and using minimal wiping debridement, it was found that HGG drops were no better than placebo in the prevention of recurrences. It therefore seems that there is little indication for the use of HGG in the treatment of corneal herpes simplex keratitis.

The influence of antibody is limited by its inability to reach replicating virus inside cells. The disruption of infected cells to express virus particles is the basis of cryosurgery that has been used prior to antibody treatment (Amoils and Maier, 1973). However, the dangers of cryosurgery restrict the application of this method. An alternative approach to the problem is the use of Fab fragments of the immunoglobulin molecule which can be split off by enzyme cleavage, and have been considered to be able to penetrate cells. However the use of such molecules (e.g. gamma-venin) in the model of established disease, i.e. disease which had existed for 48 hours prior to the introduction of treatment, was found to have no beneficial effect (Carter and Easty, 1981c).

Herpes Simplex Virus Vaccines

There has been a recent resurgence of interest in the prevention of herpes simplex virus infection by vaccination, and a number of inactivated vaccine preparations have been shown to have protective efficacy not only against primary type infections in mice and rabbits but also against the establishment of latent ganglionic infection in these animal species (Asher et al., 1978; McKendall, 1977; Walz et al., 1977). Protection against herpes keratitis with reduced disease severity has been shown in rabbits following systemic administration of live virus (Carter and Easty, 1981a), or the topical application or local injection of inactivated virus preparations (Pollikoff, 1970; Metcalf, 1980). A study by Carter et al. (1981b) demonstrated that systemic adminis-tration of a type 1 HSV subunit vaccine stimulated humoral and cellular immune responses, with good levels of protection against corneal challenge with live HSV. Humoral antibody was stimulated by one vaccination and was effectively boosted by a second vaccination (Figure 8.5). Cell-mediated immune responses were noted at this time. Along with reduced rates of viral replication which occurred in vaccinated animals, there was a reduced titre of corneal virus, and of conjunctival virus obtained by swabbing (Figure 8.6). The experimental model used was that of primary infection, and the value of the vaccine in secondary infection or recurrent disease is as yet undetermined. However, a substantial minority of populations in the developed countries exhibit no serological evidence of previous infection, and so the importance of prevention in herpetic disease, particularly at the genital site, is becoming increasingly apparent. It is considered that the selective administration of a subunit vaccine, with the prime objective of prevention of primary HSV

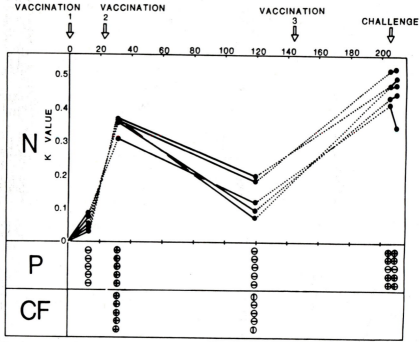

Figure 8.5. Specific antibody titres in serum taken from a group of rabbits vaccinated with herpes simplex subunit vaccine. Three vaccinations were given, and the corneas were challenged after two hundred days. Serum levels for neutralising antibody in K values (N), precipitating antibodies (P) and complement-fixing antibodies (CF) are shown.

disease at more frequent sites of infection than the eye, would be expected to provide a considerable degree of protection against ulcerative disease of the cornea, and hence would prevent the formation of the more serious forms of herpetic ocular disease. It is probable that herpes simplex vaccines will become more important in the future.

Immunopotentiation

In patients with frequent recurrences of ocular herpetic disease, there is enough indication to take steps to cut down the frequency of recurrences. One way in which this might be carried out is by the use of immunopotentiation, a means by which the systemic and local immune response directed against the virus may be enhanced. The development of immunopotentiation in the control of persistent viral disease is as yet comparatively unexplored. Levamisole is one agent that has been investigated in a number of situations. A model of chronic herpetic keratitis was developed by Smolin and his colleagues (1979), using subconjunctival corticosteroid prior and following corneal virus inoculation. In a levamisole-treated group of rabbits there was a more rapid healing of epithelial lesions than in the untreated group. It was significant that there was reduced stromal disease in the levamisole-treated group. Carter and

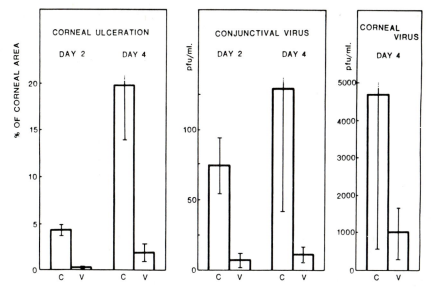

Figure 8.6.   Extent of herpetic corneal ulceration and titres of infectious virus in conjunctival swab media and in corneal extracts. Control (C); vaccinated (V) rabbits. (Mean±1 SE.)

Easty (1981*b*) have studied the influence of levamisole given orally in groups of animals with primary and secondary corneal epithelial disease. The extent of epithelial ulceration in secondary disease was reduced in levamisole-treated rabbits in contrast to the control group (Figure 8.7). However, in rabbits with primary disease, levamisole appeared to make no significant difference to the rate of virus proliferation or of healing. Similar findings were reported by Friedlander *et al.* (1978), although other workers have not identified a therapeutic effect (Kaufman and Varnell, 1977).

Levamisole has been assessed by patients with stromal disease (Kato *et al.*, 1979). It was reported that stromal oedema was cleared, and skin test reactivity to Candida and PHA increased. Sakata (1980) showed that the severity of stromal disease was reduced in experimental herpetic keratitis in levamisole-treated rabbits. Maichuk *et al.* (1980) showed reduced duration in experimental herpetic keratitis.

It is likely that in the future immunopotentiation will become a recognised treatment modality. In those patients in whom frequent epithelial disease creates a risk of developing stromal opacification, there would seem to be a potential for such modulators of the immune response. Where levamisole has been investigated in patients with infective disease, adverse reactions were a significant problem. Thus there were recognised complications including nausea, gastric intolerance, central nervous system stimulation, irritability, insomnia, a 'flu-like syndrome, skin rashes, and granulocytopenia. A high incidence of gastro-intestinal discomfort, most pronounced in the first three months of therapy, has been described with continuous administration of levamisole. It is possible that there is a potential for immune enhancement

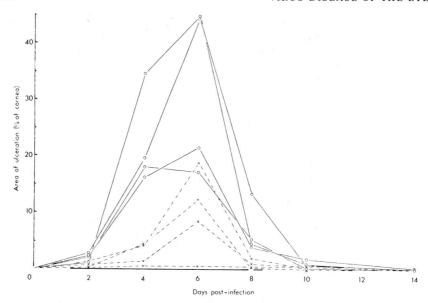

Figure 8.7. The influence of systemic levamisole on herpes virus proliferation and resolution compared with a group of controls. Both groups of animals were immune. o——o controls; x— · —x levamisole-treated.

using topical therapy. Large systemic doses of vitamin A have been reported to improve ulcerative herpetic keratitis in rabbits, though it is possible that this may have been due to the known influence of vitamin A on epithelial healing (Starr *et al.*, 1981). Nevertheless there may be a place for topical therapy.

Many therapies are available for the treatment of ulcerative herpetic keratitis (Table 8.4). The most reliable therapeutic measure is the use of the synthetic antivirals, the discovery of idoxuridine being one of the major advances in the treatment of herpes simplex virus infection. There is a continuing search for new topical and systemic antivirals. Thus Cheng (1981) has outlined the potential herpes-virus thymidine-kinase-dependent agents, which include, in addition to the presently available ACG, compounds such as 5-substituted 2′-deoxyuridine derivations, for example 5-ethyl deoxyuridine, 5-propyl deoxyuridine, 5-mercaptomethyl deoxyuridine, and E-5- (2-bromo vinyl) deoxyuridine. Other possible compounds include thymine arabinoside and 2-fluoro-5-iodo cytosine arabinoside. Other new compounds do not require the participation of virus-induced thymidine kinase; for example, phosphono-acetate and phosphonoformate, and glucose analogues such as 2-deoxyglucose. At the same time advances in delivery systems may be expected such as the use of liposomes containing IDU or other antiviral in the conjunctival sac (Smolin *et al.*, 1981).

TABLE 8.4

TREATMENT MODALITIES IN ULCERATIVE HERPETIC KERATITIS

	Advantages	Comments
Debridement	Associated with rapid resolution	Requires high level of expertise. May be associated with early recurrence
Chemical cautery debridement	Live virus is killed	Contra-indicated. May result in permanent corneal damage
Antivirals Idoxuridine (½%) drops or ointment	Highly effective therapy	May produce toxicity if used for long periods
Adenine arabinoside ointment	Highly effective therapy	Less toxic than IDU or F_3T
Trifluorothymidine drops	Highly effective antiviral Good intra-ocular penetration	May produce toxicity if used for long periods
Acycloguanosine ointment	Highly effective therapy Low toxicity level Good intra-ocular penetration	Because of low toxicity, may be used for long periods as cover for topical corticosteroid
Debridement (minimal wiping)+antiviral	Results in rapid healing	Requires expertise to debride affected epithelial cells
Cryothermy		May be associated with stromal penetration of viral antigen
Gamma globulin	Low toxicity	Not effective in established disease. Ineffective in control of steroid-enhanced ulceration
Cryothermy and immune serum	Theoretical possibility of useful therapy	Risk of stromal disease intensified
Gamma-venin (Fab fragment of IgG)	Reported to be successful in human trials	Little evidence of success in established disease in laboratory animals
Interferon	Highly successful as a prophylactic agent	Of little benefit in established disease according to evidence of clinical trials

COSTICOSTEROIDS IN HERPES SIMPLEX KERATITIS

Immunosuppressive and Anti-inflammatory Effects of Glucocorticosteroids

Despite the fact the glucocorticosteroids have been used extensively for many years as therapeutic agents in the treatment of inflammatory and immunologically mediated disease states in man, it is striking how little is known regarding the precise mechanisms of action of these agents on the various parameters of inflammatory and immunological reactivity (Fauci, 1979). Over the past years substantial advances have been made in the delineation and clarification of therapeutic mechanisms in the inflammatory and immune response in normal humans and in disease states. Difficulties have arisen in the extrapolation of the results taken from *in vitro* to the human situation, because the concentrations of corticosteroid generally employed to suppress various cell functions in these studies are usually suprapharmacologic and generally not attainable *in vivo* for any appreciable period of time. However, this may not necessarily hold for the tissues of the eye because high concentrations can be achieved following the topical introduction of corticosteroid. Several extensive reviews have emphasised that virtually every stage of the inflammatory and immunological response is subject to a greater or lesser degree of inhibition following corticosteroid application (Fauci *et al.*, 1976; David *et al.*, 1970; Gabrielsen and Good, 1967; Zurier and Weissman, 1973). There are certain aspects of the inflammatory and immune response which are differentially sensitive to corticosteroid administration, and others which are quite resistant. The most readily achieved effects are associated with leucocytes; the movement, traffic or distribution of cells is quite sensitive to their influence, while the actual functional capabilities of these cells are relatively resistant. Systemic medication results in transient lymphocytopenia and monocytopenia which are the result of redistribution out of the circulation into other body compartments. The T-lymphocyte is differentially more sensitive to this phenomenon than the B-lymphocyte. A similar redistribution occurs with eosinophils, but in contrast there is a mobilisation of neutrophils from the bone marrow reserve, an increase of circulating neutrophil half-life, and an inhibition of accumulation of cells at inflammatory sites. The mechanism of this inhibition of neutrophil accumulation is probably by an inhibition of cell adherence to endothelial surfaces, mediated most likely by a direct effect on the surface membrane configuration of the neutrophil. The redistribution phenomena associated with lymphocytes and monocytes appears to be mediated by alteration in the surface of the cells. High concentrations of corticosteroid suppress most functions of leucocytes including metabolic processes, membrane changes, synthesis of new inhibitory protein, and interference with binding of numerous factors such as antibody or complement at specific receptors on the cell surface. There is interruption of the cell-to-cell co-operation which gives rise to maximum activation, differentiation and effector function of individual populations of cells. Appreciation of the differential sensitivity and resistance of various cell types and functions to corticosteroids should allow their use in such a way that essential protective immune mechanisms are not compromised but at the same time enable the corticosteroid to inhibit those mechanisms which cause tissue damage. The cornea and the external eye should be well suited to the preferential inhibition of such tissue-damaging processes.

The corticosteroids are of considerable use in ophthalmology in the treatment of corneal inflammatory disease and uveitis. These agents interfere with the inflammation which can lead to permanent corneal scarring, but at the same time it must be remembered that their use must often influence the host in its defence against infection.

The adrenal cortex secretes three groups of adrenocortical hormones, glucocorticoids (cortisone and hydrocortisone); mineralocorticoids (deoxycortisone and aldosterone); and androgens and sex hormones. Several synthetic corticosteroids have replaced the endogenous glucocorticosteroids in clinical practice. Hydrocortisone has often been used as a reference standard of anti-inflammatory activity against which other agents are compared. Prednisolone has four times the activity of hydrocortisone when equal weights are compared, while dexamethasone and betamethasone have more than 25 times the activity of hydrocortisone (Figure 8.8). Corticosteroids are used to control corneal inflammation, and inflammatory responses in the anterior chamber. The precise mechanisms of corticosteroid action *in vivo* are probably complex even though such agents might have apparently simple effects at a cellular level. In the case of corticosteroids it is probable that there are a number of types of primary action; for instance, they kill small lymphocytes in interphase (Caron, 1967; Claman, 1972); inhibit T-cell killing of target cells *in vitro* (Cohen *et al.*, 1970); inhibit the synthesis of complement (Atkinson and Frank, 1973), lymphokines (Williams and Granger, 1969; Peter, 1971) and interferon (Mendelson and Glasgow, 1966); interfere with the migration of lymphocytes,

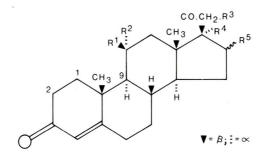

	R^1	R^2	R^3	R^4	R^5	OTHER MODIFICATIONS
BETAMETHASONE sod. phos.	HO–	H–	$-O.PO_3Na_2$	–OH	$\beta-CH_3$	$9\alpha-F$ 1=2
CLOBETASONE butyrate	O=		$-C_1$	$-O.CO.C_3H_7$	$\beta-CH_3$	$9\alpha-F$ 1=2
DEXAMETHASONE	HO–	H–	–OH	–OH	$\alpha-CH_3$	$9\alpha-F$ 1=2
FLUOROMETHOLONE	HO–	H–	–H	–OH	–H	$9\alpha-F$ 1=2
HYDROCORTISONE acetate	HO–	H–	$-O.CO.CH_3$	–OH	–H	–H
PREDNISOLONE sod. phos.	HO–	H–	$-O.PO_3Na_2$	–OH	–H	–H 1=2

Figure 8.8. The chemical formulae of the synthetic topical corticosteroids used in ophthalmology. (Courtesy, Mrs. Janet Williams.)

macrophages and polymorphs (Thompson and van Furth, 1970; Spry, 1972; de Sousa and Fachet, 1972), and impair the ability of macrophages to retain antigen on their surface. Somewhat surprisingly, there is limited evidence that on occasions immunosuppressive agents may enhance immunity by disrupting homeostatic mechanisms. For instance, antigen-antibody complexes may block the action of T-cells on target cells, and there may exist suppressor lymphocytes that inhibit the activities of either T- or B-cells. Accordingly, a selective inhibition of B-cells might, by reducing the formation of these complexes, lead to increased cytotoxic activity of T-cells, and conversely, a selective inhibition of suppressor T-cells might result in increased antibody formation by B-cells. Mechanisms such as this have been invoked to explain how highly effective immunosuppressive agents may lead to the enhancement, not suppression, of the immune response (Berenbaum, 1974).

The choice of an appropriate corticosteroid preparation must take into account the penetration of the drug into the stroma or the anterior chamber, depending on the main site of the disease. The epithelium favours the passage of lipophilic, fat-soluble, or non-polar molecules, while the stroma favours hydrophilic or water-soluble molecules. A drug, in order to have good penetrating properties, should be biphasic, but there is good experimental and clinical evidence that purely water-soluble drugs do penetrate the intact cornea. Penetration is enhanced in the inflamed eye and where the epithelium is disrupted. Preparations are available such as phosphates, alcohols and acetates, the latter being biphasic and in suspension and which must be dissolved in tears before corneal penetration may begin (Table 8.5).

The Use of Corticosteroids in Herpetic Keratitis

The early use of effective antiviral therapy in ulcerative disease can do much to prevent the onset of stromal complications in herpetic keratitis. The use of the corticosteroids in the treatment of epithelial disease is contra-indicated, and their value in the treatment of stromal disease remains somewhat controversial. Although many topical steroids are now available for the treatment of inflammatory disease of the external eye and the anterior segment, each of which has benefits over its predecessors, the complications which occur continue to provide concern for the clinician. In no part of external eye disease is this more apparent than in the treatment of stromal herpes simplex keratitis.

The effect of topical corticosteroid on the susceptibility of immune animals to re-inoculation with the HSV has been investigated by Easterbrook et al. (1973). It was demonstrated that the rate of virus isolation from previously infected rabbit corneas did not increase during simultaneous medication with corticosteroid. Following re-inoculation of virus in animals with previous experience of the corneal disease, ulcers were induced more frequently in those animals undergoing treatment with steroid than in those treated without steroid. The use of an antiviral protected the cornea against an increase in incidence of corneal disease as compared with a control group.

Using the more precise multiple inoculation model of Jones and Al Hussaini (1963) the present authors have shown a similar trend using clobetasone butyrate drops (Carter et al., 1981a). In animals which had been subjected to

TABLE 8.5

AVAILABLE CORTICOSTEROID EYE DROPS

Proprietary Name	Constituents	Concentration	Preservative
Predsol	prednisolone sodium phosphate	0·5%	benzalkonium
Predsol N	prednisolone sodium phosphate neomycin sulphate	0·5% 0·5%	thiomersal
Betnesol	betamethasone sodium phosphate	0·1%	benzalkonium
Betnesol N	betamethasone sodium phosphate neomycin sulphate	0·1% 0·5%	thiomersal
Eumovate	clobetasone butyrate	0·1%	benzalkonium
Eumovate N	clobetasone butyrate neomycin sulphate	0·1% 0·5%	benzalkonium
Maxidex	dexamethasone	0·1%	benzalkonium
Maxitrol	dexamethasone polymyxin B sulphate neomycin sulphate	0·1% 6,000 iu/ml 3·5 mg/ml	benzalkonium
FML	fluorometholone	0·1%	benzalkonium
Framycort	hydrocortisone acetate framycetin sulphate	0·5% 0·5%	
Hydrocortistab	hydrocortisone acetate	1·0%	
Sofradex	dexamethasone framycetin gramicidin	0·05% 0·5% 0·005%	

cutaneous infections six weeks previously, a dilution of 0·1 per cent induced a considerable increase of virus proliferation, which became apparent on the fourth day after the secondary infection was induced, and had considerably worsened by the seventh day (Figure 8.9). In contrast, treatment of a group of animals with primary disease did not appear to enhance the rate of virus replication. The use of 0·01 per cent and 0·001 per cent drops in immune animals did not enhance the spread of the virus in epithelium to the same extent (Figure 8.10), which supports the impression that dilute topical steroid is less likely than full-strength preparations to be associated with the formation of amoeboid type ulcers. Dilute preparations of corticosteroid, according to clinical experience, appear to be able to control and reduce cellular infiltration in the stroma. The necessity of using concomitant antiviral therapy is no longer imperative. The influence of topical corticosteroid enhancement of virus replication is not apparent until the fourth day of observation, when there is

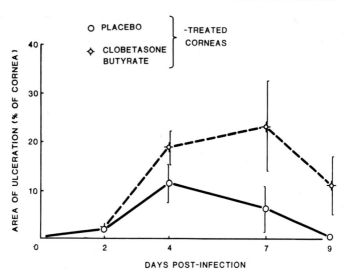

Figure 8.9. The influence of topical corticosteroid compared with placebo on virus proliferation in immune animals. Such enhancement was not apparent in non-immune animals. (Courtesy of the Editor, *British Journal of Ophthalmology*.)

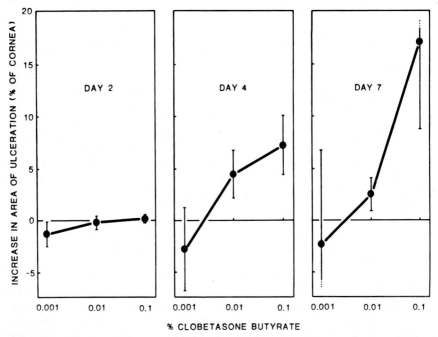

Figure 8.10. The influence of log dilutions of topical clobetasone drops on the area of corneal ulceration due to herpes simplex virus on days 2, 4 and 7. (Courtesy of the Editor, *British Journal of Ophthalmology*.)

good evidence that cellular immune mechanisms are starting to act. The delayed enhancement of virus replication in previously infected, steroid-treated animals is possibly due to the influence of the steroid on cell-mediated immune reactions rather than on humoral reactions. The influence of predni-solone drops on external eye disease, virus proliferation and latent infection has been investigated by Easty *et al.* (1983) in mice. Groups of immune mice were inoculated in the cornea with 5×10^6 pfu HSV 1 and were then treated with placebo or steroid drops. The severity of the eye disease was somewhat surprisingly more severe in the placebo-treated eyes than in those treated with steroid. However, virus isolation in the daily eye washings persisted for longer in steroid-treated eyes, and there was evidence of increased latent infection together with a greater chance of spread of such infection to non-ophthalmic parts of the trigeminal ganglion.

Laboratory studies by Cooper *et al.* (1978), who investigated the effect of prednisolone on antibody-dependent cell-mediated cytotoxicity on the growth of type 1 herpes simplex virus in human cells, supports the importance of steroid influence on immune response. In 1974 Costa and his colleagues reported that steroids could enhance the growth of herpes simplex virus in murine cells. This raised the possibility that the exacerbation of dendritic keratitis by steroids could be due to the drugs enhancing the replications of virus in the cornea. Cooper *et al.* (1978) tested this hypothesis by determining the effect of prednisolone on the growth of type 1 HSV in selected human cells, and the ability of human lymphocytes to mediate antibody-dependent cell-mediated cytotoxicity against HSV-infected fibroblasts. The experiments showed that prior treatment of human skin or corneal fibroblasts had no effect on the amount of infectious virus produced by the cells. The corticosteroid was found merely to inhibit HSV growth in PHA-stimulated lymphocytes, but this suppression occurred only if the drug was exposed to the lymphocytes within 24 hours of mitogen addition. Incubating lymphocytes with PHA for three days and then adding steroid affected neither virus growth nor the amount of uptake of 3H-thymidine following pulsing prior to the harvest. Since lymphocytes must be undergoing division to replicate HSV, and corticosteroids inhibit cell proliferation, the fact that prednisolone inhibited PHA stimulation probably explained the decreased replication of HSV in the steroid-treated lymphocytes. Steroid was found to inhibit human lymphocytes from mediating antibody-dependent, cell-mediated cytotoxicity against infected human fibroblasts. The amount of inhibition was dependent on the concentration of drug incubated with the lymphocytes. The data therefore supports a contention that the exacerbations observed when patients with dendritic keratitis are treated inadvertently with prednisolone may be due to the steroid suppressing antibody-dependent, cell-mediated cytotoxicity, and not by the promotion of virus growth in corneal epithelial cells.

An interesting model for steroid effects in herpes keratitis was described by Robbins and Galin (1975), where dextran-blue 2000 was used as a marker to determined the effect of steroids on large-molecule transfer through the cornea. In superficially scarified corneas, topically applied steroids greatly enhanced the transfer of this chromophore through the cornea in the *in vivo* state, but had little effect *in vitro*. It was concluded that the steroid effect was an active process. Since herpes simplex virus is approximately the same molecular weight and configuration as the chromophore used, the study explained one aspect of how steroids may be detrimental when used in the presence of the virus. The transfer of such large molecules was explained by the effect of steroids on the formation of mucopolysaccharides and collagen. A steroid-induced alteration of mucopolysaccharide integrity could weaken the electrostatic interaction between collagen and the surrounding mucopolysaccharides, which would compromise the relatively rigid lattice of fibrils and thus allow foreign particles easier passage through the fibrillar interstices.

Further evidence that topical steroid will not reactivate experimental herpetic ketatitis is provided by Kibrick *et al.* (1971). Bilateral herpetic keratitis was induced in rabbits and allowed to heal without treatment. After a period of between 150 and 450 days the clinically quiescent eyes were treated with topical corticosteroid. This treatment, when administered either as drops, ointment, or subconjunctivally, failed to induce a higher incidence of virus reactivation as determined by culture, than occurred in placebo-treated eyes. The data showed that topical steroid neither reactivated occult virus nor induced herpetic corneal disease. It would thus appear that it is only in the presence of active virus disease of the epithelium, that enhanced proliferation would be induced and it seems unlikely that the use of topical steroid itself acts as a trigger in the reactivation of latent disease.

The manner in which the use of topical steroid may influence the spread of virus in the epithelium and stroma is summarised in Table 8.6. It remains unclear how the virus is combated by immune processes in the cornea and what the relative importance of humoral and cell-mediated protective immune responses are. Nevertheless, there is good evidence that steroid medication can effect both arms of the immune response. The effect of local corticosteroid was examined on antibody-forming cells in the eye and draining lymph nodes by Meyer *et al.* (1975). The early reaction of the local lymph nodes and ocular tissues to the intracorneal injection of bovine gamma globulin is essentially a local response (Smolin and Hall, 1973).

TABLE 8.6

INFLUENCES ON THE EFFICACY OF CORTICOSTEROID
THERAPY IN STROMAL KERATITIS

The presence of productive virus
the presence of viral antigen
the introduction of further virus via the sensory nerve axon
the presence of immune complexes (precipitated or soluble)
    and their concentration
the nature of the inflammatory response (PMN, macrophage)
the nature of the adaptive immune responses
        humoral
        cellular
the level of involvement of the endothelium
        by inflammatory responses in the anterior seg-
        ment
        by viral antigen or productive virus.

Following the injection of bovine gamma globulin into corneal stroma, antibody-forming cell formation was not suppressed in the local ocular tissue or lymphatic nodes, but the severity of inflammatory responses in the cornea was reduced as would have been expected. Thus it is apparent that the local production of immunocompetent antibody-forming cells is not blocked by the use of topical steroid, and it therefore follows that antibody may be produced in the local tissues in spite of the use of topical steroid; it is possible that topical steroid medication would block the efferent arc of the immune response rather than the afferent arc.

Corticosteroids are known to have specific effects on lymphoid tissues and are used widely in many ocular diseases in which immunological processes play a role. Although the exact ways in which the corticosteroids achieve their anti-inflammatory activity is not understood, it is possible that they act by exerting a local anti-inflammatory effect (Zurier and Weissman, 1973), a stabilisation of the lysosomal membrane, destruction of lymphocytes, inhibition of cellular metabolism (Claman, 1972), and redistribution of lymphocytes (Claman, 1972).

Corticosteroid Management in Active Stromal Keratitis

The management of stromal keratitis with corticosteroid medication remains a dilemma for the clinician, due to the largely undetermined effects that it may have on the proliferation of virus in the keratocytes (Table 8.7). It is well known that virus or its central core may be found in the cytoplasm of keratocytes and that viral antigenic determinants may be located on the surface of these cells.

TABLE 8.7

INDICATION FOR TOPICAL CORTICOSTEROID THERAPY
IN HERPES SIMPLEX KERATITIS—STROMAL IN TYPE

Persistent stromal keratitis with threat of central corneal scarring
Early corneal vascularisation
Associated uveitis
Elevation of intra-ocular pressure
Failure of stromal disease to clear after substantial period of
    conservative treatment without topical corticosteroid.

The effects of topical steroid therapy in ulcerative disease are well known. Typically an extensive ulcer forms which may spread to take the form of a geographic or amoeboid shape. During a period of such enhanced proliferation it is predictable that a greater amount of virus will penetrate into the stroma and create a potentially dangerous situation for the future, which may not necessarily be evident during the attack of epithelial disease itself. It is often noted that major problems in the management of stromal disease occur in patients who have been aggressively treated with topical steroid during ulcerative disease at an early stage in their disease. At the same time it is increasingly evident that the severe stromal disease is now becoming less common, and it is possible that this is because of an awareness of the adverse effects of corticosteroid by practitioners.

Indications for Treatment with Topical Corticosteroid

The main indication for the use of topical corticosteroid is the development of a stromal opacity which is a threat to the vision of the patient (Table 8.7). Stromal disease can be prolonged and cause serious morbidity and psychological depression in the patient, and this also often plays a role in the decision to employ the use of corticosteroids. In kerato-uveitis or herpetic iridocyclitis, the use of topical corticosteroid becomes mandatory if there is a threat to vision or the normal physiological mechanism in the function of the eye.

Contra-indications to the Use of Topical Corticosteroid

The contra-indications to the use of corticosteroid in the treatment of stromal disease are mainly determined by the presence of active epithelial disease (Table 8.8). Where the epithelium is disrupted, either due to the use of antiviral medication, the persistence of the dendritic ulcer, or the presence of a trophic ulcer the risk of a recurrence of epithelial disease is increased. It has been our experience that complications can occur when the integrity of the epithelium is disrupted, and it is in these patients that it has proved difficult to establish control of the stromal disease because of the fear of inducing epithelial recurrence. In such patients it is advisable for the patient to be admitted to hospital so that careful monitoring will exclude the chance of these complications.

TABLE 8.8

CONTRA-INDICATIONS TO TOPICAL CORTICOSTEROID
IN HERPES SIMPLEX KERATITIS—STROMAL IN TYPE

Stromal disease in the presence of epithelial disease
   e.g. dendritic ulcer, persistent corneal erosion
Superficial stromal keratitis where keratitis is not a threat to vision
Stromal disease in infants and children
Invasion of cornea by other pathogens simultaneously.

Dosage of Corticosteroid in Stromal Herpes Keratitis

The working rule in the treatment of stromal disease is that the dosage should be that which will achieve an appropriate therapeutic effect (Table 8.9). There are a number of influences on the way in which stromal disease responds to corticosteroid, but there is little question that many types of keratitis are dose responsive, although this is not the case for all disease manifestations. Some of the factors which influence the response include the concentration, anti-inflammatory activity, and penetration. The response varies according to the type of stromal disease, and with the compliance of the patient (Table 8.10).

TABLE 8.9

PRECAUTIONS IN CORTICOSTEROID THERAPY IN STROMAL
KERATITIS

Perform regular conjunctival and lid margin cultures
Avoid if epithelial deficit present, but admit for observation
  if no alternative
Use lowest quantity which will achieve therapeutic effect
Regularly measure the intra-ocular pressure
Reduce by tapering down and avoid sudden curtailment.

TABLE 8.10

CATEGORIES OF HERPES SIMPLEX STROMAL KERATITIS AND POSSIBLE MODES OF TREATMENT

Type of disease	Clinical appearance	Diagnosis and treatment	Prognosis
Trophic ulcer	Usually central with grey, elevated border	Negative viral and bacterial culture (a) stop antivirals (b) strap lids closed (c) gel contact lens (d) conjunctival transplants (Thoft)	Trophic corneal ulcers may be persistent. Require careful follow-up and attention. Probably will cause permanent surface faceting
Stromal ghost of dendrite	Shadow of previous dendrite	No treatment; if on visual axis then employ dilute topical steroid	Gradual disappearance of scar
Disciform keratitis	Diffuse, usually central stromal haze and oedema	Usually preceded by a positive history of cold sores and/or a dendrite. Treat with the lowest steroid dilution which achieves a clinical improvement; antiviral necessary if full strength used	Classical disciform keratitis usually resolves on treatment
Wessely ring	Typical. May accompany a dendrite	Antivirals plus minimal-dose topical steroid	May be associated with the later onset of severe stromal disease
Central keratitis with vascularisation and focal infiltrates	The appearance is typical. Infiltrates yellowish and random. Excite leashes of ingrowing blood vessels	Requires full bacterial and mycotic investigation if surface of infiltrate ulcerated. Treat with antiviral, low-dose topical steroid and antibiotic	Infiltrates and vascularisation may be associated with permanent scarring, and eventual lipid deposition

TABLE 8.10 (cont.)

Limbal keratitis	Limbus-associated herpes; involves stroma, but there may be persistent overlying ulcer	Culture for herpes simplex virus. Antivirals and topical steroid	Prone to develop infiltration and vascularisation
Stromal disease with active dendrite	Dendrite may be missed without care	Culture for herpes simplex virus. Control epithelial disease with antivirals prior to the possible use of topical steroid	Extreme care is required that antiviral cover is used during steroid therapy as it is possible to induce geographical ulceration.
Kerato-uveitis (occasionally with hypopyon and secondary glaucoma)	Diffuse or limbal keratitis; large keratic precipitates which may be missed	Objective: to suppress the inflammatory reaction in the anterior chamber. Probably requires full-strength steroids plus antiviral with good penetration Check IOP regularly	May lead to prolonged morbidity. Prognosis poor
Hypopyon ulcer or abscess	Herpetic aetiology not always clear. Careful history important	Culture for HSV and bacteria. Admission. Antivirals plus antibiotics. Careful use of topical steroid when negative cultures and clinical evidence of no further deterioration	Prognosis poor
Descemetocele or perforation	Severe central stromal thinning. Shallow anterior chamber with +ve Seidel test	Culture for all organisms Admission. Antivirals and antibiotics. If perforation, bandage CL; Histoacrylate glue; conjunctival flap; emergency keratoplasty	Visual prognosis poor Keratoplasty in active herpetic keratitis carries increased risk of homograft reaction
Inactive corneal scarring reducing vision to 6/60 or less	Ensure that there is no active disease as shown by blood-vessel activity, and absence of stromal oedema and infiltrate	Planned penetrating keratoplasty. Post-op, where topical steroid is used, antiviral is necessary	Prolonged aftercare as outpatient, with frequent observations

Many cases of stromal herpes still resolve without the use of anti-inflammatory therapy, but in a number of patients it is mandatory to reduce inflammation and vascularisation, with the object of obtaining a clear cornea with a minimum amount of permanent scarring. The policy must be, therefore, to employ the minimal dosage of topical steroid that will produce a therapeutic effect. Clinical experience has shown that the use of dilute preparations reduces the incidence of complications, and at the same time achieves the therapeutic objective. Serial dilutions of prednisolone drops (0·5 per cent) can be made, and concentrations of 0·25, 0·125, 0·025 and 0·0025 per cent may all have value under differing conditions. With this in mind, the dosage of steroid is gradually increased until a therapeutic effect is obtained following which, once inflammation has been suppressed, the therapy is tailed off over a period of four or more weeks to prevent further exacerbation. Patients should be seen at regular intervals and careful records kept of the inflammatory disease; if possible the patient should be seen by the same observer on each occasion.

Once steroid medication has been introduced, taking the patient off such therapy may become a significant problem. The more serious cases of herpetic keratitis with stromal involvement may become worse on sudden curtailment, with a rebound of inflammation. In the patient in whom therapy has been maintained for months or even years with a potent steroid it may prove virtually impossible to curtail therapy and it is questionable whether it should be attempted. However, although the dilemma encountered in making appropriate decisions in these cases is now becoming rare, they can still be a trap for the unwary.

The use of steroids in the management of stromal herpes keratitis demands a measure of expertise which is not always understood. Similar to the use of systemic steroids in management of many inflammatory diseases, their use increases with experience, and topical steroid should only be introduced under the guidance of a specialist in external ocular disease.

Where no response is obtained with the use of dilute preparations, and it is necessary to increase the concentration of the drops, or introduce them more frequently, it becomes necessary to cover their use with an antiviral. Indeed one of the most important uses of antiviral therapeutic agents is in their preventative role against recurrence when corticosteroid is necessary. In such cases, toxicity is seldom seen, and according to clinical experience it is possible to continue such medication for long periods without the appearance of the typical signs. Difficulties may be encountered where the steroid is tapered off or curtailed, when the toxicity syndrome becomes apparent after a long delay. From this it would appear that the manifestations of toxicity are suppressed by the steroid. The toxic effects which eventually become manifest may occasionally present a greater hazard than the original disease process.

In ophthalmology there is a continuing requirement for a non-steroid anti-inflammatory preparation which does not carry the unwanted side-effects of the corticosteroids. It is important that new therapeutic agents should be tested in the laboratory to identify a concentration which does not result in the enhancement of virus proliferation. Such studies are best carried out in laboratory immune animals with secondary herpes simplex keratitis. Other drugs such as flurbiprofen (Trowsdale *et al.*, 1980) have been investigated but no advantages over topical corticosteroid have yet been realised.

Treatment Problems in Herpes Simplex Keratitis

Certain clinical manifestations of herpes simplex keratitis can present especially difficult problems for the inexperienced. Bilateral disease is comparatively rare as herpetic eye disease is characteristically unilateral. The incidence is generally thought to be between 1 and 3 per cent. There is a tendency for the patients to be younger and to be atopic. The latter group are particularly liable to develop bilateral primary blepharoconjunctivitis. The use of topical steroid in atopic subjects is tempting, as many of them have allergic eye disease. However, this is beset with potential risk once latency has become established. It is therefore important that caution is observed in the management of bilateral disease, particularly when associated with allergic eye disease, when corticosteroid must be avoided.

Where stromal disease is associated with epithelial disease, either as a dendritic ulcer or as a persistent erosion, the use of topical corticosteroid must be avoided. It is vital that the epithelium is allowed to regenerate, reducing the chances of the recurrence of a particularly severe type.

The management of a geographic ulcer in itself can present problems. Geographic ulcers may occur in patients who have been treated in error by an untrained practitioner, or following keratoplasty, where no antiviral cover has been used. It is often necessary to admit patients with severe disease of this type so that steroid can be either reduced or stopped, and intensive antiviral therapy introduced. Caution must be observed in the postoperative graft, as over-zealous reduction of topical steroid can result in a serious rebound of inflammation, and to lasting damage of the donor tissue.

The treatment of herpetic uveitis can also present complex problems. Uveitis of this nature can present in isolation, occasionally in children who had had a severe attack of primary disease. It may not be associated with a previous history of epithelial or stromal disease. It is particularly resistant to topical corticosteroid therapy, and may often require rather prolonged instillations. The use of a topical antiviral of good penetration and low toxicity should be employed where it is clearly known that the uveitis is due to herpes simplex virus. On occasions uveitis may occur in one eye and stromal disease in the other. It is in these patients that careful use of topical steroid with frequent follow-up is needed.

The Surgery of Herpetic Keratitis

The indications for surgical intervention in herpetic keratitis result from failure in medical treatment. The use of tarsorrhaphies or conjunctival flaps is now less frequent, and with improving results following keratoplasty, the latter procedure is carried out in the majority of patients requiring emergency or cold surgery. Thus stromal abscesses which fail to respond to medical therapy can be treated with penetrating keratoplasty, although when the eye is highly inflamed there seems little doubt that there is an increased risk of an early graft rejection episode. Where surgical procedures are carried out in the presence of inactive stromal disease the results are more encouraging.

Lamellar grafts are associated with a high incidence of recurrence (65 per cent: Rice and Jones, 1973). Herpes virus particles in the host stroma deep to lamellar grafts can be demonstrated by electron-microscopy. It has been considered that an improved success rate can be obtained using a penetrating keratoplasty, where the rate is said to reach 78 per cent. Rice and Jones (1973) reported that the success rates in active and inactive disease are approximately the same. Thirty-five per cent of those receiving lamellar grafts developed recurrences of epithelial keratitis, in contrast to which 9 per cent of eyes receiving penetrating grafts developed recurrent ulcerative disease. Pollack and Kaufman (1972) experienced a considerable difference in success rates following keratoplasty in active and inactive disease. Of their twenty clinically active cases, 45 per cent achieved clear grafts, while in inactive disease clear grafts were obtained in all the patients.

Although the use of a graft as a therapeutic measure in active disease can be valuable, it has been the experience of many surgeons that the incidence of rejection episodes in this group is high. Nevertheless, where a corneal perforation is threatened, reversal of this situation has a beneficial influence on patient morale and reduces a prolonged period of morbidity. Patients may be able to return to full activity with the possibility of a further penetrating keratoplasty in the future.

Witmer (1981) has referred to the poor results of lamellar keratoplasty in herpetic keratitis. He reported a recurrence of ulcerative disease in 53 per cent of patients with penetrating keratoplasties, which was considerably reduced by the concomitant use of trifluorothymidine therapy. Foster (1981) has recently reported a series of keratoplasties performed in several categories of disease. Transplantation for herpes simplex keratitis in eyes that were not heavily vascularised, or not inflamed or ulcerated, was highly successful. Chronic or recurrent 'immune' disciform oedema in the stroma gave satisfactory results. Where keratoplasties were performed for the establishment of the integrity of the globe the results were less satisfactory, and were routinely associated with clouding of the tissue. Foster suggests that management of such perforations or impending perforations with lamellar patch grafts or with cyanoacrylate tissue adhesive, with later penetrating keratoplasty for visual rehabilitation, is highly successful. Where there is associated disease such as the sicca syndrome, atopy or ocular rosacea, poor results were reported.

The difficulties which can be encountered with severe atopic disease as a background in herpetic keratitis have been emphasised by Easty et al. (1975). Figure 8.11 demonstrates severe graft failure occurring in a patient with adult eczema and gross elevation of serum IgE levels. Subjects with atopic disease of the tarsal plates present a bad risk, and are prone to prolonged epithelial erosions, and to epithelial recurrences of ulcerative herpetic disease. It is considered that penetrating keratoplasties should be avoided in highly atopic subjects because of the extremely poor results which can be anticipated. However, where closely matched tissue using HL-A tissue types have been used, together with systemic immunosuppressives, considerable success has been achieved in a small group of subjects (Figure 8.12). The complications encountered in penetrating keratoplasty are tabulated (Table 8.11).

The prognosis and management of corneal transplantation for herpetic

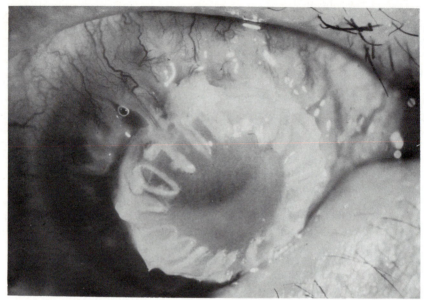

Figure 8.11. Acute graft failure in a highly atopic individual with herpetic keratitis and threatened perforation. Due to the failure of a preliminary graft, virgin silk sutures were used on the second occasion in an attempt to provoke rapid healing of the interface.

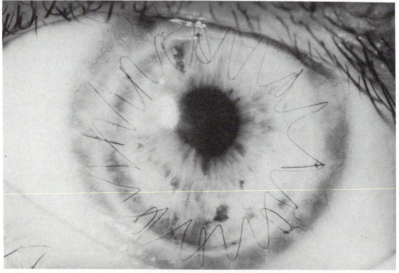

Figure 8.12. The opposite eye of the patient shown in Figure 8.11; systemic immunosuppressive therapy resulted in a transparent graft.

TABLE 8.11

COMPLICATIONS IN KERATOPLASTY FOR HERPES SIMPLEX KERATITIS

Complication	Identification	Treatment
EARLY		
Sutures eroding through	Slit-lamp examination	Shortening. Gel contact lens
Immediate endothelial decompensation	Failure of graft to dehydrate	Later regraft
Immediate postoperative inflammation	Slit-lamp examination Maximal on day 5	Intensive topical corticosteroid to re-establish endothelial privilege
Epithelial toxicity	Slit-lamp microscopy Prolonged use of antivirals pre- or post-operation	Cut dosage of antiviral. Change to less toxic antiviral
Persistent central erosion	Staining with rose bengal	Avoid prolonged antiviral therapy. Use of gel continuous wear CL
INTERMEDIATE OR LATE		
Recurrence of epithelial disease	Slit-lamp appearance is not always diagnostic; cultures are important	Antiviral therapy. Reduction or cessation of corticosteroid
Recurrence of stromal disease	Usually follows further dendrite	Corticosteroid with antiviral cover
Recurrence of uveitis	May be associated with endothelial decompensation. KP distributed on donor and recipient	Controlled use of corticosteroid plus antivirals
Homograft rejection	Classical appearance of endothelial line of lymphocytes, with loss of endothelial function	Topical corticosteroid with antiviral cover

keratitis have been discussed by Cobo *et al.* (1981). Postoperative management consisted of cycloplegics and high-dose topical corticosteroid without antiviral cover. Episodes of allograft rejection were treated with subconjunctival injection of dexamethasone or betamethasone and intensive topical dexamethasone therapy without antiviral cover. However, episodes of epithelial recurrence were treated with antiviral in the usual way. Out of a total of 132 keratoplasties, a survival rate of clear grafts was 64 per cent at two years. Allograft rejection accounted for 64 per cent of cloudy grafts. The survival rate by life-table analysis showed that 69 per cent of keratoplasties were clear at 2 years in uninflamed eyes, compared to 44 per cent in eyes which were actively inflamed at the time of surgery. The degree of vascularisation was closely related to the tendency to undergo rejection. Thirty-two per cent of eyes undergoing allograft rejection developed epithelial herpetic recurrences within 4 months, as opposed to a recurrence rate of 6 per cent at 4 months in eyes which were uncomplicated by allograft rejection. Neither group, however, received antiviral cover.

The mechanism of disease recurrence in either stroma or epithelium, in patients who have undergone lamellar keratoplasty *vis a vis* those who have undergone penetrating keratoplasty, is interesting. It can be speculated that a lamellar graft would provide a layer of corneal tissue which is separate from the recipient at the interface, where a wall of scar tissue forms. It seems unlikely that the donor tissue would be invaded by sensory neurons until at least a period of 12 months has passed. Recurrence of stromal disease is therefore likely to be due to presence of virus in the recipient which spreads into the donor tissue. Recurrence of epithelial disease would seem due to the spread of virus into the recipient cornea, where it is likely that the dendrite spreads on to the donor tissue. The stromal disease which follows is often directly related to the epithelial disease pattern in its own topography. In penetrating keratoplasty, where the barrier between the donor and recipient is complete and there is interruption of the sensory innervation, the risks of virus penetration into the new tissue is less. This may account for the accepted view that stromal disease rarely recurs following penetrating keratoplasty, although it is encountered following an episode of epithelial disease.

Where the cornea has active herpetic disease in the stroma together with uveitis and generalised inflammation of the anterior segment, it is wise to avoid continuous suturing with 10 monofilament nylon materials. Interrupted sutures avoid difficulties associated with eroding through of continuous sutures, and thereby avoids the risk of vascularisation and rejection episodes. It is important that the knots of interrupted sutures are buried during the surgery for the same reason.

Where the graft is performed for irreversible scarring following previous herpetic stromal disease with a persistent stromal opacity, continuous sutures may be used with a buried knot. Where suture erosions occur a contact lens is easily applied; this creates a more comfortable situation for the patient and at the same time seems to prevent the ingrowth of new vessels.

The use of topical corticosteroid in the management of keratoplasty can be critical in deciding the eventual outcome of the graft. The objective is to reduce the inflammatory responses that are non-specific, are induced by the corneal grafting procedure itself and are responsible for the loss of the privileged situation of the anterior chamber. Such responses would be greater where the eye is already suffering active inflammatory disease. These responses include the appearance of polymorphonuclear leucocytes at the limbus and possibly in the recipient cornea, the break-down of the blood-aqueous barrier, the production of prostaglandins from the ocular tissues together with other inflammatory mediators. It is the aim of the early use of corticosteroid to re-establish the privilege of the corneal endothelium in an attempt to inhibit or reduce the sensitisation of T-cell subsets. Thus, contact between this important cell layer and immunologically competent lymphocytes is required before an adaptive or specific immune response can be directed against these cells. Antibody formation may be necessary for this process of cell recognition. Lymphocyte co-operation or inhibition may take place, traffic of cells through the eye, and eventual proliferation are all steps which occur prior to the mounting of a homograft reaction. It is considered that the exposure of the endothelial layer during the immediate postoperative period is likely to be a time of sensitisation, although rejection episodes are generally delayed well after the operative procedure. The response to corticosteroid is measured by the reduction of limbal vascularisation, the vessels becoming narrowed and eventually closing, and the disappearance of circulating cells in the anterior chamber.

There is a risk of severe recurrence of epithelial disease during keratoplasties performed for HSK undergoing treatment with corticosteroid, a risk which can be reduced by the use of topical antiviral therapy. However, the consequence of this can be a considerable degree of toxicity to the donor corneal epithelium, and so the dosage should be cut accordingly. It is to be hoped that acyclovir will prove to be less toxic than the other antivirals and therefore be of value in the long term.

The many postoperative complications following keratoplasty (Table 8.11) are now well known and will not be elaborated upon. Where the chances of success are small in patients with severe pre-operative corneal vascularisation or active inflammation, there is an indication for the use of typed and matched tissue, using HL-A antigens. There is little doubt on a theoretical basis that close matching of donor with recipient must help to improve the prognosis, a fact which is clearly indicated when autologous tissue is used for the transplant, where the need for topical corticosteroid is considerably reduced. Other risk factors include the presence of circulating antibody to HL-A antigens which can occur following a blood transfusion, or a pregnancy. These antibodies can now be identified and there is some evidence that they should be assessed in serum prior to keratoplasty, and if found to be present, then the tissue antigens against which these antibodies are directed should be avoided.

It is because of the increased risk of a graft rejection episode following keratoplasty in HSK that constant vigilance must be maintained for this in the first months of postoperative care. It is essential that the patient be told of the possible modes of presentation so that action can be taken immediately and advice sought at the earliest opportunity. It is not always easy to determine whether anterior-segment inflammation results from a recurrence of inflammation due to reactivation of herpetic disease in the uvea or in the recipient stroma, or whether the reaction is a true homograft rejection reaction. Where there is a typical lymphocyte line originating at a leash of blood vessels the diagnosis presents little difficulty as this appearance is a classical one which is accepted as a homograft reaction (Figure 8.13). Where keratitic precipitates are found in both the donor and recipient, then it is possible that they are due to a recurrence of uveitis. Dependent upon the nature of the inflammatory stimulus is clearly the mode of treatment; thus, in rejection, aggressive use of topical steroid must be maintained for a period and then tapered down; in the case of recurrence of herpetic disease, the dosage of steroid is considerably less. It is considered that antiviral cover should be used in both these situations.

One of the major difficulties which arise in patients with herpetic keratitis following keratoplasty is with epithelial regeneration. Thus if a patient has been treated for a considerable time with antivirals prior to surgery, the recipient epithelium regenerates and spreads on to the donor tissue slowly, and at times a persistent erosion may develop at the centre of the new tissue. The use of antivirals following keratoplasty has therefore been thought to be

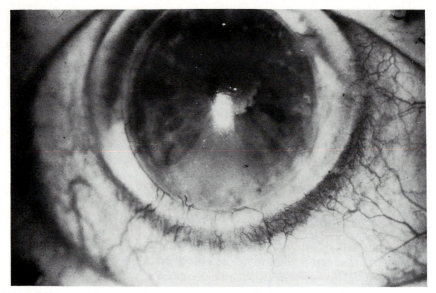

Figure 8.13. Early homograft reaction in a patient with herpes simplex keratitis. Oedema is apparent in the lower part of the tissue and a line of lymphocytes was visible on the endothelium with the slit lamp.

contra-indicated, but at the same time recurrence of epithelial disease is a significant cause of corneal graft failure in these patients. On occasions where a penetrating keratoplasty has failed, it has been possible to carry out successful grafts using immunosuppression for short-term intervals. Thus in patients with severe atopy and gross elevation of serum IgE, where the risks of epithelial and stromal recurrence and of a homograft reaction are high, the use of immunosuppressive dosages of corticosteroid and other immunosuppressive reagents for periods of 2-3 weeks following keratoplasty have, on occasions, been found to give successful results where the prognosis has been poor. The objective is to reduce the necessity for intensive topical corticosteroid. It is aimed at allowing the cornea to regain its privilege by reducing non-specific immunological reactions induced by surgery. These reactions include increased permeability of the blood vessels of the iris and ciliary body, the triggering of the complement cascade, the excitation and degranulation of mast cells in the anterior uvea, and the attraction of PMN into the corneal limbus, ciliary body, and iris. This therapy probably reduces the sensitisation of lymphocytes, lymphocyte proliferation and differentiation. Non-specific immune mechanisms would also be suppressed.

Summary

Corneal grafts for herpetic keratitis present a number of hazards for the unwary. It is preferable not to operate on patients with active inflammatory disease in view of the increased rate of complications involving sutures, and the homograft reaction. It is important to the clinician that he does not forget that the patient he is treating is herpetic, which is only too easy in patients who have been referred, or in whom previous grafts have been performed. The modifications which must be considered in the postoperative treatment include frequent observation, carefully controlled use of topical corticosteroid, and use of antiviral cover in controlled dosage in order to avoid epithelial disease recurrence. Culture of the conjunctival sac for virus and bacteria should be regularly performed because corticosteroid and antivirals have immunosuppressive properties. The dosage of corticosteroid should be tapered down to dilutions which may be used for long periods without so much risk of exacerbating disease recurrence in the epithelium. At the same time, tapering down prevents rebound of inflammation which can be associated with graft rejection and failure. Eroding continuous sutures, or prominent knots disturb epithelial regeneration; this may be helped by the use of bandage gel contact lenses for short periods.

OTHER SURGICAL TREATMENTS

Other aids in the management of the more severe complications of herpetic keratitis are available. Thus, bandage contact lenses (permanent corneal membrane; Sauflon, 85) which contain 79·4 per cent water may be effectively employed to help the resolution of chronic trophic corneal erosions. They can also be used in the postoperative phase of the corneal graft where suture ends are prominent, or where a continuous suture has eroded to form elevated loops, both of which invite the ingrowth of new vessels into the cornea. The tendency towards neovascularisation can be prevented with the use of a bandage contact lens at this stage. It is important to be aware that secondary invaders can contaminate such lenses, and it is therefore necessary to take regular cultures to exclude pathogenic bacteria in the conjunctival sac.

Where trophic ulcers defy treatment by strapping the lids closed with tape or the use of a bandage lens, Thoft (1982) has recommended the use of autotransplants of conjunctival tissue from the opposite eye, which are introduced into the bulbar conjunctiva of the affected eye close to the limbus. It is recommended that four transplants are made, and it has been reported that erosions may heal following the introduction of healthy conjunctival tissue, which then acts as a source of cells which eventually become transformed to corneal epithelial cells on reaching the limbus. Tarsorrhaphies and conjunctival flaps are now rarely performed.

Where an acute perforation has occurred in the absence of dense cellular infiltration, the use of histoacrylate glue can be helpful; this measure seals the rupture and reformation of the anterior chamber. An elective keratoplasty can be performed when the inflammatory response in the cornea and the anterior segment has died down.

The treatment of herpes simplex keratitis presents the ophthalmologist with many problems. It is often however those cases where the initial or early treatment has been ill-considered that the more severe manifestations of disease occur, and in future these complications will become less frequent. It is to be hoped that the development of non-steroidal anti-inflammatory agents in the next decade will not have the adverse influence on virus proliferation of present-day corticosteroid therapy, and that inflammatory disease of the corneal and anterior segment may be treated without the fear of causing more severe disease processes.

REFERENCES

ABEL, R., KAUFMAN, H. E. and SUGAR, J. (1975). Effect of intravenous adenine arabinoside on herpes simplex keratouveitis in humans. In: *Adenine Arabinoside: an Antiviral Agent*, p. 393. Eds. D. Pavan-Langston, R. A. Buchanan and G. A. Alford. New York: Raven Press.

ALLEN, J. C. and SZJNADER, E. (1976). Neutral red treatment of herpes simplex in rabbits. *Invest. Ophthal.*, **15**, 142–143.

AMOILS, S. P. and MAIER, G. (1973). Cryosurgery and immunotherapy in herpes keratitis. *Brit. J. Ophthal.*, **57**, 809–14.

ASHER, L. V. S., WALZ, M. A. and NOTKINS, A. L. (1978). Effect of immunisation on the development of latent ganglionic infection in mice challenged intravaginally with herpes simplex virus types 1 and 2. *Amer. J. Obstet. Gynecol.*, **131**, 788.

ATKINSON, J. P. and FRANK, M. M. (1973). Effect of cataract therapy on serum complement components. *J. Immunol.*, **111**, 1061–66.

BAKHLE, Y. S., SEARS, M. L. and PRUSOFF, W. H. (1965). Radioactive idoxuridine administered into the conjunctival sac of the rabbit: a study of metabolism and tissue distribution. *Arch. Ophthal.*, **73**, 248–52.

BAUBLIS, J. V., WHITLEY, R. J., CH'IEN, L. T. and ALFORD, C. A. (1975). Treatment of cytomegalovirus infection in infants and adults. In: *Adenine Arabinoside: an Antiviral Agent*, p. 247. Eds. D. Pavan-Langston, R. A. Buchanan and G. A. Alford. New York: Raven Press.

BAUER, D. J. (1980*a*). Laboratory studies on acyclovir. In: *Developments in Antiviral Therapy*, p. 43. Eds. L. H. Collier and J. Oxford. London: Academic Press.

BAUER, D. J. (1980*b*). The chemotherapy of herpes virus infections. In: *Recent Advances in Clinical Virology*, No. 2. Ed. A. P. Waterson. London: Churchill Livingstone.

BAUER, D. J., COLLINS, P., TUCKER, W. E. and MACKLIN, A. W. (1979). Treatment of experimental herpes simplex keratitis with acycloguanosine. *Brit. J. Ophthal.*, **63**, 429–35.

BERENBAUM, M. C. (1974). Comparison of the mechanisms of action of immunosuppressive agents. *Progr. Immunol.*, **5**, 233.

BIRON, K. K. and ELION, G. B. (1979). Sensitivity of varicella zoster virus *in vitro* to acyclovir. *19th Interscience Conference on Antimicrobial Agents and Chemotherapy. Abstract No 249*. Boston.

BONAMOUR, D. and DUGARRE, L. J. (1959). Local gammaglobulin in ocular therapeutics. *Bull. Soc. Ophtal. Paris.*, **5–6**, 438–41.

BRIGDEN, D., FOWLE, A. and ROSLING, A. (1980). Acyclovir, a new antiherpetic drug; early experience in man with systemically administered drug. In: *Developments in Antiviral Therapy*, p. 53. Eds. L. H. Collier and J. Oxford. London: Academic Press.

BURNETT, J. W. and KATZ, S. L. (1963). A study of the use of 5-iodo-2'-deoxyuridine in cutaneous herpes simplex. *J. Invest. Derm.*, **40**, 7–8.

BURNS, R. P. (1963). A double-blind study of IDU in human herpes simplex keratitis. *Arch. Ophthal.*, **70**, 318–24.

CALABRESI, P., CARDOSO, S. S., FINCH, S. C., KLIGERMAN, M. M., VON ESSEN, C. F.,

CHU, M. Y. and WELCH, A. T. (1961). Initial studies with 5-iodo–2'-deoxyuridine. *Cancer Res.*, **21**, 550–9.

CARON, G. A. (1967). Prednisolone inhibition of DNA synthesis by human lymphocytes induced *in vitro* by phytohemagglutinin. *Int. Arch. Allergy*, **32**, 191–200.

CARTER, C. A. and EASTY, D. L. (1981*a*). Experimental ulcerative herpetic keratitis. I. Systemic immune responses and resistance to corneal infection. *Brit. J. Ophthal.*, **65**, 77–81.

CARTER, C. A. and EASTY, D. L. (1981*b*). The influence of levamisole in ulcerative disease of the cornea in the experimental animal. (*Unpublished results.*)

CARTER, C. A. and EASTY, D. L. (1981*c*). Experimental ulcerative herpetic keratitis. III. Evaluation of hyperimmune gammaglobulin therapy. *Brit. J. Ophthal.*, **65**, 392–5.

CARTER, C. A., EASTY, D. L. and WALKER, S. R. (1981*a*). Experimental ulcerative herpetic keratitis. II. Influence of topical corticosteroid in immunised rabbits. *Brit. J. Ophthal.*, **65**, 388–91.

CARTER, C. A., HARTLEY, C. E., SKINNER, G. R. B., TURNER, S. P. and EASTY, D. L. 1981*b*). Experimental ulcerative herpetic keratitis. IV. Preliminary observation on the efficacy of a herpes subunit vaccine. *Brit. J. Ophthal.*, **65**, 679–82.

CHENG, Y. C. (1981). Molecular basis and pharmacological consideration of selective antiherpetic agents. In: *Herpetic Eye Diseases*, p. 237. Ed. R. Sundmacher. Munich: J. F. Bergmann Verlag.

CHIN, E. N. (1978). Treatment of herpes simplex keratitis with idoxuridine and vidarabine: a double-blind study. *Ann. Ophthal.*, **10**, 1171–4.

CLAMAN, H. N. (1972). Corticosteroids and lymphoid cells. *New Engl. J. Med.*, **287**, 388–97.

COBO, L., COSTER, D. J., RICE, N. S. C. and JONES, B. R. (1981). Prognosis and management of corneal transplantation for herpetic keratitis. In: *Herpetic Eye Diseases*, p. 435. Ed. R. Sundmacher. Munich: J. F. Bergmann Verlag.

COHEN, I. R., STAVEY, L. and FELDMAN, M. (1970). Glucocorticoids and cellular immunity *in vitro*. Facilitation of the sensitisation phase and inhibition of the effector phase of lymphocyte antifibroblast reaction. *J. Exp. Med.*, **132**, 1055–70.

COLLINS, P. and BAUER, D. J. (1979). The activity *in vitro* against herpes virus of 9-(2-hydroxyethoxymethyl) guanine (acycloguanosine), a new antiviral agent. *J. Antimicrob. Chemother.*, **5**, 431–6.

COLLUM, L. M. J., BENEDICT-SMITH, A. and HILLARY, I. B. (1980). Acyclovir in dendritic corneal ulceration. In: *The Cornea in Health and Disease.* Ed. P. Trevor-Roper. RSM International Congress Series No 40. London: RSM/Academic Press.

COOPER, J. A. D., DANIELS, C. A. and TROFATTER, D. P. (1978). The effect of prednisolone on antibody-dependent cell-mediated cytotoxicity and the growth of type 1 herpes simplex virus in human cells. *Invest. Ophthal. Vis. Sci.*, **17**, 381–384.

CORWIN, M. E., OKUMUTO, M., THYGESON, P. and JAWETZ, E. (1963). A double-blind study of the effect of 5-iodo-2'-deoxyuridine on experimental herpes simplex keratitis. *Amer. J. Ophthal.*, **55**, 225–29.

COSTA, J., YEE, C., TROOST, T., MANSON, T. and RABSON, S. (1974). Effect of dexamathasone on herpes simplex virus type 2 infection *in vitro*. *Nature*, **252**, 745–6.

COSTER, D. L., JONES, B. R. and FALCON, M. C. (1977). Role of debridement in the treatment of herpetic keratitis. *Trans. Ophthal. Soc. U.K.*, **97**, 314–317.

COSTER, D. L., JONES, B. R. and McGILL, J. I. (1979). Treatment of amoeboid herpetic ulcers with adenine arabinoside or trifluorothymidine. *Brit. J. Ophthal.*, **63**, 418–21.

COSTER, D. J., McKINNON, J. R., McGILL, J. I., JONES, B. R. and FRAUNFELDER, F. T. (1976). Clinical evaluation of adenine arabinoside and trifluorothymidine in the treatment of corneal ulcers caused by herpes simplex virus. *J. Infect. Dis.*, Suppl. A., **133**, 173–7.

COSTER, D. J., WILHELMUS, K. R., MICHAUD, R. and JONES, B. R. (1980). A comparison of acyclovir and idoxuridine as treatment for ulcerative herpetic keratitis. *Brit. J. Ophthal.*, **64**, 763–5.

DAVID, D. S., GRIECO, H. and CUSHMAN, P., JR. (1970). Adrenal glucocorticoids after twenty years. A review of their clinical relevant consequences. *J. Chron. Dis.*, **22**, 637–711.

DELAMORE, I. W. and PRUSOFF, W. H. (1962). Effect of 5-iodo-2′-deoxyuridine on the biosynthesis of phosphorylated derivatives of thymidine. *Biochem. Pharmacol.*, **11**, 101–12.

DE MIRANDA, P., KRASNY, H. C., GOOD, S., PAGE, D. A., CREACH, T. H. and ELION, G. B. (1978). Metabolic disposition of 9-(2-hydroxymethyl) guanine (BW 248 U) in different species. *18th Interscience Conference on Antimicrobial Agents and Chemotherapy. Atlanta, Abst. 66.*

DE SOUSA, M. and FACHET, J. (1972). The cellular basis of mechanism of action of cortisone acetate on contact sensitivity to oxazolone in the mouse. *Clin. Exp. Immunol.*, **10**, 673–84.

EASTERBROOK, M., WILKIE, J., COLEMAN, V. and DAWSON, C. R. (1973). The effect of topical corticosteroids on the susceptibility of immune animals to reinoculation with *Herpes simplex*. *Invest. Ophthal.*, **12**, 181.

EASTY, D. L., ENTWHISTLE, C., FUNK, A. and WITCHER, J. (1975). Herpes simplex keratitis and keratoconus in the atopic patient: a clinical and immunological study. *Trans. Ophthal. Soc. U.K.*, **95**, 267–76.

EASTY, D. L., TULLO, A., SHIMELD, C., HILL, T. J. and BLYTH, W. (1983). The influence of prednisolone on external eye disease, virus proliferation and latent infection in an animal model of herpes simplex keratitis. *International Herpesvirus Workshop, Oxford*, p. 177.

EL KORASHY, H. S. (1942). Herpes simplex (febrilis) of cornea. *Bull. Ophthal. Soc. Egypt*, **35**, 112–115.

FALCON, M. G. and JONES, B. R. (1979). Acycloguanosine: antiviral activity in the rabbit cornea. *Brit. J. Ophthal.*, **63**, 422–4.

FALCON, M. G., JONES, B. R., WILLIAMS, H. P., WILHELMUS, K. and COSTER, D. J. (1981). Adverse reactions in the eye from topical therapy with idoxuridine, adenine arabinoside and trifluorothymidine. In: *Herpetic Eye Diseases*, p. 263. Ed. R. Sundmacher. Munich: J. F. Bergmann Verlag.

FAUCI, A. S. (1979). Immunosuppression and anti-inflammatory effects of glucocorticoids. *Monogr. on Endocr.*, **12**, 440–65.

FAUCI, A. S., DALE, D. C. and BALOW, J. E. (1976). Glucocorticosteroid therapy; mechanism of action and clinical considerations. *Ann. Intern. Med.*, **84**, 304–15.

FIELD, H. J. (1981). The clinical implications of acyclovir-resistant mutants of herpes simplex virus. In: *Herpetic Eye Diseases*. Ed. R. Sundmacher. Munich: J. F. Bergmann Verlag.

FOSTER, C. (1981). Penetrating keratoplasty for herpes simplex keratitis. In: *Herpetic Eye Diseases*, p. 425. Ed. R. Sundmacher. Munich: J. F. Bergmann Verlag.

FRIEDLAENDER, M. H., SMOLIN, G. and OKUMOTO, M. (1978). The treatment of herpetic reinfection with levamisole. *Amer. J. Ophthal.*, **86**, 245–49.

FULHORST, H. W., RICHARDS, A. B., BOWBYES, J. and JONES, B. R. (1972). Cryotherapy of epithelial herpes simplex keratitis. *Amer. J. Ophthal.*, **73**, 46–51.

GABRIELSEN, A. E. and GOOD, R. A. (1967). Chemical suppression of adoptive immunity. *Advanc. Immunol.*, **6**, 91–229.

GASSET, A. R., AKABOSH, I. and TAKASHI, P. (1976). Teratogenicity of adenine arabinoside (Ara A). *Invest. Ophthal.*, **15**, 556–557.

GORDON, Y. J., LAHAV, M., PHOTION, S. and BECKER, Y. (1977). Effect of phosphono-acetic acid in the treatment of experimental HSK. *Brit. J. Ophthal.*, **61**, 506–509.

GUNDERSEN, T. (1936). Herpes corneae: With special reference to its treatment with strong solution of iodine. *Arch. Ophthal.*, **15**, 225–49.

HALL-SMITH, S. P., CORRIGAN, M. J. and GILKES, M. J. (1962). Treatment of herpes simplex with 5-iodo-2'-deoxyuridine. *Brit. Med. J.*, **2**, 1515–16.

HART, D. R. L., BRIGHTMAN, V. J. F., BRADSHAW, G. A., PORTER, G. T. J. and TULLY, M. J. (1965). Treatment of human herpes simplex keratitis with idoxuridine. *Arch. Ophthal.*, **73**, 623–34.

HERRMANN, E. C. JR. (1961). Plaque inhibition test for detection of specific inhibition of DNA containing viruses. *Proc. Soc. Exp. Biol. (N.Y.)*, **107**, 142–5.

IBRAHAM, A. (1967). Evaluation of IDU in the treatment of dendritic ulcer. *Bull. Ophthal. Soc. Egypt*, **60**, 245–249.

ISAACS, A. and LINDENMANN, J. (1957). Virus interference. I. The interferon. *Proc. Roy. Soc. B.*, **147**, 258–67.

ITOI, M., GEFTER, J. W., KANEKO, N., ISHII, Y., RAMRER, R. M. and GASSET, A. R. (1975). Teratogenicities of ophthalmic drugs. I. Antiviral ophthalmic drugs. *Arch. Ophthal.*, **93**, 46–51.

JEPSON, C. N. (1964). Treatment of herpes simplex of the cornea with IDU. *Amer. J. Ophthal.*, **57**, 213–17.

JONES, B. R. and AL HUSSAINI, M. K. (1963). Therapeutic considerations in ocular vaccinia. *Trans. Ophthal. Soc. U.K.*, **83**, 613–31.

JONES, B. R., COSTER, D. J., FALCON, M. F. and CANTELL, K. (1976). Clinical trials of topical interferon therapy of ulcerative viral keratitis. *J. Infect. Dis.*, **133**, Suppl. A. 93–5.

JONES, B. R., COSTER, D. J., FISON, P. N., THOMPSON, G. M., COBO, L. M. and FALCON, M. G. (1979). Efficacy of acycloguanosine (Wellcome 248 u) against herpes simplex corneal ulcers. *Lancet*, **1**, 243–4.

JONES, B. R., COSTER, D. J., WILHELMUS, K. R. and MICHAUD, R. (1980). Acyclovir (Zovirax); an effective antiviral for herpetic keratitis. In: *The Cornea in Health and Disease*. Ed. P. Trevor-Roper. RSM International Congress Series No 40. London: RSM/Academic Press.

JUEL-JENSEN, B. E. and MACCALLUM, F. O. (1964). Treatment of herpes simplex lesions of the face with idoxuridine: Results of a double-blind controlled trial. *Brit. Med. J.*, **2**, 987–988.

JUEL-JENSEN, B. E. and MACCALLUM, F. O. (1965). Herpes simplex lesions of the face treated with idoxuridine applied by spray gun: Results of a double-blind controlled trial. *Brit. Med. J.*, **1**, 901–3.

JUEL-JENSEN, B. E. and MACCALLUM, F. O. (1972). *Herpes Simplex Varicella and Zoster: Clinical Manifestations and Treatment*. London: Wm. Heinemann Medical Books.

KATO, F., OHNO, S. and MATSUDA, H. (1979). The effect of levamisole in herpetic stromal keratitis. *Jap. J. Clin. Ophthal.*, **33**, 375.

KAUFMAN, H. E. (1962). Clinical cure of herpes simplex keratitis by 5-iodo-2'-deoxyuridine. *Proc. Soc. Exp. Biol. (N.Y.)*, **109**, 251–2.

KAUFMAN, H. E., ELLISON, E. D. and TOWNSEND, W. M. (1970). The chemotherapy of herpes iritis with adenine arabinoside and cytarabine. *Arch. Ophthal.*, **84**, 783–7.

KAUFMAN, H. E. and HEIDELBERGER, C. (1964). Therapeutic antiviral action of 5-trifluoromethyl-2'deoxyuridine in herpes simplex keratitis. *Science*, **145**, 585–6.

KAUFMAN, H. E., MUDD, S., VARNELL, E. D. and ENGLESTEIN, J. (1975). The effect of non-specific immune stimulation on the recurrence rate of herpetic keratitis in rabbits. *Invest. Ophthal.*, **14**, 469–471.

KAUFMAN, H. E., NESBURN, A. B. and MALONEY, E. D. (1962). IDU therapy of herpes simplex. *Arch. Ophthal.*, **67**, 583–91.

KAUFMAN, H. E. and VARNELL, E. D. (1977). Lack of levamisole effect in experimental herpes keratitis. *Invest. Ophthal.*, **16**, 1148–1150.

KIBRICK, S. and KATZ, A. S. (1970). Topical idoxuridine in recurrent herpes simplex. *Ann. N.Y. Acad. Sci.*, **173**, 83–89.

KIBRICK, S., TAKAHASHI, G. H. and LEIBOWITZ, H. M. (1971). Local corticosteroid therapy and reactivation of herpetic keratitis. *Arch. Ophthal.*, **86**, 694–698.

KLIGMAN, A. M. (1965). Topical pharmacology and toxicology of dimethyl sulphoxide. I and II. *J. Amer. Med. Ass.*, **193**, 796–804, 923–28.

LAHAV, M., DUEKER, D., BHATT, P. N. and ALBERT, D. M. (1975). Photodynamic inactivation in experimental herpetic keratitis. *Arch. Ophthal.*, **93**, 207–214.

LAIBSON, P. R., HYNDIUK, R., KRACHMER, J. H. and SCHULTZ, O. (1975). Ara-A and IDU therapy of human superficial herpetic keratitis. *Invest. Ophthal.*, **14**, 762–763.

LAIBSON, P. R. and KRACHMER, J. H. (1975). Controlled comparison of adenine arabinoside and idoxuridine therapy of human superficial dendritic keratitis. In: *Adenine Arabinoside: an Antiviral Agent*, p. 323. Eds. D. Pavan-Langston, R. A. Buchanan and G. A. Alford. New York: Raven Press.

LAIBSON, P. R. and LEOPOLD, I. H. (1965). An evaluation of double-blind IDU therapy in 100 cases of herpetic keratitis. *Trans. Amer. Acad. Ophthal. Otolaryng.*, **68**, 22–34.

LANGSTON, R. H. S., PAVAN-LANGSTON, D. and DOHLMAN, C. H. (1974). Antiviral medication and corneal wound healing. *Arch. Ophthal.*, **92**, 509–513.

LULY, J. P., JOHNSON, T., BUCHANAN, R., CH'IEN, L. T., WHITLEY, R. and ALFORD, C. (1975). Adenine arabinoside therapy of varicella-zoster virus infections: Summary of Phase II studies. In: *Adenine Arabinoside: an Antiviral Agent*, p. 225. Eds. D. Pavan-Langston, R. A. Buchanan and G. A. Alford. New York: Raven Press.

LUNTZ, M. H. and MACCALLUM, F. O. (1963). Treatment of herpes simplex keratitis with 5-iodo-2'-deoxyuridine. *Brit. J. Ophthal.*, **47**, 449–56.

MACCALLUM, F. O. and JUEL-JENSEN, B. E. (1966). Herpes simplex virus skin infection in man treated with idoxuridine in dimethyl sulphoxide. Results of a double-blind controlled trial. *Brit. Med. J.*, **2**, 805.

McGILL, J. I., COLLINS, P., CANTELL, K., JONES, B. R. and FINTER, N. (1976). Optimal schedules for use of interferon in the corneas of rabbits with herpes simplex keratitis. *J. Infect. Dis.* (Suppl A) **133**, 13–17.

McGILL, J. I., COSTER, D., FRAUENFELDER, T., HOLT WILSON, A. D., WILLIAMS, H. and JONES, B. R. (1975). Adenine arabinoside in management of herpetic keratitis. *Trans. Ophthal. Soc. U.K.*, **95**, (2) 246–9.

McGILL, J. I., HOLT WILSON, A. D., McKINNON, J. R., WILLIAMS, H. P. and JONES, B. R. (1974). Some aspects of the clinical use of trifluorothymidine in the treatment of herpetic ulceration of the cornea. *Trans. Ophthal. Soc. U.K.*, **94**, 342–352.

McGILL, J. I. and OGILVIE, M. (1980). Viral drug resistance in herpes simplex ulceration. In: *The Cornea in Health and Disease*. Ed. P. Trevor-Roper. RSM International Congress Series No 40. London: RSM/Academic Press.

McGILL, J. I. and TORMEY, P. (1981). The clinical use of acyclovir in the treatment of herpes simplex corneal ulceration. In: *Herpetic Eye Diseases*, p. 319. Ed. R. Sundmacher. Munich: J. F. Bergmann Verlag.

McKENDALL, R. R. (1977). Efficacy of herpes simplex virus type 1 immunisation in protecting against acute and latent infection by herpes simplex virus type 2 in mice. *Infection & Immunity*, **16**, 217–19.

MACKENZIE, A. D. (1964). A comparison of IDU solution, IDU ointment, and carbolisation in the treatment of dendritic corneal ulcer. *Brit. J. Ophthal.*, **48**, 274–276.

MAICHUK, Y. F., KAZACHENKO, M. A., KLADOVA, L. A., MIKULI, S. G., ORLOVSKAYA, L. E. and POSDNIAKOV, V. I. (1980). Levamisole in the treatment of ophthalmic herpes and prevention of recurrences. (Eng. Abstr.) *Vestn. Oftal.*, **97**, 36–9.

MANTEI, N., SCHWARZSTEIN, M., STREULI, M., PANEM, S., NAGATA, S. and WEISSMANN, C. (1980). The nucelotide sequence of a cloned human leukocyte interferon with DNA. *Gene*, **10**, 1–10.

MARKHAM, R. H. C., CARTER, C., SCOBIE, M. A., METCALF, C. and EASTY, D. L. (1977). Double-blind clinical trial of adenine arabinoside and idoxuridine in herpetic corneal ulcers. *Trans. Ophthal. Soc. U.K.*, **97**, 333–340.

MENDELSON, J. and GLASGOW, L. A. (1966). The *in vitro* and *in vivo* effects of cortisol on interferon production and action. *J. Immunol.*, **96**, 345–52.

METCALF, J. J. (1980). Protection from experimental ocular herpetic keratitis by a heat-killed virus vaccine. *Arch. Ophthal.*, **98**, 893–96.

MEYER, R. F., SMOLIN, G., HALL, J. M. and OKUMOTO, M. (1975). Effect of local corticosteroids on antibody-forming cells in the eye and draining lymph nodes. *Invest. Ophthal.*, **14**, 138–144.

NESBURN, A. B., ROBINSON, C. and DICKINSON, R. (1977). Adenine arabinoside effect on experimental idoxuridine-resistant herpes simplex infections. *Invest. Ophthal.*, **15**, 302–304.

NORTH, R. D., PAVAN-LANGSTON, D. and GEARY, P. (1976). Herpes simplex virus types 1 and 2: Therapeutic response to antiviral drugs. *Arch. Ophthal.*, **94**, 1019–21.

O'BRIEN, W. J. and EDELHAUSER, H. F. (1977). The corneal penetration of trifluoro-thymidine, adenine arabinoside and idoxuridine: a comparative study. *Invest. Ophthal.*, **16**, 1093–1103.

O'DAY, D. M., JONES, B. R., POIRIER, R., PILLEY, S., CHISHOLM, I., STEELE, A. and RICE, N. S. C. (1975). Proflavine photodynamic viral inactivation in herpes simplex keratitis. *Amer. J. Ophthal.*, **79**, 941–948.

O'DAY, D. M., POIRIER, R. H., JONES, D. B. and ELLIOTT, J. H. (1976). Vidarabine therapy of complicated herpes simplex keratitis. *Amer. J. Ophthal.*, **81**, 642–49.

PATTERSON, A., FOX, A. D., DAVIES, G., MAGUIRE, C. et al. (1963). Controlled studies of IDU in the treatment of herpetic keratitis. *Trans. Ophthal. Soc. U.K.*, **83**, 583–591.

PAVAN-LANGSTON, D. (1975). Clinical evaluation of adenine arabinoside and idoxuridine in the treatment of ocular herpes simplex. *Amer. J. Ophthal.*, **80** (3), 495–502.

PAVAN-LANGSTON, D. (1977). Trifluorothymidine and idoxuridine therapy of ocular herpes. *Amer. J. Ophthal.*, **84**, 818–25.

PAVAN-LANGSTON, D. and DOHLMAN, C. H. (1972). A double-blind clinical study of adenine arabinoside therapy of viral keratoconjunctivitis. *Amer. J. Ophthal.*, **74**, 81–8.

PAVAN-LANGSTON, D., DOHLMAN, C. H. and GEARY, P. A. (1973). Intraocular penetration of Ara-A and IDU: therapeutic implications in clinical herpetic uveitis. *Trans. Amer. Acad. Ophthal. Otolaryng.*, **77**, 455–66.

PETER, J. B. (1971). Cytotoxins produced by human lymphocytes inhibition by anti-inflammatory steroids and anti-malarial drugs. *Cell. Immunol.*, **2**, 199–202.

POLLACK, F. and KAUFMAN, H. E. (1972). Penetrating keratoplasty in herpetic keratitis. *Amer. J. Ophthal.*, **73**, 908–913.

POLLIKOFF, R. (1970). Topical vaccine therapy in herpetic keratitis. *Lancet*, **1**, 1064.

PRUSOFF, W. H. (1959). Synthesis and biological activities of iododeoxyuridine, an analogue of thymidine. *Biochim. Biophys. Acta (Amst.)*, **32**, 295.

RAPP, F. and VANDERSLICE, D. (1964). Spread of zoster virus in human embryonic lung cells and the inhibitory effect of iododeoxyuridine. *Virology*, **22**, 321–30.

RICE, N. S. C. and JONES, B. R. (1973). Problems of corneal grafting in herpetic keratitis. In: *Corneal Graft Failure*, p. 221. Amsterdam: Elsevier, North Holland.

ROBBINS, R. M. and GALIN, M. A. (1975). A model for steroid effects in herpes keratitis. *Arch. Ophthal.*, **93**, 828–830.

SAKATA, H. (1980). Effectiveness of levamisole on experimental stromal herpes simplex keratitis. *Folia Ophthal. Jap.*, **31**, 308.

SCHAEFFER, H. J., BEAUCHAMP, L., DE MIRANDA, P., ELION, G. B., BANER, D. J. and COLLINS, P. (1978). 9-(2-hydroxyethoxymethyl) guanine activity against viruses of the herpes group. *Nature*, **272**, 583.

SHIOTA, H., INOUE, S. and YAMANE, S. (1979). Efficacy of acycloguanosine against herpetic ulcers in rabbit cornea. *Brit. J. Ophthal.*, **63**, 425–28.

SIDWELL, R. W., DIXON, G. J., SELLERS, S. M. and SCHABEL, F. M. (1968). *In vitro* antiviral properties of biologically active compounds. II. Studies with influenza and vaccinia viruses. *Applied Microbiol.*, **16**, 370–92.

SLOAN, B. J., MILLER, F. A., EHRLIAN, J., McLEAN, I. W. and MACHAMER, H. E. (1969). Antiviral activity of 9-8-D-arabino-furanosyladine. IV. Activity against intra-cerebral herpes simplex virus infections in mice. In: *Antimicrobial Agents and Chemotherapy, 1968*. Bethesda: Research Studies Press.

SMOLIN, G. and HALL, J. (1973). Afferent arc of the corneal immunologic reaction. II. Local and systemic response to bovine gamma-globulin. *Arch. Ophthal.*, **90**, 231–4.

SMOLIN, G., OKUMOTO, M., FEILER, S. and CONDON, D. (1981). Idoxuridine-liposome therapy for herpes simplex keratitis. *Amer. J. Ophthal.*, **91**, 220.

SMOLIN, G., OKYMOTO, M. and FRIEDLAENDER, M. (1979). The treatment of herpes simplex keratitis with levamisole. In: *Immunology and Immunopathology of the Eye*, p. 226. Eds. Silverstein and O'Connor. New York: Masson.

SPRY, C. J. H. (1972). Inhibition of lymphocyte recirculation by stress and cortico-trophin. *Cell. Immunol.*, **4**, 86–92.

STARR, M. B., DAWSON, C. R., BRIONES, O. and OH, J. (1981). Vitamin A in experimental herpetic keratitis. *Arch. Ophthal.*, **99**, 322–6.

SUGAR, J., VARNELL, E., CENTIFANTO, Y. and KAUFMAN, H. E. (1973). Trifluorothymi-dine treatment of herpetic iritis in rabbits and ocular penetration. *Invest. Ophthal.*, **12**, 532.

SUNDMACHER, R., CANTELL, K., HANG, P. and NEUMANN HAEFELIN, D. (1978). Role of debridement and interferon in the treatment of dendritic keratitis. *Albrecht v Graefes Arch. Klin. Exp. Ophthal.*, **207**, 77–82.

SUNDMACHER, R., NEUMANN-HAEFELIN, D. and CANTELL, K. (1981). Therapy and prophylaxis of dendritic keratitis with topical human interferon. In: *Herpetic Eye Diseases*. Ed. R. Sundmacher. Munich: J. F. Bergmann Verlag.

TAYLOR, J. L. and O'BRIEN, W. J. (1981). The cytotoxicity of nucleoside antivirals to epithelial cells of ocular origin. In: *Herpetic Eye Diseases*, p. 269. Ed. R. Sundmacher. Munich: J. F. Bergmann Verlag.

THOFT, R. A. (1982). Indications for conjunctival transplantation. *Ophthalmology*, **89**, 335–340.

THOMPSON, J. and FURTH, R. van (1970). The effect of fluorocorticosteroids on the kinetics of mononuclear phagocytes. *J. Exp. Med.*, **131**, 429–42.

TROBE, J. D., CENTIFANTO, Y., ZAM, Z. S., VARNELL, E. and KAUFMAN, H. E. (1976). Anti-herpes activity of adenine arabinoside monophosphate. *Invest. Ophthal.*, **15**, 196–199.

TROWSDALE, M. D., DUNDEL, E. C. and NESBURN, A. B. (1980). The effect of flurbiprofen in herpes keratitis in rabbits. *Invest. Ophthal. and Vis. Sci.*, **19**, 267.

TULLO, A. B., SHIMELD, C., HILL, T. J., BLYTH, W. and EASTY, D. L. The influence of topical corticosteroid on the establishment of latency in herpes simplex keratitis in immune mice. (*In preparation.*)

VAN BIJSTERVELD, O. P. and POST, H. J. (1980). Trifluorothymidine and adenine arabinoside in the treatment of dendritic keratitis. In: *Herpetic Eye Diseases*. Ed. R. Sundmacher. Munich: J. F. Bergmann Verlag.

WALZ, M. A., PRICE, R. W., HAYASHI, K., KATZ, B. J. and NOTKINS, A. L. (1977). Effect of immunisation on acute and latent infection of vagino-uterine tissue with herpes simplex virus types 1 and 2. *J. Infect. Dis.*, **135**, 744–52.

WELLINGS, P. C., AWDRY, P. N., BORS, F. H., JONES, B. R., BROWN, D. C. and KAUFMAN, H. E. (1972). Clinical evaluation of trifluorothymidine in the treatment of herpes simplex corneal ulcers. *Amer. J. Ophthal.*, **73**, 932–42.

WHITCHER, J. P., DAWSON, C. R., HOSHIWARA, I., DAGHFOUS, T., MESSADI, M., TRIKI, F. and OH, J. O. (1976). Herpes simplex keratitis in a developing country. *Arch. Ophthal.*, **94**, 587–592.

WILHELMUS, K. R., COSTER, D. J. and JONES, B. R. (1981). Acyclovir and debridement in the treatment of ulcerative herpetic keratitis. *Amer. J. Ophthal.*, **91**, 323–7.

WILLIAMS, T. W. and GRANGER, G. A. (1969). Lymphocyte *in vitro* cytotoxicity: correlation of depression with release of lymphotoxin from human lymphocytes. *J. Immunol.*, **103**, 107–8.

WITMER, R. (1981). Results of keratoplasty in metaherpetic keratitis. In: *Herpetic Eye Diseases*, p. 419. Ed. R. Sundmacher. Munich: J. F. Bergmann Verlag.

YAMAGUCHI, K., OKUMOTO, M., STERN, G., FRIEDLAENDER, M. and SMOLIN, G. (1979). Idoxuridine and bacterial corneal infection. *Amer. J. Ophthal.*, **87**, 202–5.

ZURIER, R. B. and WEISSMAN, G. (1973). Anti-immunologic and anti-inflammatory effects of steroid therapy. *Med. Clin. N. Amer.*, **57**, 1295–1307.

CHAPTER NINE

Ocular Disease in Varicella Zoster Infections

VARICELLA ZOSTER

Biological Characteristics

Varicella zoster is caused by a DNA virus with a size and structure similar to that of HSV, as seen by EM preparations of vesicular fluid or infected tissues from humans, and from tissue culture (Figure 9.1). It can be seen in the cell nucleus as a particle with a dense central core 30–50 nm in diameter surrounded by an oval membrane, the protein coat or capsid, which is 95 nm in diameter. The capsomeres are similar in appearance to those described for HSV. Like HSV the particle may acquire a second membrane from the inner nuclear membrane before or during its exit to the cytoplasm, when it then becomes mature. The extracellular mature particles from vesicular fluid are about 150–200 nm in diameter. Extracellular open envelopes and disrupted capsids are also noticeable.

No susceptible animal is yet available, and therefore tissue-culture studies have provided much of the information with regard to the spread of the virus. Epithelial, glial and fibroblastic tissues taken from humans support propagation. Human embryonic skin, lung and kidney grafted on to the chorio-allantois of hens eggs or maintained in organ culture *in vitro* are also suitable for culture of the virus. The cells used for routine isolation may be primary human amnion, human embryo lung fibroblasts and human thyroid. In contrast to HSV, the cycle of replication is longer. An interval of 8–16 hours occurs between the inoculation of the virus from vesicular fluid and the first evidence of growth. A focal lesion is produced which extends radially as a result of progressive infection of contiguous cells. Giant multinucleated cells occur, due to the fusion of infected cells which can be shown to contain eosinophyllic type A inclusions.

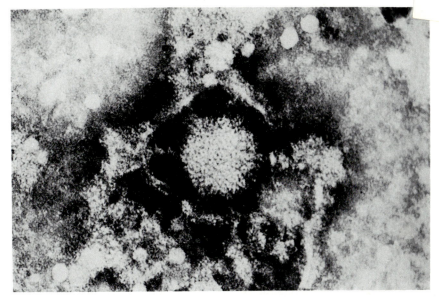

Figure 9.1. Electron micrograph of varicella zoster virus. The capsomers are easily seen (×200 000). (Courtesy, Dr. Gordon Skinner.)

Laboratory Diagnosis

Where rapid tests are required, EM and immunofluorescence can be used. Complement fixation can be carried out using fluid taken from vesicles. Complement fixation tests for serum antibody in convalescent serum will take 24 hours. Isolation in tissue culture gives a positive answer in between 48 and 72 hours, but is unlikely to be positive once scabs have formed. There appears to be one antigenic type of varicella zoster agent. The tests available include precipitating, complement fixing, fluorescent and neutralising antibody tests.

Varicella zoster virus (Herpes virus varicellae), is the aetiological agent of two diseases in man, varicella and herpes zoster. Varicella (chickenpox) is a ubiquitous, contagious, generalised exanthematous disease of seasonal epidemic propensities that follows primary exposure of a susceptible individual, most often a child. Herpes zoster (shingles) is an endemic sporadic disease, most frequent in elderly people, and characterised by the appearance of a unilateral, painful vesicular eruption localised to the dermatome innervated by a specific dorsal root or extramedullary cranial ganglion. In contrast to varicella, which follows primary exogenous contact with the causative organism, zoster reflects endogenous activation of a viral infection that has survived in latent form following an attack of varicella. Although the two disease entities are generally considered to be distinct, the patient with zoster may develop a disseminated varicelliform eruption, and conversely and rarely, the patient with varicella may exhibit concentration of lesions somewhat reminiscent of zoster.

Varicella remains one of the more prominent diseases caused by viruses in childhood for which no effective vaccine has yet been obtained. The prevalence of its delayed manifestation herpes zoster is increasing in the developed countries, due to the growing numbers of elderly in the populations and to the increasing use of immunosuppressive therapy together with cytotoxic agents, both of which adversely influence the host defence mechanisms.

Herpes zoster was described in premedieval times, but varicella was not differentiated from smallpox (variola) until the end of the nineteenth century. The infectious nature of varicella was demonstrated in 1875 by Steiner, who induced the disease in volunteers by inoculating vesicular fluid from patients with chickenpox. Kundratitz was able to transmit organisms from patients with zoster to induce varicelliform cutaneous lesions in 1925. It was therefore surmised that there was a relationship between varicella and zoster, and this was supported by the observation that children who had been in contact with patients with zoster occasionally acquired varicella. The School Epidemics Committee of Great Britain in 1938 were able to link 18 outbreaks of varicella with exposure to patients suffering from zoster. Tyzzer (1906) and Lipschutz (1921) were able to describe independently the histopathological lesions in varicella and zoster and it became apparent that there was considerable similarity between the two conditions. Garland (1943) suggested that zoster might reflect a reactivation of a latent varicella virus, a mechanism which now can be seen to be similar to the mechanism thought to occur in recurrence of the herpes simplex virus in clinical disease.

Transmission

The disease may rarely be transferred from a pregnant mother to the fetus near term, the disease manifesting within 10 days of birth. Meyers (1974) collected details from 43 cases of congenital varicella reported in the literature since 1878, and noted a fatality rate of 10 per cent. In 46 mothers who developed varicella in the last 17 days of pregnancy 24 per cent of newborn infants developed overt signs of varicella. Although it had been suggested that varicella in the early stages of pregnancy may lead to congenital malformations, in a prospective study in the United Kingdom the incidence of congenital abnormality did not differ from a control group (Manson et al., 1960).

Postnatal transmission in the past has been thought to be due to droplet infection, but spread occurs also by direct contact. The duration of infectivity of infected droplets is probably fairly limited. Infection occurs in the immunoincompetent host for a period of 7 days, in contrast to a normal immunocompetent host where the crop of lesions will last for a period of 4–5 days. Tyzzer (1906) observed that the lesions first affect the endothelium of the capillaries of the skin and suggested that a viraemia occurs in the prodromal period. A typical case is probably infectious for 1–2 days prior to the appearance of the generalised eruption, and for 4–5 days thereafter, until the last crop of vesicles has evolved to the purulent and crusted state. Lesions may not be confined to the skin only but may be found in the respiratory, urinary and gastro-intestinal tracts.

The individual with herpes zoster is infectious and can induce infection as varicella in a susceptible host by transmission of the virus. The mechanism is not clearly understood but is probably similar to that of varicella. A significant proportion of patients with zoster have diffuse cutaneous lesions in a chicken-pox-like distribution which would reflect a transient viraemia. Thirty-three per cent of patients in a survey carried out in Sweden demonstrated cutaneous lesions in addition to the lesions confined to the cutaneous dermatome (Oberg and Svedmyr, 1969), and 16 per cent of a group of patients in England developed widely distributed lesions (Juel-Jensen and MacCallum, 1972).

Pathogenesis and Immunity

The mode of entry of the virus into the host in varicella is not known, and its route can only be surmised from the patterns of events in other virus diseases. It is thought that the virus enters through exposed mucous membranes of the oropharynx, the upper respiratory tract, the conjunctiva or the skin, although the latter would seem unlikely. Having entered the host virus replication occurs intracellularly at the site of entry, with subsequent cycles of replication occurring in the local cells eventually leading to dissemination via the blood stream or the lymphatics. Information gathered from the pattern of growth curves *in vitro* suggest that multiple cycles of proliferation occur during a long incubation period. Non-specific host immune responses occur at the early stages of the development of disease, but later specific immune responses manifest. However, the rate of proliferation of virus overwhelms the initial immune response, and the viraemia induces prodromal symptoms, followed by the appearance of the cutaneous lesions. The viraemia is probably cyclical, reflected by successive crops of cutaneous vesicles. Finally the cutaneous disease is terminated by specific immune responses in immunocompetent hosts.

Assumption and surmise also prevail in explaining the immunopathogenesis of zoster. In a majority of cases the virus is thought to be present in the body following an initial attack of varicella probably during infancy or childhood. It is not known whether the interim infection is persistent or latent. In persistent infections it is thought that virions are constantly being elaborated, while in latent infections the viral genome persists without virus replication. Herpes zoster must reflect an episode of renewed virus replication in a partially immune host as a consequence of a previous attack of varicella. Epidemiological evidence that cases of zoster occur sporadically with no temporal or spatial contact with varicella supports the contention that reactivation is endogenous and is not related to the transmission of virus from one infected host to another. It is thought that the virus persists in a quiescent state in sensory ganglia. It is possible that many sensory ganglia may harbour the virus following varicella, and when systemic immune protection mechanisms fall below a certain threshold the virus may replicate and produce selective involvement in a sensory ganglion. Virions are then transported antidromically down a sensory nerve and released around the nerve endings in the skin where the characteristic clusters of lesions are produced. The fact that a viraemia may occur simultaneously is confirmed by the presence of a varicelliform eruption at the same time as an eruption typical of zoster. Pathological changes have long been known to occur in the posterior root ganglion, and VZ virus has been demonstrated in affected nervous elements using electron microscropy and specific immunofluorescent techniques (Esiri and Tomlinson, 1972; Ghatak and Zimmerman, 1973). However, it has not proved possible to isolate live virus from dorsal root ganglia obtained randomly at autopsy from varicella-immune adults (Weller, 1976).

Because of the spontaneous nature of zoster it has proved difficult to investigate the humoral and cell-mediated immune responses which may contribute in the process which triggers virus replication to the extent that clinical disease occurs. It is postulated that these parameters may fall to threshold levels but it is practically impossible to demonstrate such a pre-eruptive change in the clinical field. Comparisons have been made between varicella and zoster and it has been possible to demonstrate differences in antibody responses in the two diseases. In an immunoresponsive host, zoster attacks terminate when reactivated defence mechanisms exceed the hypothetical threshold level. When these levels subsequently decline, a further attack may ensue. Specific antibody, as determined by a number of techniques, may show a marked secondary rise after an attack of zoster, but differences in the response shown by immunoglobulin subclasses have been reported. There are difficulties in the interpretation of paired sera, as it is not clearly known when the peak titres of antibody levels occur in relation to the clinical disease during which serum antibody levels do not always show a rise in titre, presumably because this may have already taken place during the prodromal stage of the disease. Although it might not have been expected, a rise in IgM-specific antibody has been reported (Ross and McDaid, 1972), while a rapidly migrating IgG subclass antibody with specificity against varicella zoster virus antigen was found in patients recovering from zoster, but not in patients after an attack of varicella (Leonard et al., 1970). It was postulated that the host response might not be complete following varicella, but was complete following zoster. In this way, following varicella, a failure to eliminate the virus could be hypothesised which allowed the presentation of disease recurrence in the form of an attack of zoster. Differences in antibody responses have also been reported by Palusuo (1972) using a platelet aggregation technique; such a method was able to demonstrate specific antibody following zoster but not after an attack of varicella. The pathological significance of such anomalous findings are difficult to explain.

Cell-mediated reactions following varicella zoster infections have been defined, but there remain many problems which need to be further investigated. Russell et al. (1972) were able to demonstrate that lymphoblastic transformation to specific antigen was depleted following such infections in zoster patients, and suggested that a transient depletion of cell-mediated reactions might be the trigger for the recurrence of viral activity. However, Jordan and Merrigan (1974) demonstrated that such deficits returned to normal in the convalescent period following the eruption. Thus if a state of immuno-unresponsiveness existed, it was repaired rapidly following the infection. It remains significant that attacks of zoster occur in immunosuppressed patients and patients with acquired deficiency associated with malignancies and with Hodgkin's disease, where evidence for immunodeficiency has been identified by Gold and Nankervis (1973). The influence of several immune factors on the course of disseminated zoster was studied by Stevens and Merigan (1972). Host immune parameters including quantitative immunoglobulins, circulating lymphocyte counts, delayed hypersensitivity to multiple skin-test antigens, and lymphocyte transformation to phytohaemagglutinin did not correlate with dissemination of the disease. Development of specific complement-fixing antibody was delayed in some patients with disseminated disease. The interferon content in vesicles was low early in the disease in patients with localised and disseminated zoster, and then rose abruptly to a peak value as pustulation and crusting occurred. Titres in patients with localised disease rose earlier than in patients with disseminated disease. The finding suggested that there were at least two host factors whose interaction might determine host responses to zoster; the first was local interferon production which was possibly produced by sensitised lymphocytes, and the second was humoral antibody acting to prevent or shorten dissemination of local disease. The elapsed time between an attack of varicella and zoster is thought to be an important determinant in the pathogenesis of zoster; there appears to be a gradual decay with advancing years in those responses which serve to contain the virus, and they theoretically may become depressed to an extent which eventually allows reactivation of latent VZ virus. Recently, antibody-dependent cell cytotoxicity against VZ-infected human fibroblasts, using human effector peripheral blood monocytes and human serum, has been reported (Souhami et al., 1983). Investigations in patients with various manifestations of varicella zoster infection in the future may prove interesting.

Varicella

The prodromal symptoms in adults occur as a fever accompanied by malaise 2 days before the appearance of the rash. In children the early symptoms are mild and the appearance of the rash may be the first evidence of illness.

The lesions develop as small, irregular, rose-coloured macules in the centre of which there appears a vesicle containing clear fluid. The vesicle may either rupture or the contents may become purulent. Concurrent lesions may have reached different stages of development. Successive crops of new lesions may occur over a period of 2–4 days so that at the climax of the exanthem, there may be in any one area cutaneous lesions represented by early immature lesions, or mature purulent or ruptured vesicles. The lesions first appear on the scalp and then on the trunk, with little involvement of the extremities. Involvement of the mucous membrane of the oropharynx and the vagina may occur, and it is also possible that lesions may occur in the respiratory and gastro-intestinal tracts.

The illness is benign in the immunocompetent subject and is accompanied by mild malaise, pruritus and fever for 2–3 days. These symptoms may be more marked in adults where varicella pneumonia is a common complication. Secondary bacterial infection of the cutaneous lesions occurs frequently. In the immunodeficient or the immunosuppressed host the symptoms may be more severe, as are the clinicopathological responses. In such patients there may be involvement of the gastro-intestinal tract, the respiratory tract and the liver and spleen.

Ocular Manifestations

Vesicular lesions in the conjunctiva are rarely seen in varicella, but occasionally small, papular, phlyctenulae-like lesions occur on the margins of the lids, the conjunctiva or the limbus. The latter may develop into ulcers with excavated edges and associated with a considerable inflammatory reaction in the lids. The cornea may show a superficial punctate keratitis and a marginal keratitis in the presence of limbal pustules. Central corneal lesions may rarely develop as a disciform keratitis. Formation of a descemetocele has been reported associated with iridocyclitis terminating in phthisis bulbi (Ellenberger, 1952).

Dendritic figures have been recorded in patients with a recent history of varicella infections (Yuchida *et al.*, 1980). The lesions occurred approximately four months after the appearance of varicella cutaneous lesions, while the disciform keratitis which had already developed was undergoing treatment with topical dexamethasone drops, together with idoxuridine and atropine. The appearances were similar to those previously described by Nesburn *et al.* (1974). It seems probable that the occurrence of these lesions is associated with the use of topical corticosteroid, prescribed for the stromal kerato-uveitis. Varicella zoster is frequently difficult to isolate from the cornea (Yuchida *et al.*, 1980). However, immunofluorescence on scrapings from the epithelial lesions demonstrated that there was positive fluorescence for varicella zoster virus. Positive serum antibody was found in one of the two patients, which was compatible with varicella, but the absence of positive antibody findings in the other patient could not be adequately explained.

Corneal involvement may occur late in the disease, weeks or months after resolution of the exanthem, when a shallow ulcer can occur. Lesions such as small blebs in the presence of stromal keratitis with corneal oedema have been described. Such lesions tend to remain localised and cause the formation of small, permanent scars. Disciform keratitis may occur which shows little difference compared with that due to herpes simplex keratitis, but responds well to the use of topical corticosteroid.

Herpes Zoster

The varicelliform eruption in zoster is unilateral and initially sharply limited in a band or patchlike distribution to the dermatome supplied by a specific dorsal root or extramedullary cranial nerve ganglion. Within the dermatome the lesions may be profuse or they may be limited to a few scattered vesicles that on occasions may be easily missed. The dermatomes commonly affected are those of the fifth cranial nerve and the trunk where the ganglia that are involved extend from the third dorsal to the second lumbar segments. Lesions therefore rarely involve the extremities. A prodromal symptom before the appearance of the rash may be pain and paraesthesia in the involved dermatome. The lesions appear to occur in successive crops; they may take longer to resolve than in varicella and virus may be recovered up to a week after the onset of the eruption. The scabs are non-infectious and may persist for up to two weeks after the end of the vesicular phase. In many cases secondary infection is inevitable and may cause persistent purulent ulceration in the dermatome, which delays the onset of scab formation and eventual healing. Involvement of the central nervous system can occur in association with the cutaneous eruption and a spinal fluid pleocytosis is common. Motor

paralysis may occur though it is uncommon and is not associated with a fatal outcome.

Herpes Zoster Ophthalmicus

Involvement of the first division of the fifth cranial nerve is commonly seen in elderly patients in ophthalmology. The vesicular eruption extends from the brow into the parietal region well above the hairline. The attack is preceded by a neuralgic pain localised to the same dermatome, and is characteristically associated with the appearance of a variable number of vesicles which eventually form scabs. The lesions may be sparse or plentiful, and on occasions may form a diffuse scab so that the multifocal nature of the original infection is no longer visible. In many patients the frontal nerves are involved, but in a proportion of patients the nasociliary branch is involved so that the eruption extends on to the side of the nose (Figure 9.2 and 9.3). It is rare to see extension of the lesions across the midline, but more than one dermatome can be involved and it is not uncommon for the maxillary division of the fifth nerve to be involved at the same time as the first division. The attack is accompanied by a pyrexia and malaise and often by extreme discomfort. The periorbital tissues become oedematous to such an extent that the lids become closed on the side of the lesion, from where the oedema may spread to the other side so that the patient may be incapacitated by this enforced lid closure. Rarely, the cutaneous eruption may be persistent and lead to deep ulceration of the skin,

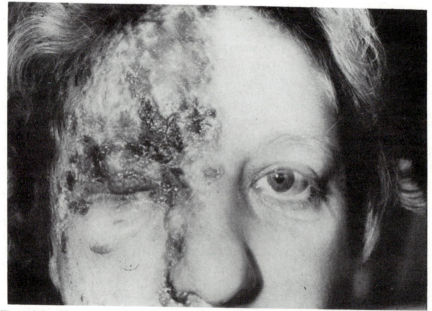

Figure 9.2. Herpes zoster ophthalmicus affecting the nasociliary branch of the ophthalmic division of the trigeminal nerve, together with frontal nerve involvement. (Courtesy, Mr. Ron Marsh.)

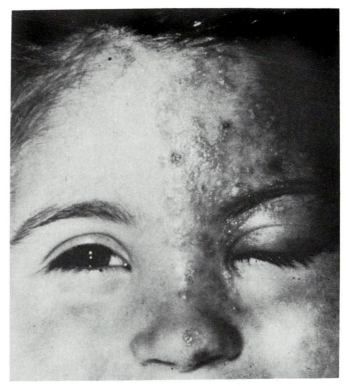

Figure 9.3.   Herpes zoster ophthalmicus in an 11-year-old girl. It is uncommon to see herpes
zoster at this age.

producing an appearance of gangrenous ulceration. In the severe case, such as
occurs in the immunocompromised host, there may be loss of hair and brow
together with necrosis of the skin and orbital tissues.

The incidence of herpes zoster ophthalmicus in communities is not clearly
known. In 1981, 63 new cases were seen during a 6-month period, out of a
total of 7,113 emergency patients. Five of these patients required admission
(Vernon, 1982, personal communication).

Ocular Involvement

The effects of infection with the zoster virus on the eye and the orbital
contents may be mild or severe, and may affect most of the tissues (Figure 9.4).
Ocular involvement is often, but not inevitably, associated with involvement
of the nasociliary nerve. The severity of the ocular disease does not necessarily
seem to be related to the severity of the cutaneous eruption, and it is
remarkable that mild cutaneous disease may be accompanied by severe and
persistent ocular disease.

Herpes zoster ophthalmicus is a disease in which the symptoms and signs
may range from the trivial to the devastating (Marsh, 1976; Table 9.1). The

TABLE 9.1

THE OCULAR MANIFESTATIONS OF HERPES ZOSTER OPHTHALMICUS

Site of disease	Diagnosis; classification	Treatment
The cutaneous eruption	Variable; may be subtle	Topical corticosteroid and antibiotic combination
Post-herpetic neuralgia	Can be the most significant problem; components: hypersensitivity to light touch, long-lasting neuralgia	Cold packs Vibration Phenytoin, sodium valproate, carbamazepine, clonazepam, tricyclic antidepressants, substituted phenothiazines. Amitriptyline (best tricyclic in pain conditions). Mianserin (tetracyclic). Sympathetic blockade
Scarring of lids trichiasis, entropion	Manifestations which can be easily overlooked	Careful attention to the lid margins, and appropriate action
Keratoconjunctivitis sicca	Use corneal stain	Tear substitutes
Neurotrophic keratopathy	Test for presence	Take care with use of corticosteroid
Scleritis	Nodular, diffuse, associated with keratitis	Minimal amount of topical corticosteroid which will control the inflammation
Corneal disease	Subtypes: epithelial, dendritic, persistent erosion, mucous plaque keratopathy, punctate stromal keratitis, diffuse keratitis with involvement of endothelium, focal stromal keratitis, persistent central corneal scarring with lipid deposition, diffuse corneal scarring, detachment of Descemet's membrane, central and peripheral corneal melt and secondary infective disease	Where epithelial deficits, regular culture for bacteria. Careful use of topical corticosteroid; the rebound phenomenon is a cause for serious disease. Care with topical steroid where cornea is anaesthetic
Corneal melting syndrome	May be associated with rheumatoid arthritis or occur in isolation; peripheral or central	Treat with caution, avoiding corticosteroid. Anticollagenases; tarsorrhaphy; penetrating keratoplasty for central thinning and perforation
Vasculitis	Sectorial atrophy of iris, retinal vasculitis, optic atrophy (? ischaemic), anterior segment necrosis	
Cranial nerve palsies	III, IV and VI cranial nerves	
Central nervous involvement	Progressive hemiplegia should be regarded as viral in origin until proved otherwise	

inflammatory changes induce diseases which can be separated from those caused by nerve damage, and tissue scarring. These inflammatory changes may be expressed in the form of nummular, disciform and mucous plaque keratitis, or indirectly as vasculitis in cases of episcleritis, scleritis, iritis, papillitis, or proptosis with occasionally third-nerve palsy (Marsh, 1976; Marsh et al., 1977). Nerve damage may result in neuroparalytic keratitis, ocular muscle palsy, and neuralgia. Tissue scarring in the skin of the lids and conjunctiva can be associated with severe neuralgia, exposure keratitis, trichiasis, lid-margin deformity and anomalies in the tear film. The ocular complications can be considered in three phases: acute, chronic and relapsing. Most patients who develop a systemic varicelliform eruption in addition to an attack of ophthalmic zoster should be investigated for systemic immunodeficiency, as a proportion suffer from one of the reticuloses, malignant tumours, or may indeed be receiving systemic immunosuppressives (Stevens and Merrigan, 1972).

The lids may show changes which may be caused by the vesicular eruption producing distortion of the lashes and aberrant growth, so that ingrowth towards the surface of the cornea can be a hazard in convalescent patients. Patients in whom a tarsorrhaphy has been necessary at some stage in their treatment may suffer from similar problems, inexpert surgery leading to inclusion of lashes between the adherent lid margins which can become a permanent irritant in an already critical situation. It is not uncommon for aberrant lash growth to follow the opening of tarsorrhaphy. Persistent spastic entropion may result in irritation of the globe, often caused by the blepharospasm induced by ocular and cutaneous post-herpetic neuralgia. It is rarely possible to obtain a satisfactory view of the upper tarsal plates at the height of the attack due to the acute oedema of the periorbital tissues, the reaction generally being non-specific, with the appearance of follicles in the lower fornix with hyperaemia in both the upper and the lower tarsal plates. The preauricular gland is palpable.

The changes in the bulbar conjunctiva in the acute phase consist of hyperaemia and oedema. In the delayed complications of the disease the conjunctiva may show hyperaemia associated with the nodular episcleritis or scleritis which may be one of the more common inflammatory sequelae. The scleritis may be diffuse or nodular and can be missed when the reaction is present in the upper part of the globe when it lies hidden beneath the upper lid. A thorough search of this region is important following HZO as such reactions can often explain persistent symptoms.

Corneal disease may take many different forms and can provide considerable problems in management. Herpes zoster dendritic keratitis has been described by Pavan-Langston and McCulley (1973). The dendritic figures are often subtle and may be multiple and small (Plate II*b*). Their significance is two-fold in that their presence is an indicator of ocular involvement, which has importance in determining a long-term prognosis, and at the same time should not be interpreted as demonstrating an associated attack of herpes simplex keratitis. Marsh et al. (1976) have described two distinct types of epithelial disease, an early dendritic form, and a delayed form characterised by corneal mucous plaques that may take a dendritiform pattern. The plaques are

PLATE II

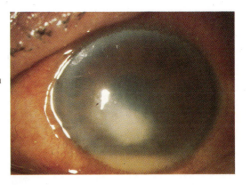

(a) Herpetic keratitis abscess with hypopyon uveitis.

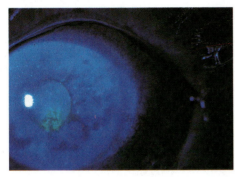

(b) Small dendritic ulcer in a patient with herpes zoster ophthalmicus.

(c) The end result in a patient with herpes zoster ophthalmicus, and disseminated varicella. He was immunodeficient, suffering from Hodgkin's disease, and had undergone treatment with radiotherapy and cytotoxic drugs. There was anterior segment necrosis, and vasculitis affecting the periorbital tissues.

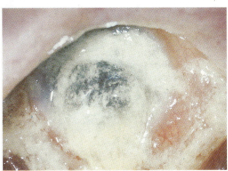

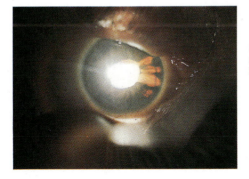

(d) Sectorial iris atrophy following herpes zoster ophthalmicus, demonstrated by slit-lamp transillumination through the pupil.

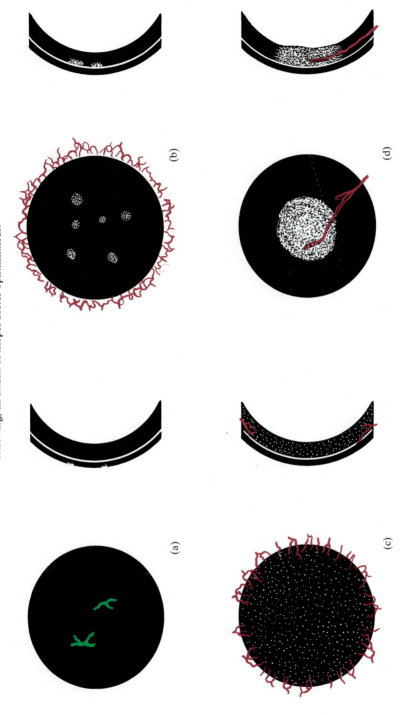

Figure 9.4. Schematic representation of the categories of corneal disease which can be seen in association with, or following, an attack of herpes zoster ophthalmicus.

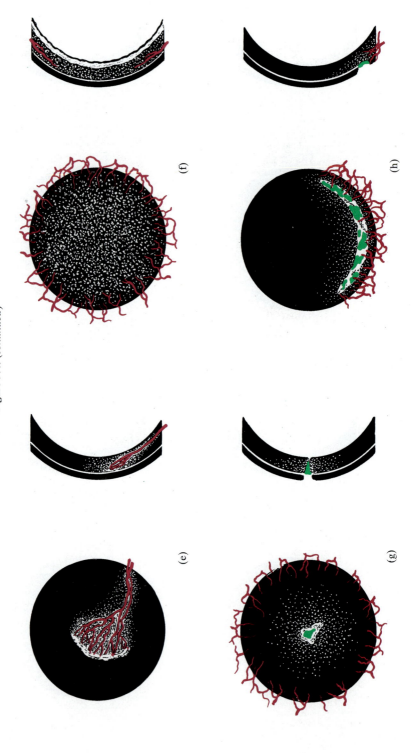

Figure 9.4. (*continued*)

(e)

(f)

(g)

(h)

Figure 9.4. (*continued*)

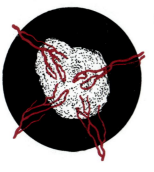

(j)

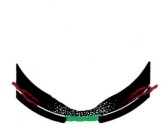

(i)

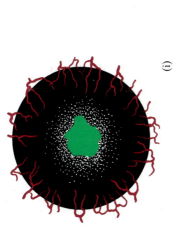

(a) Small dendritic figures
(b) Superficial stromal punctate keratitis
(c) Diffuse keratitis with stromal thickening and mild
infiltration
(d) Disciform opacity with vascularisation
(e) Permanent central corneal scar with lipid deposition and
vascularisation
(f) Diffuse stromal opacification and thickening, with
endothelial detachment
(g) Central corneal perforation in association with
anaesthesia and disciform keratitis
(h) Peripheral corneal melting syndrome associated with
rheumatoid arthritis on occasions
(i) Persistent central erosion
(j) Acute stromal abscess following cessation of topical
corticosteroid.

composed of mucus that is adherent to swollen, degenerating epithelial cells. The clinical differentiation between epithelial lesions in zoster and herpes simplex keratitis is considered essential, since topically applied corticosteroid is contra-indicated in epithelial disease due to herpes simplex, but is often indicated in the management of herpes zoster. Prior to reports of pure zoster-induced dendritic epithelial lesions, there have been accounts of a number of cases of suspect combined zoster and herpes simplex keratitis (Acers and Vaile, 1967; Giles, 1969; Sugar, 1971; Forrest and Kaufman, 1976). Although coincident disease may remain a possibility (Marsh *et al.*, 1976) it appears to be more likely that epithelial disease mimicking dendritic ulceration is due to replication of the varicella-zoster organism rather than a combined infection. Thus, in a review of 500 cases of ocular zoster seen by Marsh and his colleagues, only two cases of virologically proven herpes simplex dendritic keratitis could be found, whereas the incidence of dendritiform epithelial changes in this group was of the order of 13 per cent overall. In contrast to herpes simplex keratitis in which the ulcer presents a fine lacy appearance, with or without terminal end bulbs, the acute lesion in zoster is small, often stellate with a simple raised contour, and is situated usually in the periphery of the cornea. The delayed corneal lesion, which is due to the laying down of a mucous plaque, presents a coarse, elevated appearance, with obvious grey-white plaques (Figure 9.5). Rose bengal in herpes simplex infection stains the edge of the ulcer, while fluorescein stains the base of the ulcer. Zoster ulcers stain sparingly with rose bengal and fluorescein. In the case of the delayed mucous

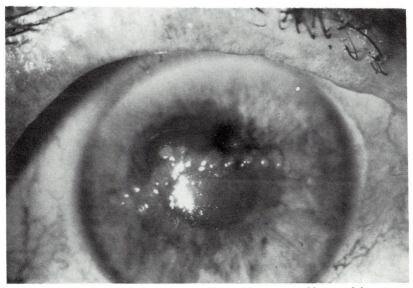

Figure 9.5. Mucous plaque deposits in a patient with a recent history of herpes zoster ophthalmicus.

plaque lesion, there is brilliant staining of the whole lesion with rose bengal, and sparse staining with fluorescein.

The stroma of the cornea may be affected in a large number of ways following an attack of herpes zoster ophthalmicus. The manifestations present a similar degree of variability as in the case of stromal herpes simplex keratitis. It nevertheless remains possible to distinguish several syndrome complexes which are characteristic and may allow the observer to determine the aetiology of the condition in the absence of the appropriate history. The common post-zoster pattern of corneal disease is the appearance of *punctate stromal opacities* which are situated in the superficial stromal layers (Figure 9.6). They are irregular in diameter and may be associated with cellular infiltration in their locality as determined with a high magnification on the slit-lamp microscope. A *focal keratitis* which may often extend into the centre of the cornea may initially bear similarities to a typical disciform keratitis as seen in herpes simplex keratitis, but later it may lead to permanent superficial stromal scarring with superficial stromal vascularisation (Figure 9.7). The surface overlying the inactive keratitis may be irregular or faceted, which may cause greater visual disturbance than the opacity itself.

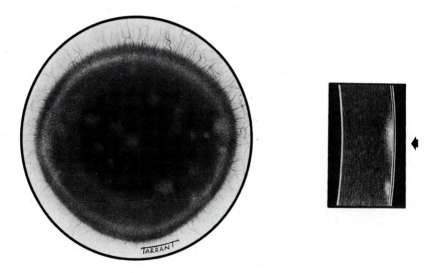

Figure 9.6.   Punctate stromal opacities in a patient with a history of herpes zoster ophthalmicus. (Courtesy, Professor Barrie Jones.)

Vascular responses occur in stromal disease, but are not specific in appearance. Vascular arcades often originate as a narrow band at the limbus branching out in the shape of a fan to eventually reach the periphery of a central corneal lesion. A characteristic deposit with the crystalline appearance of cholesterol may be seen at this edge, which may be the cause of the visual loss. Fluorescein angiography of corneal vessels in zoster keratitis demonstrate

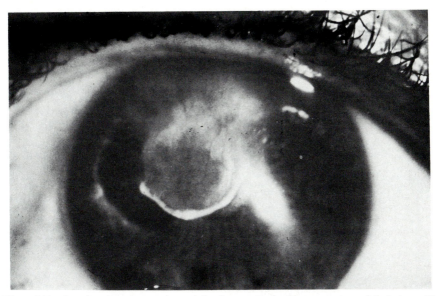

Figure 9.7.   Inactive central corneal scar following an attack of herpes zoster ophthalmicus with ocular involvement. There is lipid deposit at the edge of the scar which is vascularised.

an early and profuse loss of dye at the apex of the arcade, which is prominent in the region of lipid deposit, and it is possible that it originates from the intravascular compartment rather than from changes in the stroma alone. The permeability of these peripheral vessels would be expected to be pronounced during active inflammatory disease, and it is best explained by the presence of a hyperlipidaemia occurring during this time with a consequent 'overflow' of serum lipid into the stroma, forming a permanent deposition.

Focal keratitis presents a changing clinical pattern over a period of time, and careful attention should be paid to the interpretation of the clinical activity at the time of observation, as this largely determines the treatment of the condition. Disease activity is assessed according to the usual signs employed in the assessment of those patients with herpes simplex keratitis. The stroma may be thickened as shown by the use of the narrow beam of the slit-lamp; cellular infiltrates of various types may be seen which may be focal, diffuse and in one plane of the stroma, or closely related to the apices of ingrowing blood vessels. The blood vessels show activity which may often be difficult to determine without considerable clinical experience. The changes to be noted would include the appearance of hairpin bends at the apices of the vascular arcades which may not necessarily have reached the main focus of inflammatory disease, dilatation of the vascular systems, the presence of an extensive complex of vessels through which the circulation of blood is rapid, and the presence of inflammatory cells in the immediate neighbourhood of the proliferating vessels.

A *diffuse herpes zoster keratitis* can be recognised in which there is

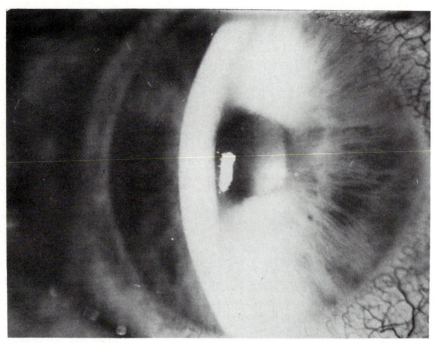

Figure 9.8. Diffuse stromal keratitis with mild cellular infiltration and stromal oedema following herpes zoster ophthalmicus six months after presentation. A sectorial defect in the iris indicated clearly the origin of the lesion.

generalised oedema of the stroma in association with mild cellular infiltration (Figure 9.8). The course may be mild and easily controlled with topical treatment with anti-inflammatory therapy. A *diffuse keratitis* with a more severe prognosis may occur in which the cellular infiltration is accompanied by oedema and vascularisation. The stromal oedema may be persistent and resistant to topical therapy, leading to the formation of a widely disseminated scar with permanent vascularisation and on occasions the separation of the endothelium with considerable disruption of the anterior chamber (Figure 9.9).

The presence of corneal anaesthesia following herpes zoster ophthalmicus has a bearing on the clinical course and the treatment which is chosen. In the presence of corneal anaesthesia, a disturbance of the integrity of the epithelium may lead to a *corneal erosion* which provides great difficulties in treatment, and may often seem to resist almost any form of therapy offered. The erosions develop from the coalescence of small abrasions, or may be induced by the use of an eye pad. The initial appearance may be seemingly benign, but if not treated immediately, may lead to a chronic lesion which defies all approaches to profitable management. Chronic erosions develop a heaped-up edge of inert epithelium with a deposit of mucus on the base. There is an associated area of stromal oedema and infiltration beneath, and a few blood vessels may encroach toward the central lesion. The edge of the ulcer develops a rolled appearance

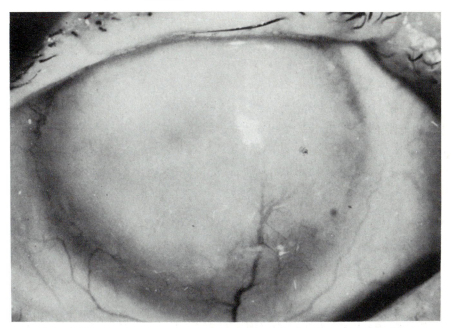

Figure 9.9. Diffuse corneal scarring and vascularisation following herpes zoster ophthalmicus. There was gross corneal thickening and on keratoplasty it was found that Descemet's membrane and the endothelium had become detached from the rest of the stroma.

and thereafter resists almost all attempts to change its natural course, which is, however, towards resolution, although over a period of months (Figure 9.10). These erosions are not entirely confined to patients who suffer from HZO, but occur in patients with corneal anaesthesia from a number of causes, such as section of the first division of the trigeminal nerve for neuralgia, or following keratoplasty, where corneal anaesthesia is one factor in the aetiology of the original condition. On clinical grounds it would seem that in addition to the presence of an anaesthetic cornea, the presence of mucus deposition is important in its induction. Mucoid discharge in the conjunctival sac should therefore be recorded and regarded as an adverse sign. The persistence of erosions creates a serious risk of secondary infection and cognisance of this must be taken in regard to management.

Keratitis leading to *corneal perforation* is a rare complication in HZO. The perforation may not only occur in association with a chronic central erosion, but may also occur at an early stage of treatment with corticosteroid in the presence of corneal anaesthesia. Similar disease has been seen where herpes zoster ophthalmicus has occurred in patients with rheumatoid arthritis. Such patients are occasionally at risk of spontaneous peripheral corneal melting syndrome occurring inside the limbal margin. The precise mechanism of this has not yet been elicited, but there is a possibility that the presence of virus antigen in the corneal stroma plays some part in the aetiology. We have seen

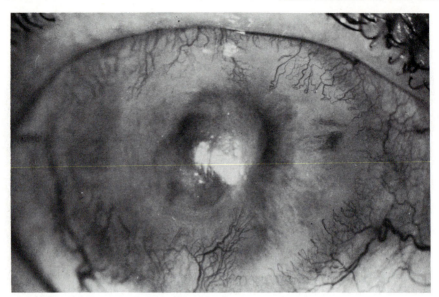

Figure 9.10.   An area of central corneal thinning is present just below and temporal to the visual axis. There is an associated epithelial deficit. The deficit eventually resolved with the help of a continuous-wear contact lens and regular observation.

patients with severe rheumatoid arthritis in whom corneal melting was apparently triggered by an attack of herpes zoster ophthalmicus with ocular disease. The patients suffered from both peripheral and central melting with eventual loss of the anterior chamber due to diffuse thinning and perforation. On replacement of the corneal tissue with a 13-mm transplant there was no recurrence of the melting process, which indicated the possible importance of the varicella zoster virus triggering the syndrome. However, although this is an attractive hypothesis, no evidence of the organism could be found on electron-microscopy of the disc of corneal tissue taken from the recipient. At the same time, previous experience in the peripheral corneal melting syndrome has shown high recurrence in patients who have undergone replacement of corneas following perforation, indicating that the immune mechanism involved is different, or that the same antigen exists in the donor as well as in the recipient cornea. Similar observations have been made by Mondino *et al.* (1978) where peripheral corneal ulcerations were reported following HZO (Figure 9.11).

Patients undergoing treatment with immunosuppressive or cytotoxic agents have long been known to be at risk of infective disease particularly with viral agents such as the varicella zoster virus. Similarly, patients with blood dyscrasias with secondary cell-mediated immunodeficiency are liable to develop a severe form of herpes zoster infection. A patient with Hodgkin's disease undergoing treatment with radiotherapy and chemotherapy developed an extremely severe eruption over the left side of the forehead with keratitis and uveitis. The eye became completely immobile with total ophthalmoplegia.

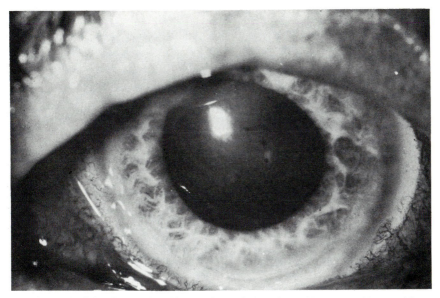

Figure 9.11.   Peripheral corneal melting syndrome in a patient with a recent history of herpes
zoster ophthalmicus. He also had inactive rheumatoid arthritis.

In addition to the HZO there was a severe generalised varicella eruption. Eventually the corneal endothelium lost all function and the cornea became grossly oedematous. The immobility of the eye was associated with poor lid closure, which compounded the effect of secondary infection associated with peripheral corneal melting. At the end of three weeks the eye perforated and eventually was removed (Plate IIc).

Atrophic changes may occur in the iris following corneal disease, the pigment epithelium becoming affected in the first instance, with eventual involvement of the sphincter pupillae. The atrophy may be subtle and only become visible by careful transillumination of the iris using a small central coaxial beam with the slit-lamp microscope (Figure 9.12 and Plate IId). The initial changes appear as specks but as the process develops, they increase in size and may coalesce to form a diffuse atrophy of a sector of iris tissue. The changes are mostly confined to the pigment epithelium, and there is often little abnormality to be seen in the stroma of the iris, apart from surface pigment mottling which is probably due to migration of pigment granules from the pigment epithelium. Where there is severe intra-ocular disease, the iris atrophy may be diffuse, with considerable effects on the size of the pupil, which can be unresponsive to light stimulation. Where sectorial atrophy has occurred, the pupil may be distorted, and the whole appearance may bear close similarities to the iris changes found following attacks of angle-closure glaucoma. Using fluorescein angiography it is possible to show that the sectorial atrophy is associated with local areas of ischaemia which precisely match the atrophic sectors, which supports the idea that in addition to perineural immune

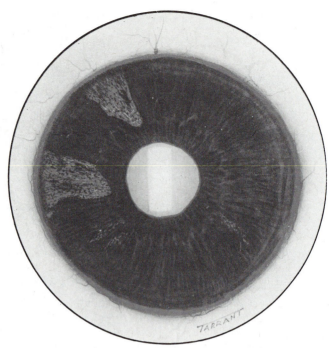

Figure 9.12. Iris atrophy associated with previous herpes zoster ophthalmicus. There is sectorial atrophy of the pigment epithelium. The stromal appearance is normal using indirect illumination.

responses, there are also changes in blood vessels which are probably secondary to previous vasculitis (Marsh *et al.*, 1974).

Where the initial attack of HZO was mild with minor involvement of the skin, the diagnosis of recurrent keratitis may not be obvious to the clinician, and it is particularly in such cases that confusion between keratitis due to varicella zoster and that due to herpes simplex virus may occur. The presence of sectorial atrophy can be helpful in arriving at the correct diagnosis, and if the diagnosis continues to remain unclear, iris angiography can be helpful, because the atrophy which may occasionally accompany herpes simplex keratitis is associated with patent iris vessels in contrast to the situation in varicella zoster infection. The pathogenesis of the often prolonged sequelae which occur in the eye following herpes zoster ophthalmicus is unclear. Figure 9.13 summarises some of the possible mechanisms involved in the production of disease of the anterior segment.

Herpes zoster ophthalmicus has been associated with diverse manifestations in the posterior pole, including papillitis, choroiditis, and retinal haemorrhage (Edgerton, 1945). There have been reports of a secondary granulomatous angitis rather than perineuritis, and some cases have been histologically confirmed (Kolodny *et al.*, 1968; Rosenblum and Hadfield, 1972). Evidence has also been recorded in a biopsy of the temporal artery (Victor and Green, 1976). Hesse (1977) reported a patient who developed retinal involvement

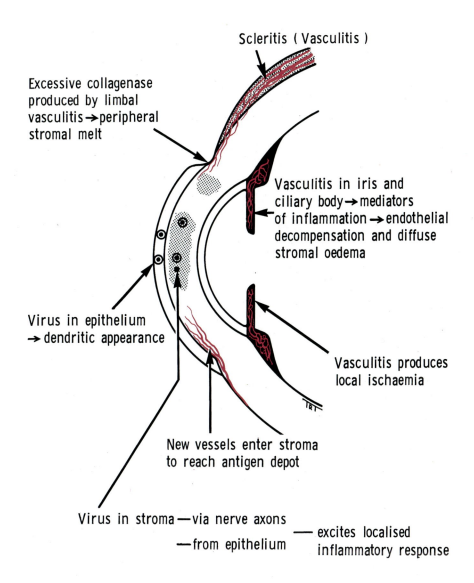

Figure 9.13. Immunopathogenesis of anterior segment disease resulting from herpes zoster ophthalmicus with ocular involvement.

following HZO, where fluorescein angiography revealed that the venous system was primarily involved in the vascular inflammation.

In 1968, a survey of 21 eyes by Naumann *et al.*, revealed considerable perivascular cuffing with lymphocytes, with striking infiltration of the long posterior ciliary nerves. Retinal thrombophlebitis may lead to severe subhyaloid and vitreous haemorrhage.

Treatment

Ophthalmic zoster is often a sadly neglected disease in ophthalmology because of its many facets of presentation, its chronicity in certain patients, and its severity in others. On occasions the original attack of zoster may be forgotten and the condition treated as herpes simplex virus disease, when the treatment regime can produce more severe disease due to the toxic effects that follow the use of antiviral therapy in the long term.

Many patients who suffer from ophthalmic zoster are elderly, frail and infirm, and therefore need immediate admission. However, once admitted it should be remembered that such cases represent a source of infection for those who have not previously contracted the disease, and there is therefore a necessity for barrier nursing and for isolation. It is important that infants and children should be kept away from these patients, together with nursing staff with a negative history of varicella. The secondary infection which can often occur provides a further source of bacteria, representing a hazard to those awaiting intra-ocular surgery as well as for those in whom surgical procedures have been carried out.

Post-herpetic neuralgia is a poorly understood and somewhat neglected complication which is only too common in many elderly patients. The pain is usually severe in the first 2 weeks, and then it may regress. Drugs such as Distalgesic, Fortral or DF118 can be tried, but if no therapeutic effect is obtained, resort should be made to stronger analgesics such as pethidine. In post-herpetic neuralgia, there may be paraesthesia or a constant ache, often located to a maximal area of pain with the original dermatomal distribution of the eruption. Patients may complain particularly of pain around the eyebrow, about the inner third. The incidence of severe neuralgia is of the order of 7 per cent. Antidepressants can be useful for the depression which often occurs following an attack, and amitriptyline has proved to be particularly useful. Where secondary infection of the skin or the eye occurs, topical application of antibiotics is clearly indicated. Antibiotic/steroid combinations as ointments have proved to be useful in the treatment of the skin eruption, seeming to prevent the formation of the severe crusts which are a frequent consequence of the condition. The good response of the skin eruption to the use of topical steroid is paradoxical, in view of the known tendency for patients who are either immunodeficient or undergoing treatment with immunosuppressive drugs to develop more severe forms of zoster attacks. Calamine lotion is not indicated, as it appears to perform no useful function and may help to prolong the discomfort of the patient (Figure 9.14).

The use of topical corticosteroid/antibiotic combinations in the eye during the acute phase of the condition has been recommended where the lid vesicles are discharging and forming crusts, and even though there may be a

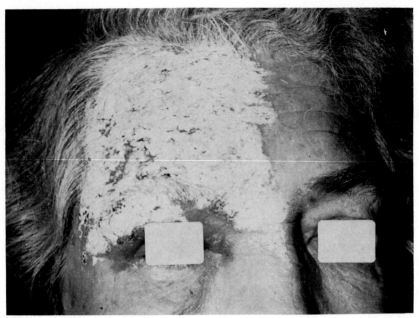

Figure 9.14. Treatment with calamine of the cutaneous eruption in herpes zoster ophthalmicus does not seem to perform any useful function, and there is the risk of contamination of vesicles. The use of antibiotics or antibiotic/steroid combinations is thought to reduce the severity of the crusts. (Courtesy, Mr. Ronald Marsh.)

mucopurulent conjunctivitis (Marsh, 1976). It would be clearly important to exclude secondary invaders by conjunctival swabbing prior to the initiation of topical steroid therapy, so that the appropriate antibiotic may be chosen for any pathogenic organisms which might be found. Antibiotic therapy remains important in the treatment in the various manifestations of corneal hypo-aesthesia but the same antibiotic should not be employed for long periods in view of the risk of inducing resistant organisms.

The use of topical corticosteroid is one of the anchors in successful management of the anterior-segment complications in HZO. The various forms of keratitis can be treated with steroid without the fears which beset the clinician in the management of herpes simplex keratitis, although topical steroid can occasionally lead to more serious complications by indirect routes. It must be emphasised that once steroids have been started and maintained for a length of time, it may prove difficult to terminate the therapy without exciting a severe rebound or recurrence of stromal inflammation which can prove more severe than the original attack (Plate IIIa). Thus, careful tapering off of therapy, through dilutions of steroid with reduction in the rate of instillation, can help to prevent what can often seem to be a catastrophic loss of vision long after the original disease has regressed. In the early treatment of corneal disease, the principles which apply to the treatment of herpes simplex keratitis should also apply to the treatment of zoster. The minimal dosage of topical therapy which is successful in achieving a therapeutic effect should be used. The use of potent steroid in the initial management may result in rapid clearing of the stroma, but in the long term it may prove difficult to taper the therapy off. In contrast, where less potent steroids such as prednisolone drops (0.5, 0.25, 0.125 and 0.05 per cent) are employed less difficulty can be encountered in weaning the patient off therapy.

Disease in the corneal stroma probably represents the immunological response to the presence of viral antigen which has become trapped in the tissue. It seems evident that there is also a second element in ocular disease, taking the form of a vasculitis which may affect the sclera or the iris. Frequently the iritis may be accompanied by a rise in the intra-ocular pressure, and it is in these conditions that the use of the more potent corticosteroid preparations such as dexamethasone and betamethasone are helpful. It may on occasions be impossible to see why the intra-ocular pressure becomes elevated in HZO as the causes may be single or multiple, as in other inflammatory disease of the anterior segment, and it is important to carry out a complete examination in order to define the mechanisms early in the disease process. This must include the use of gonioscopy for examination of the angle of the anterior chamber. Although in many patients corticosteroid usage can result in a reduction of pressure, on occasions the elevation may persist, when a secondary response resulting from the steroid itself must be considered. If such is the case, the steroid should be terminated for a period and the intra-ocular pressure monitored during this interval. If the pressure shows a tendency to fall, dilute steroid preparations should be employed, or alternatively those preparations which have a lesser tendency towards inducing a rise of pressure in positive responders, such as clobetasone butyrate, or fluorometholone drops should be used. The scleritis in zoster can prove extremely persistent and refractory to treatment, and because of this, secondary cataract formation may occur if the patient is not kept under adequate supervision.

The use of systemic steroid has been claimed to have advantages for the patient in that it has been thought to result in less severe post-herpetic neuralgia (Scheie, 1970), but the evidence for this is unconvincing, and on clinical grounds it would seem to be unacceptable in view of the serious disease which can occur in immunosuppressed patients. In patients who have presented with the more serious forms of the disease, such as those with proptosis, third-nerve palsies, or ischaemic optic neuropathy, consideration of such therapy must be balanced against theoretical possibilities that further deterioration can be induced. Since it has not proved possible to perform useful therapeutic trials to compare such therapeutic models in the more serious forms of HZO, it would seem that conservative management would be the treatment of choice. On occasions where there is persistent, unremitting scleritis which fails to respond to topical corticosteroid, the use of systemic prostaglandin antagonists has been shown to have some therapeutic effect (Watson et al., 1966).

Damage to the mechanisms which operate to produce a stable precorneal tear film may occur in HZO. Artificial tears can help to prevent the formation of dry spots, while the use of mucolytic agents such as acetylcysteine can be helpful in reducing the formation of mucous plaque.

The formation of a large, persistent corneal erosion in the presence of corneal anaesthesia can be troublesome, and is associated with mucus deposition in the base of the ulcer. It is helpful to remove the plaque in such cases, and thereafter the use of a high-water-content contact lens can be of considerable aid. However, such lenses in the presence of corneal anaesthesia are not without risk of inducing secondary infection or perforation, and it is important that follow-up is maintained until the epithelium has regenerated to cover the eroded area. At the same time, the understanding and co-operation of the patient must be obtained, and an explanation alerting him to the symptoms and signs suggestive of secondary corneal infection should be provided.

The value of topical or systemic antiviral therapy in herpes zoster infection remains unclear. Trials using intravenous cytosine arabinoside have been carried out (Pierce and Jenkins, 1973) which not unexpectedly provided unclear results in view of the difficulties in obtaining suitable control patients. These difficulties were highlighted by a study in which those on placebo showed as much improvement as those undergoing treatment with cytosine arabinoside (Stevens et al., 1973; Wellings, 1979). Cytosine arabinoside has been utilised systemically for varicella or zoster in patients undergoing immunosuppression. Controlled trials have revealed little evidence that the source of zoster has been improved (Merigan, 1981).

Adenine arbinoside given intravenously has been investigated. Adenine arabinoside was given at the dose of 10 mg per kg for seven days. The effects on the healing of the rash, post-herpetic neuralgia, and the development of ocular complications were studied in 24 patients. The trial was randomised in accordance with three criteria: the severity of the rash, the length of time that the rash had existed before treatment, and whether ocular complications were apparent at presentation or not. Although clinically there appeared to be a more rapid healing of the rash and quicker resolution of conjunctival hyperaemia, with a lesser chance of the development of episcleritis and with postponement of corneal sensitivity loss, these effects were not statistically significant (Marsh et al., 1981a). There is a real hope that systemic treatment with acyclovir as tablets, which is now undergoing clinical trials, will prove to be beneficial in all forms of herpes zoster.

The effect of levamisole, which restores T-cell and macrophage function, has also been investigated in a double-blind controlled trial in ophthalmic zoster (Marsh et al., 1981b). In forty-seven patients who were assessed in this trial, the only statistically significant finding in favour of levamisole was a more rapid resolution of mucus in the tear film. There was less rapid healing of the rash in the levamisole patients than in those taking the placebo. There were a significant number of adverse reactions. In particular, levamisole did not influence the severity or duration of post-herpetic neuralgia. It has a number of recognised complications, including nausea, gastric intolerance, central nervous stimulation, irritability, a 'flu-like syndrome, skin rashes and granulocytopenia.

The influence of topical acyclovir in herpes zoster disease of the eye has been investigated by McGill (1981). In fifteen out of eighteen patients treated with topical acyclovir the ocular disease subsided after a short course of treatment, and lasting ocular damage was minimised. There were no recurrences after treatment had been stopped. Herpes zoster kerato-uveitis, which can persist for months, also quickly resolved. When steroids were added to the regime, treatment was prolonged and the disease recurred once therapy was stopped. This suggests that non-productive viral antigen still existed within the deeper tissues.

The influence of interferon in ophthalmic zoster has been investigated by Sundmacher *et al.* (1981). In a placebo-controlled trial to evaluate the effect of systemic interferon while employing topical corticosteroids for zoster keratitis and iritis, no major difference could be found in the incidence of epithelial virus disease, iritis, or nummular keratitis. It was concluded that systemic interferon therapy starting at the sixth day of the illness did not improve the course of the disease. There was an impression that additional interferon exerted some positive effects which were shown by a quicker improvement of iritis and a less sudden appearance of corneal opacities. Intramuscular leucocyte interferon appeared to shorten the course of zoster in immunosuppressed individuals (Merigan *et al.*, 1978).

Local treatment of the cutaneous eruption is considered to be valuable by Juel-Jensen and MacCallum (1972). Success or failure in any treatment will rest on its ability to shorten the spells of pain – both the acute pain early in the disease and the persistent neuralgia which is one of the most harrowing aspects. The uncomplicated zoster eruption may be treated by the continuous application of idoxuridine in dimethylsulphoxide (DMSO). A piece of lint is cut to the shape of the lesion, thoroughly soaked in a 40 per cent solution of idoxuridine in DMSO, and applied to the lesion. Two larger pieces of lint are then applied over the first piece and taped into position. The procedure is continued for four days and more solution of antiviral is applied every visit. It is considered that such treatment curtails the duration of pain in zoster. Juel-Jensen and MacCallum (1972) reported a significant reduction in pain in a placebo-controlled trial investigating the value of such methods. Few adverse complications have been noted due to the use of DMSO there being no evidence of systemic toxicity in a large number of patients. There also is no evidence of ocular damage, although it is essential that the IDU/DMSO solution must not be introduced into the eye. Where treatment is started too late, the results have not been successful and persistent pain has remained. Failures were those in whom the eruption had existed for at least one week before treatment was initiated. Benefit to patients can only be obtained by following the method of application as originally described.

The treatment of the corneal disease with topical antivirals would seem logical where there is evidence of epithelial disease in the early stages, and even where there is no such evidence it would not be harmful to instil drops as a prophylactic against proliferation of the virus in the epithelium. Where it is not possible to examine patients because of the considerable lid oedema present, it would seem that antiviral therapy is justified. However, where the ocular disease is delayed and there is stromal keratitis, prolonged treatment with antiviral agents can be damaging both to the epithelium of the cornea and to the conjunctiva.

Persistent scarring in the corneal stroma may be helped with a corneal graft.

Because the disease is one predominantly found in the aged, the clinical indications are comparatively rare. Keratoplasty is carried out as an emergency if perforation, often the result of injudicious use of topical corticosteroid, has occurred. Occasionally following severe disease the endothelium may become separated or detached from the stromal layer, producing pronounced corneal oedema. Corneal anaesthesia is an added hazard which can mitigate against a successful keratoplasty. It is therefore the impression that the success rate in HZO for keratoplasty is not high, and unless there are good indications it would seem inadvisable to perform such procedures. Figure 9.15 demonstrates a successful keratoplasty in a patient with diffuse corneal opacification following herpes zoster ophthalmicus.

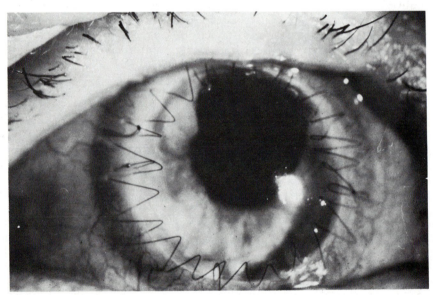

Figure 9.15.   Successful corneal transplant in a patient with diffuse corneal opacification and a secondary cataract due to herpes zoster ophthalmicus.

There are many forms of zoster keratitis, as has already been pointed out. A corneal melting process can be set up in the centre of the cornea or at the periphery. When there is corneal anaesthesia it is particularly important that care be taken in the use of topical steroid, as on occasions sudden perforation has occurred. Peripheral melting syndromes, particularly in association with rheumatoid arthritis, can be extremely difficult to treat. Central melting syndrome has also been recorded in association with rheumatoid arthritis. Whether the melting process is related to the rheumatoid arthritis or to the fact that many of the patients are on low dosages of immunosuppressive and anti-inflammatory drugs is not clear. The treatment modes advocated for the peripheral corneal melting syndrome are probably indicated also in the treatment of melting diseases associated with herpes zoster ophthalmicus.

Thus l-cysteine or acetyl cysteine drops should be tried because of their anti-collagenolytic activity. Because cases are rare it is impossible to know whether limbectomy, which has been advocated for the treatment of peripheral corneal melting syndrome, can be expected to be helpful. In such cases careful supervision is the most important step that can be taken. Admission is often necessary to ensure that the therapy given will not lead to a worsening of the disease. Gel contact lenses can be used on in-patients and frequently on monitored out-patients too, but it must be remembered that lenses have been known to be associated with secondary corneal infection. Success has been experienced with a central melting syndrome associated with a persistent corneal erosion which eventually epithelialised with a continuous-wear contact lens. Where the melting process carries on relentlessly, a large anterior segment graft can be carried out, although the success of such procedures has not been impressive. However, it is unlikely that the central melting process recurs in the donor tissue, in contrast to peripheral corneal melting syndromes, either associated with other diseases or in isolation, where the donor disc can be attacked and destroyed by a process which appears to be exactly similar to the one preceding the keratoplasty. There is a valuable place for the use of histoacrylate glue, given in the immediate treatment of corneal perforation. Careful application can result in a reformation of the anterior chamber, which allows time for donor corneal tissues to be obtained. It is also possible that the melting process will resolve, and regeneration of stromal tissue occur, so that a keratoplasty is no longer required.

In conclusion, the treatment of both the rash and the ocular disease in herpes zoster ophthalmicus can give rise to serious problems. It remains to be seen whether the use of topical or systemic preparations of the more recent antivirals will be effective in reducing the severity of both the skin eruption and the post-herpetic neuralgia. At the present time it is considered that careful application of idoxuridine with dimethylsulphoxide does have a beneficial effect on the rash. It is vital that secondary infection is prevented, and at the same time steps should be taken to reduce the inflammatory response by using topical application of a corticosteroid to the eruption. Where eye disease occurs it is important to assess the intra-ocular pressure at regular intervals. In many cases of kerato-uveitis a rise may occur. Patients may also undergo a pressure response following the use of topical corticosteroid. It follows that short-term topical antibodies should be used in these patients. In keratitis there is a rapid response to corticosteroid, with clearing of the stroma. Once corticosteroids have been introduced it is essential to monitor the patient closely, and also to taper down steroid by dilution over many weeks, as it is felt by many that a more serious keratitis may result from a rebound of inflammation on sudden curtailment of steroid therapy. In the case of iritis with sectorial atrophy of the iris, aggressive treatment with corticosteroid is not often necessary. Patients with zoster uveitis do not appear to get posterior synechiae.

REFERENCES

ACERS, T. E. and VAILE, V. (1967). Coexistent herpes zoster and herpes simplex. *Amer. J. Ophthal.*, **63**, 992–3.

EDGERTON, A. E. (1945). Herpes zoster ophthalmicus. Report of cases and review of literature. *Amer. J. Ophthal.*, **34**: July, Aug.

ELLENBERGER, C. (1952). Case of phthisis bulbi due to chickenpox. *Arch. Ophthal.*, **47**, 352–53.

ESIRI, M. M. and TOMLINSON, A. H. (1972). Herpes zoster: Demonstration of virus in trigeminal nerve and ganglion by immunofluorescence and electron microscopy. *J. Neurol. Sci.*, **15**, 35–48.

FORREST, W. M. and KAUFMAN, H. E. (1976). Zosteriform herpes simplex. *Amer. J. Ophthal.*, **81**, 86–8.

GARLAND, J. (1943). Varicella following exposure to herpes zoster. *New Engl. J. Med.*, **228**, 336–37.

GHATAK, N. R. and ZIMMERMAN, H. M. (1973). Spinal ganglion in herpes zoster: A light and electron microscopic study. *Arch. Path.*, **95**, 411–5.

GILES, C. L. (1969). Coexisting herpes zoster and herpes simplex ocular involvement. *Eye, Ear, Nose Thr. Monthly*, **48**, 216–8.

GOLD, E. and NANKERVIS, G. A. (1973). Varicella-zoster viruses. In: *The Herpesviruses*, p. 327. Ed. A. S. Kaplan. New York: Academic Press.

HESSE, R. J. (1977). Herpes zoster ophthalmicus associated with delayed retinal thrombophlebitis. *Amer. J. Ophthal.*, **84**, 329–31.

JORDAN, G. W. and MERRIGAN, T. C. (1974). Cell-mediated immunity to varicella-zoster virus: *in vitro* lymphocyte responses. *J. infect. Dis.*, **130**, 495–501.

JUEL-JENSEN, B. E. and MacCALLUM, F. O. (1972). *Herpes Simplex Varicella and Zoster: Clinical Manifestations and Treatment*. London: Wm. Heinemann Medical Books.

KOLODNY, E. H., REIBEIZ, J. J. CAVINESS, V. S. and RICHARDSON, E. P. (1968). Granulomatous angiitis of the central nervous system. *Arch. Neurol.* **19**, 310.

KUNDRATITZ, K. (1925). Experimentelle libertragung von Herpes Zoster auf den Menschen und die Beziehungen von Herpes Zoster zu Varicellen. *Mschr. Kinderheilk.*, **29**, 516.

LEONARD, L. L., SCHMIDT, M. J. and LENNETTE, E. H. (1970). Demonstration of viral antibody activity in two immunoglobulin G subclasses—patients with varicella-zoster infection. *J. Immunol.*, **104**, 23–7.

LIPSCHUTZ, B. (1921). Untersuchungen uber die Atiologie der Krankheiten der Herpesgruppe (Herpes zoster, Herpes genitalis, Herpes febrilis). *Arch. Derm. Syph. (Berl.)*, **136**, 428.

McGILL, J. (1981). Topical acyclovir in herpes zoster ocular involvement. *Brit. J. Ophthal.*, **65**, 542–550.

MANSON, M. M., LOGAN, W. P. D. and LOY, R. M. (1960). *Rubella and other infections during pregnancy*. Report 101, pp 1–101. London: Her Majesty's Stationery Office.

MARSH, R. J. (1976). Current management of ophthalmic herpes zoster. *Trans. ophthal. Soc. U.K.*, **96**, 334–7.

MARSH, R. J., DULLEY, B. and KELLY, V. (1977). External ocular motor palsies in ophthalmic zoster: a review. *Brit. J. Ophthal.*, **61**, 677–682.

MARSH, R. J., EASTY, D. L. and JONES, B. R. (1974). Iritis and iris atrophy in herpes zoster ophthalmicus. *Amer. J. Ophthal.*, **78**, 253–261.

MARSH, R. J., FRAUNFELDER, F. T. and McGILL, J. I. (1976). Herpetic corneal epithelial disease. *Arch. Ophthal.*, **94**, 1899–1902.

MARSH, R. J., LAIRD, R., ATKINSON, A. and STEELE, A. McD. (1981*a*). A controlled trial of intravenous therapy with adenine arabinoside (Ara-A) in ophthalmic zoster. In: *Herpetic Eye Diseases*. Ed. R. Sundmacher. Munich: J. F. Bergmann Verlag.

MARSH, R. J., OLSEN, L., WEATHERHEAD, R. and JONES, B. R. (1981*b*). A double-blind controlled trial of therapy with levamisole in ophthalmic zoster. In: *Herpetic Eye Diseases*. Ed. R. Sundmacher. Munich: J. F. Bergmann Verlag.

MERIGAN, T. C. (1981). Systemic application of antivirals for herpes infections A247. In: *Herpetic Eye Diseases*. Ed. R. Sundmacher. Munich: J. F. Bergmann Verlag.

MERIGAN, T. C., RAND, K. H., POLLARD, R. B. *et al.* (1978). Human leukocyte interferon for the treatment of herpes zoster in patients with cancer. *New Engl. J. Med.*, **298**, 981–7.

MEYERS, J. D. (1974). Congenital varicella in term infants: Risk reconsidered. *J. infect. Dis.*, **129**, 215–7.

MONDINO, B. J., BROWN, S. I. and MONDZELEWSKI, J. P. (1978). Peripheral corneal ulcers with herpes zoster ophthalmicus. *Amer. J. Ophthal.*, **86**, 611–4.

NAUMANN, G., GASS, J. D. M. and FONT, R. L. (1968). Histopathology of herpes zoster ophthalmicus. *Amer. J. Ophthal.*, **65**, 533–41.

NESBURN, A. B., BORIT, A., PENTELEI-MOLNAR, J. and LAZARO, R. (1974). Varicella dendritic keratitis. *Invest. Ophthal.*, **13**, 764–70.

OBERG, G. and SVEDMYR, A. (1969). Varicelliform eruptions in herpes zoster—some clinical and serological observations. *Scand. J. infect. Dis.*, **1**, 47.

PALUSUO, T. (1972). Varicella and herpes zoster: Differences in antibody response revealed by the platelet aggregation technique. *Scand. J. infect. Dis.*, **4**, 83.

PAVAN-LANGSTON, D. and McCULLEY, J. P. (1973). Herpes zoster dendritic keratitis. *Arch. Ophthal.*, **89**, 25–9.

PIERCE, L. E. and JENKINS, R. B. (1973). Herpes zoster ophthalmicus treated with cytarabine. *Arch. Ophthal.*, **89**, 21–24.

ROSENBLUM, W. I. and HADFIELD, M. G. (1972). Granulomatous angiitis of the nervous system in cases of herpes zoster and lymphosarcoma. *Neurology (Minneap.)*, **22**, 348–54.

ROSS, C. A. C. and McDAID, R. (1972). Specific IgM antibody in serum of patients with herpes zoster infections. *Brit. med. J.*, **4**, 522–3.

RUSSELL, A. S., MAINI, R. A., BAILEY, M. and DUMONDE, D. C. (1972). Cell mediated immunity to varicella-zoster antigen in acute herpes zoster (shingles). *Clin. exp. Immunol.*, **14**, 185–7.

SCHEIE, H. G. (1970). Herpes zoster ophthalmicus. *Trans. ophthal. Soc. U.K.*, **90**, 899.

SCHOOL EPIDEMICS COMMITTEE OF GREAT BRITAIN. (1938). *Epidemics in Schools*. Medical Research Council, Special Report, Series No 227, London: His Majesty's Stationery Office.

SOUHAMI, R. L., BABBAGE, J. and SIGFUSSON, A. (1983). Antibody dependent cell cytotoxicity against varicella zoster infected human fibroblasts. *International Herpesvirus Workshop, Oxford*, p. 111.

STEINER, (1875). Zur Inokulation der varicellen. *Wien. med. Wschr.*, **25**, 306.

STEVENS, D. A., JORDAN, G. W., WADDELL, T. F. and MERIGAN, T. C. (1973). Adverse effect of cytosine arabinoside on disseminated zoster in a controlled trial. *New Engl. J. Med.*, **289**, 873–8.

STEVENS, D. A. and MERIGAN, T. C. (1972). Interferon, antibody and other host factors in herpes zoster. *J. clin. Invest.*, **51**, 1170–8.

SUGAR, H. S. (1971). Herpetic keratouveitis. Clinical experiences. *Ann. Ophthal.*, **3**, 355.

SUNDMACHER, R., NEUMANN-HAEFELIN, D. and CANTELL, K. (1981). Trials with interferon in ophthalmic zoster. In: *Herpetic Eye Diseases*. Ed. R. Sundmacher. Munich: J. F. Bergmann Verlag.

TYZZER, E. E. (1906). The history of skin lesions in varicella. *Philipp. J. Sci.*, **1**, 349.

VICTOR, D. I. and GREEN, W. R. (1976). Temporal artery biopsy in herpes zoster ophthalmicus with delayed arteritis. *Amer. J. Ophthal.*, **82**, 628–30.

WATSON, P. G., LOBASCHER, D. J., SABISTON, D. W., LEWIS-FANING, E., FOWLER, P. D. and JONES, B. R. (1966). Double blind trial of treatment of episcleritis-scleritis with oxyphenbutazone or prednisolone. *Brit. J. Ophthal.*, **50**, 463–81.

WELLER, T. H. (1976). Varicella-herpes zoster virus. In: *Viral Infections of Humans*, p. 457. Ed. A. S. Evans. Chichester: John Wiley & Sons.

WELLINGS, P. C. (1979). Assessment of cytosine arabinoside in the management of herpes zoster ophthalmicus. *Trans. Ophthal. Soc. N.Z.*, **31**, 64–68.

YUCHIDA, Y., KANKKO, M. and HAYASHI, K. (1980). Varicella dendritic keratitis. *Amer. J. Ophthal.*, **89**, 259.

CHAPTER TEN

The Adenoviruses

ANDREW TULLO

THE adenoviruses are a large, important group of DNA viruses which infect man and other species. Thirty-five immunologically distinct serotypes have been described among those of human origin, and they most commonly cause upper respiratory, ocular and gastro-intestinal disease.

The virus particle (70–80 nm diameter) has a DNA core surrounded by a capsid of 252 capsomeres arranged to form a icosahedron (Figure 10.1). Two hundred and forty of the capsomeres are known as hexons, each having six neighbouring capsomeres. The hexons are associated with the common group antigen, which enable the complement fixation test and the immunofluorescence test to distinguish the particle as an adenovirus. The type specificity, as determined by neutralisation tests, is a property of another hexon-associated antigen. The 12 capsomeres at the apices of the icosahedron are called pentons, each consisting of a base and fibre. The haemagglutination properties of the virus relate to the fibre. This latter function was used by Rosen (1960) to subdivide the human adenoviruses into three main sub-groups (Table 10.1).

TABLE 10.1

GROUPING OF ADENOVIRUSES

Serotypes	Haemagglutination Property
Group I 3, 7, 11, 14, 21	agglutinate rhesus monkey, but not rat RBC
Group II 8, 9, 10, 13, 19, 30	agglutinate rat, but not rhesus monkey RBC. (Also only group which agglutinate human group 'O' RBC)
Group III 1, 2, 4, 5, 6	partially agglutinate rat RBC only

This classification can be used to emphasise some clinical and epidemiological features of the more common serotypes causing eye disease. For example, it is the serotypes of Group II which are most frequently associated with the more severe ocular disease of epidemic keratoconjunctivitis (EKC).

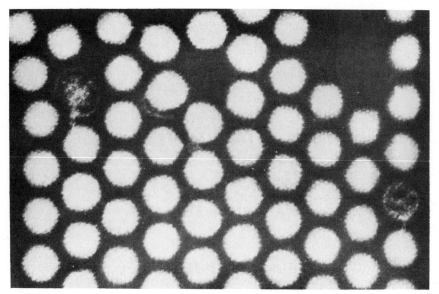

Figure 10.1. Electron micrograph of a negatively stained preparation of adenovirus. Virions (70–80 nm diameter) show the icosahedral arrangement of capsomeres (× 120 000).

Hybridisation of different types has been achieved experimentally (Golden *et al.*, 1971) and the appreciation recently that there are circulating strains which display marked cross-reactivity to neutralising antibody (Hierholzer and Rodriguez, 1981) suggest that this process may occur spontaneously, perhaps during simultaneous outbreaks of two types (Schaap *et al.*, 1979).

The development of new techniques is providing the basis for more detailed classification of the adenoviruses (Wadell, 1979), which by generally concurring with each other emphasise how the molecular biology of adenoviruses can be seen to influence their clinical and epidemiological features. One such relatively recent introduction to the study of viruses has been the method of restriction site mapping of DNA. Bacterial endonucleases are used to cleave the viral DNA and the fragments are subsequently separated by gel electrophoresis. Such a process is likely to form a more fundamental basis for classification than the present serological methods of neutralisation and haemagglutination which rely on antigenic determinants representing less than 1 per cent of the virus genome (Wadell and de Jong, 1980). Restriction endonuclease analysis may also show up differences between isolates with different biological activities but which are serologically identical (Wadell and Varsanyi, 1978).

History

The first description of a member of this group of viruses was made by Rowe *et al.* in 1953. Isolation of other immunologically distinct types followed rapidly, and by the time 12 types had been described, the term adenovirus had been adopted, the first isolation having been made from human adenoidal tissue. Since then, outbreaks of disease caused by these agents have been reported regularly, not least by ophthalmologists, and an impressive literature has accumulated. The numbered serotypes which are known to cause spontaneous infections of the eyes are: 1, 2, 3, 4, 5, 6, 7, 8; and less commonly 9, 10, 11, 13, 14, 15, 19, 20, 21, 22, 23, 24, 29 (Bell *et al.*, 1960; *British Journal of Ophthalmology*, 1977). Yet other serotypes have been shown to produce disease when introduced into the eyes of volunteers (Locatcher-Khorazo and Seegal, 1972*a*).

The term epidemic keratoconjunctivitis (EKC) was introduced by Hogan and Crawford in 1942 following particularly large and severe epidemics of eye disease on the west coast of America. The condition also acquired the name at that time of 'shipyard eye'. Similar outbreaks had been reported previously in several European and Asian countries under a variety of different names (Locatcher-Khorazo and Seegal, 1972*b*), following the first report by Fuchs in 1889. The early descriptions of clinical details can hardly be improved (Swanzy, 1915).

When the causative organism of such outbreaks was identified as adenovirus type 8 in 1955 (Jawetz *et al.*) this serotype rapidly gained notoriety for the ease with which it could be spread, especially from and within eye units (Thygeson, 1957; Davidson, 1964; Barnard *et al.*, 1973).

Until recently, ocular infection by adenovirus type 8 was synonymous with EKC, but now other serotypes belonging to Rosen's haemagglutination Group II are recognised as being capable of causing similarly severe disease, namely types 10, 19, 10/19*, and 10/19/13/30* (Zografos, 1977; Desmyter *et al.*, 1974; Tullo and Higgins, 1979; Schaap *et al.*, 1979). The more recent outbreaks, including those caused by type 8, have been smaller than those previously reported. This may reflect a greater awareness amongst ophthalmologists of the potential hazard these serotypes present to themselves and their patients. Alternatively it may be that there is a reduction in the virulence of currently circulating strains.

Epidemiology

It is difficult to make an accurate estimation of the incidence of eye disease caused by adenoviruses. Some cases are treated by general practitioners and others are probably trivial or transient so that medical advice is not sought. In those presenting to an eye unit, investigation may be carried out with a varying degree of thoroughness and even when the cause of probable viral conjunctivitis is actively sought there are cases which escape diagnosis. Isolation of the virus becomes unlikely if swabs are taken when infectivity is falling off, and paired samples of serum must be taken at optimum times to produce diagnostic results. Records at the Bristol Eye Hospital suggest that possible viral conjunctivitis affects up to 6 per cent of patients attending the casualty department and that in 21 per cent of these an adenovirus is the causal agent (Tullo, 1980).

Despite the lack of pathognomonic features of adenovirus eye infection, the combination of clinical and epidemiological findings may produce a charac-

---

* These recently identified intermediate types have now been allocated the separate identity of Adenovirus type 37 (deJong *et al.*, 1981).

teristic picture. The term epidemic keratoconjunctivitis (EKC) is used to describe outbreaks where there is clustering of cases, typically around and within a hospital eye department. A significant degree of corneal involvement is implied by this term.

In the Western world, antibodies to serotypes causing EKC are rare in the normal population (Barnard *et al.*, 1973; Tullo and Higgins, 1979). Apart from the inherent pathogenicity of Group II adenoviruses for the eye, spread in the community is clearly aided by absence of type-specific antibody in the population. However, in the Orient, type 8 infection is encountered commonly in children, producing a systemic upset with absent or transient eye involvement. This early endemic exposure produces an immunity of up to 33 per cent in the adult population and consequently explosive outbreaks of eye disease in adults are rare (Jawetz *et al.*, 1956). A 33-year-old man was recently seen in Bristol, who had developed a sore eye during his flight home from a two-week holiday in Hong Kong. He was observed to develop a bilateral keratoconjunctivitis and adenovirus type 8 was cultured from eye swabs. There was no cross-infection at the hospital during five visits, although his wife developed a similar condition. This case provides a good example of the potential source of a hospital-based outbreak in the West, where the level of immunity is low. An outbreak of EKC caused by adenovirus type 8 was observed in 1975 in a Vietnamese refugee camp in Florida. Interestingly, it was the refugee children who made up over half the cases, and unlike the typical juvenile infection in the Orient, systemic symptoms were uncommon. Unfortunately, equipment was not available to record the degree of ocular involvement (Zweighaft *et al.*, 1977).

Pharyngoconjunctival fever (PCF) is another clinico-epidemiological entity, consisting of a classical triad of non-purulent follicular conjunctivitis, pharyngitis and pyrexia. This condition is highly infectious and is most likely to spread in schools and swimming baths (Ormsby and Aitchison, 1955). Corneal involvement is uncommon and if present is only transient. It has been largely identified with type 3 infection, though it is also a common result of infection by type 7. Both these serotypes belong to Group I of Rosen's classification.

Group III consists of those serotypes which are usually considered to be endemic. However, type 4 has shown the capacity for causing outbreaks of disease. As such, it is best known for outbreaks of upper respiratory tract infection (acute respiratory disease) in military recruits (Hilleman and Werner, 1954). However, it may also cause outbreaks of conjunctivitis. One such outbreak was shown to be related to a contaminated swimming pool (d'Angelo *et al.*, 1979). A recent hospital-based (nosocomial) outbreak has occurred (Levandowski and Rubenis, 1981). Another was a community outbreak in the Bristol area which demonstrated some unusual features (Tullo and Higgins, 1980). 113 cases of follicular conjunctivitis were seen over a six-month period; 15 per cent had associated respiratory-tract symptoms and 20 per cent had corneal disease. Unlike classical EKC or PCF, this outbreak was evenly distributed throughout the community, apart from 9 cases of probable infection at the Eye Hospital. It is clear that this particular strain of adenovirus had a true predilection for the eye. The typical history was of spontaneous onset, and only 13 per cent of patients gave a history of contact with another person with signs or symptoms of conjunctivitis. This suggests that close contact with an infected eye was not a prerequisite for transmission of the virus. The possibility of asymptomatic ocular carriage acting as a reservoir of adenovirus infection has been raised (O'Day *et al.*, 1976). However, asymptomatic respiratory carriage would provide even greater opportunity for dissemination of adenovirus type 4, which commonly infects the respiratory tract. The source of isolated and community outbreaks of eye disease may well be the gastro-intestinal tract (Jones, 1962). It has also been proposed that chronic ocular infection (Pettit and Holland, 1979) and even the genital tract (Schaap *et al.*, 1979; Harnett and Newnham, 1981; Tullo, 1981) could be the source of some outbreaks.

Study of the distribution of antibodies to adenovirus in the population indicates that children are exposed early in life to the common endemic types of lower pathogenicity, e.g. types 1, 2, 5 and 6, which usually result in respiratory-tract and gastro-intestinal infection (Fox *et al.*, 1977), but can also produce eye infection. When conjunctivitis in children is associated with a sore throat, adenoviruses are commonly responsible (Gigliotti *et al.*, 1981).

This EKC, PCF and conjunctivitis caused by the endemic serotypes, make up a spectrum of disease that can be produced when adenoviruses infect the eye.

The pattern of adenoviral eye disease has been considered in the Bristol area over a period of nine years. The total number of 426 cases have been presented according to Rosen's classification (Tullo, 1980), but are presented here according to type only (Figure 10.2). Three separate outbreaks caused by

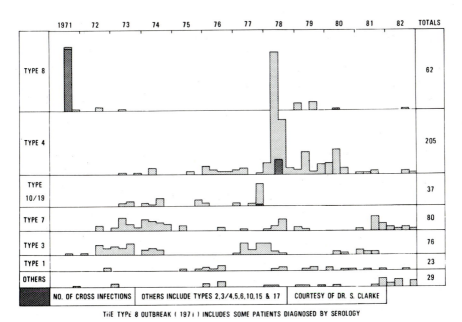

Figure 10.2. Distribution of adenoviruses isolated from eye swabs in the Bristol area, 1971–1982.

types 8, 10/19 and 4 are included. The predominance of Group II serotypes as a cause of outbreaks is also shown in a similar Australian study (Irving *et al.*, 1981).

Clinical Features

The condition of adenovirus eye infection is usually an acute, self-limiting follicular keratoconjunctivitis; signs may range from a transiently red eye with trivial soreness, to a severe keratitis with uveitis producing pain and photophobia. Rarely, chronic keratitis (Boniuk *et al.*, 1965) and chronic conjunctivitis (Darougar *et al.*, 1977) have been reported. There are no pathognomonic signs of adenovirus eye disease, and the similarity with other infections, such as the follicular keratoconjunctivitis of primary herpes simplex and chlamydial infection, may make diagnosis difficult (Darougar *et al.*, 1978). Rarely, Stevens-Johnson syndrome results from ocular adenovirus infection (Kiernan *et al.* 1981).

Children and young adults are most commonly affected, both sexes equally. There is no overall seasonal variation in the incidence of infections. The incubation period is from 2–14 days, while a person with overt disease may remain infectious for a further 10–14 days.

A review of experimental and clinical observations indicates that a number of factors influence the development of signs and symptoms in a person at risk of infection (Table 10.2).

TABLE 10.2

FACTORS INFLUENCING THE RISK OF OCULAR INFECTION OF A PERSON EXPOSED TO AN ADENOVIRUS

SEROTYPE	Certain serotypes have a predilection for the eye (Group II); amongst serologically identical types there may be differences in the genome.[1]
INOCULUM	The size of the inoculum is important;[2] inhibiting factors may play a part.[3]
TRAUMA	Self-inflicted by rubbing; iatrogenic by applanation; removal of a foreign body; experimental.[4]
IMMUNITY	Previous exposure to a serotype confers immunity to that serotype.

1. Wadell and Varsanyi, 1978.   3. Golden *et al.*, 1971.
2. Jawetz, 1962.   4. Bietti and Bruna, 1957.

Symptoms

The rapid onset of symptoms or soreness and watering are typical. A foreign-body sensation is a frequent accompaniment in the more severe cases of infection seen in EKC. Asymptomatic carriage even of epidemic strains has been demonstrated (O'Day *et al.*, 1976), so that irritation of the eye from other causes and consequent rubbing may produce an epithelial foothold for an inoculum of virus (Bietti and Bruna, 1957).

The corneal involvement and especially anterior uveitis, which may occur in EKC produces photophobia and pain. Blurring of vision occurs in association with corneal stromal involvement, and central scarring can cause lasting visual disturbance.

While the second eye is affected in a proportion of patients, involvement is almost always less than in the first eye, and may be trivial.

A patient with the pharyngitis, conjunctivitis and pyrexia of PCF may also have myalgia, stomach pains and diarrhoea; although EKC is more specifically an ocular condition, malaise may accompany the marked soreness and pain around the eye.

Signs

While it has been stated that the adenovirus produces no pathognomonic ocular signs, summation of the features of an eye under scrutiny may enable adenovirus infection to be put at the top of a list of differential diagnoses.

Follicular conjunctivitis is by far the commonest clinical finding of eyes infected by adenoviruses. The degree of the follicular response is variable, and occurs most markedly in the lower palpebral conjunctiva and fornix. The papillary response, most marked in EKC, is found predominantly in the upper tarsal conjunctiva, and is most marked in those patients complaining of a foreign-body sensation. The plica may be particularly hyperaemic. The petechial haemorrhages seen on the everted lid in some cases (Laibson *et al.*, 1970) appear to stem from the central vessels of the papillae (Figure 10.3). More profuse subconjunctival haemorrhages, both bulbar and in the lower fornix, may also occur, typically in EKC, and serve as a reminder that such lesions are not pathognomonic of an enterovirus infection (Aoki *et al.*, 1980).

Exudation resulting in inflammatory membrane formation (Dawson *et al.*, 1970) may occur, especially from a severe papillary response, and in a young adult this is a useful clue to the aetiology (Figure 10.4). Conjunctival scarring occurs in the severest cases of EKC, particularly when preceded by an inflammatory membrane (Figure 10.5; Dawson *et al.*, 1972).

Chemosis, when present, is not usually a prominent feature. There may be sufficient lid swelling to produce a slight ptosis. Lymphadenopathy of pre-auricular and submandibular glands is probably present in approximately two-thirds of cases (Table 10.3), but can be easily missed (Laibson *et al.*, 1968).

TABLE 10.3

DISTRIBUTION AND FREQUENCY OF SIGNS DURING THE COURSE OF
ADENOVIRUS 10/19 INFECTION IN 19 PATIENTS.

Site	Sign	Number of patients in whom present (and %)	
Conjunctiva	Follicles	18	(95)
	Papillae	18	(95)
	Chemosis	5	(26)
	Inflammatory membrane	7	(37)
	Scarring	7	(37)
	Punctate epithelial keratitis	8	(42)
Cornea	Subepithelial lesions	11	(58)
	Disciform keratitis	1	(5)
Regional glands	Lymphadenopathy	7	(37)

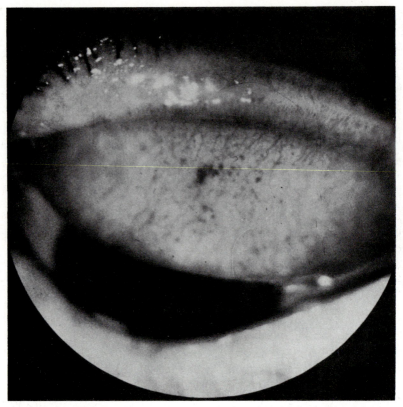

Figure 10.3. Petechial haemorrhages in conjunctivitis due to adenovirus type 4.

Keratitis

Corneal involvement in adenovirus infection is the most important factor in determining the severity of the acute and the longer-term symptoms. Keratitis has been observed in infections with types 3, 4, 5, 7, 9, 11, 19, 21 and 10/19 (Laibson, 1975; Darougar *et al.*, 1978; Tullo and Higgins, 1979). The evolution of corneal lesions, notably those caused by adenovirus type 8 infections, have been carefully documented (Dawson *et al.*, 1970; Jones, 1958). The first sign is a diffuse punctate epitheliopathy, best demonstrated with rose bengal stain, which appears within a few days of the onset of symptoms. These lesions may resolve without trace. Alternatively, a more focal keratitis develops and, typically at around three weeks, early discrete anterior stromal opacities become discernible (Figure 10.6). A transient intra-epithelial stage without staining may be observed. It is proposed that the punctate subepithelial lesions are an immunopathological phenomenon resulting from the interaction of viral antigen and antibody in the anterior stroma, with the cornea acting as a blotter (Jones, 1958). At the time of infection, the virus becomes established in corneal epithelial cells (Dawson *et al.*, 1972), and although virus can seldom be

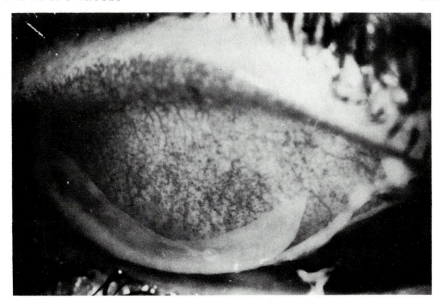

Figure 10.4. Membrane formation in a young adult with adenoviral conjunctivitis.

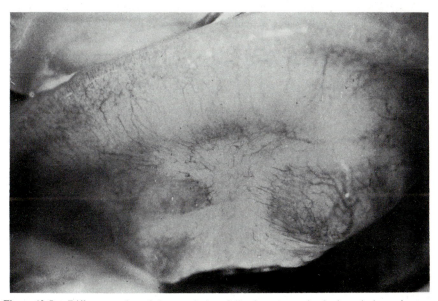

Figure 10.5. Diffuse scarring of the tarsal plate following an attack of adenoviral membranous conjunctivitis.

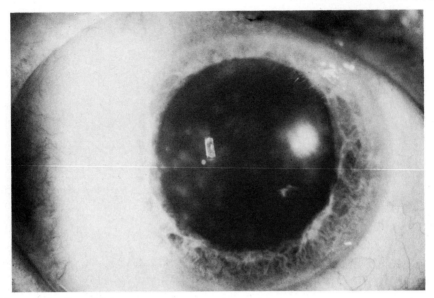

Figure 10.6. Superficial stromal punctate keratitis caused by adenoviral infection. The opacities are demonstrated by a limbal scattering technique.

isolated from the eye after 10–14 days of the infection, this does not exclude the continued production of viral antigen (Periera, 1972). Persistent adenovirus antigen has been demonstrated in experimental keratitis in rabbits (Schwartz *et al.*, 1979) and histology of corneal opacities indicates that they are composed of polymorphs and mononuclear cells (Lund and Stefani, 1978). In patients with epithelial erosions, the condition rarely progresses to stromal disease (Laibson, 1975). This suggests that the epithelium is important in facilitating a continuing antigenic stimulus. Once antibody has diffused into the stroma and encountered viral antigen, it seems likely that at a critical point antigen/antibody complexes precipitate out, attracting complement and a subsequent cellular infiltrate.

The small discrete anterior stromal opacities are the hallmark of adenovirus keratitis. They may vary in number from less than ten to over one hundred, and are more numerous in the first affected eye. Initially the distribution of the lesions is most likely to be uniform, but on follow-up it has been noted that they are more likely to persist in the upper peripheral cornea (Tullo and Higgins, 1979).

When lesions occur in the paracentral cornea, disturbance of vision may occur. The author has recorded visual symptoms eighteen months after infection with adenovirus type 10/19, and noted stromal opacities elsewhere in the cornea in another patient eight years after infection with adenovirus type 8, though it has been stated that both symptoms and signs may be permanent (Laibson, 1975).

Disciform keratitis has been observed alone and in the presence of discrete stromal opacities (Bietti and Bruna, 1957) and associated with a demonstrable rise in antibody titre to adenoviruses from paired serum samples (Tullo and Higgins, 1979).

Dendritiform epithelial defects in the absence of any evidence of herpes simplex have been noted in adenovirus disease of the eye (Tullo and Higgins, 1980) and represent areas of healing ulceration.

Other uncommon signs include anterior uveitis (Barnard et al., 1973) and raised intra-ocular pressure (Hara et al., 1980).

Treatment

There is no established treatment of acute adenovirus infection of the eye, though it is the usual practice to prescribe antibiotic drops which may alleviate symptoms. No antiviral agent has, as yet, been shown to have any significant effect (Dudgeon et al., 1969; Pavan-Langston and Dohlman, 1972). The use of topical immunoglobulins or interferon remains a possibility for treating viral disease, although if shown to be effective, the delay in obtaining laboratory confirmation of the diagnosis would limit the usefulness of these expensive measures. There is no doubt that topical steroids are very effective in clearing stromal opacities, but treatment must be monitored carefully. Apart from the usual attendant risks of the use of steroids, a rebound phenomenon may take place when treatment is stopped, leading to persistent corneal lesions (Tullo and Higgins, 1979). It is known that use of steroid early in the disease may suppress the appearance of stromal opacities (Laibson et al., 1970); however, they tend to appear on stopping treatment and their presence may ultimately be prolonged. As most infections are self-limiting and many corneal lesions may produce no symptoms, the only specific indication for the use of topical steroids is when the vision of the affected eye is compromised after resolution of the acute stage.

The most important measure in the management of adenovirus eye infection is the prevention of spread. This involves advice to the patient on how long they are likely to remain infectious, and the common-sense precautions they should take in the prevention of spread of virus. The greatest onus of responsibility lies with those who are consulted by patients suffering from possible adenovirus eye infection. Cross-infection still occurs most frequently in Eye Hospitals and units, and in treatment centres in industry where ocular trauma is common. Precautions include a high index of suspicion of any follicular keratoconjunctivitis, thorough hand-washing immediately after examining patients, avoidance of the use of tonometers and contact lenses, and their routine disinfection (Clarke et al., 1972).

REFERENCES

AOKI, K., KATO, M., OHTSUKA, H., TOKITA, H., OBARA, T., NAKAZONO, N., SAWADA, H. and ISHII, K. (1980). Clinical and etiological study of viral conjunctivitis 1974–1978, Sapporo, Japan. Jap. J. Ophthal., 24, 149–159.

BARNARD, D. L., DEAN HART, J. C., MARMION, V. J. and CLARKE, S. K. R. (1973). Outbreak in Bristol of conjunctivitis caused by adenovirus type 8, and its epidemiology and control. Brit. Med. J., 2, 165–169.

BELL, S. D. (Jr.), ROTA, T. R. and McCOMB, D. E. (1960). Adenovirus isolated from Saudi Arabia: six new serotypes. *Amer. J. Trop. Med.*, **9**, 523–526.

BIETTI, G. B. and BRUNA, F. (1957). Epidemic keratoconjunctivitis in Italy: some contributions to its clinical aspects, epidemiology and etiology. (*Amer. J. Ophthal.*, **43**, Part II. 50–57.

BONIUK, M., PHILLIPS, C. A., and FRIEDMAN, J. B. (1965). Chronic adenovirus type 2 keratitis in man. *New Engl. J. Med.*, **273**, 924–925.

British Journal of Ophthalmology (1977). Editorial. Adenovirus keratoconjunctivitis. **61**, 73–75.

CLARKE, S. K. R., DEAN HART, J. C. and BARNARD, D. L. (1972). The disinfection of instruments and hands during outbreaks of epidemic keratoconjunctivitis. *Trans. Ophthal. Soc. U.K.*, **92**, 613–617.

D'ANGELO, L. J., HIERHOLZER, J. C., KEENLYSIDE, R. A., ANDERSON, L. J., and MARTONE, W. J. (1979). Pharyngoconjunctival fever caused by adenovirus type 4; a report of a swimming pool related outbreak with recovery of the virus from the pool water. *J. Infect. Dis.*, **140**, 42–47.

DAROUGAR, S., PEARCE, R., GIBSON, J. A. and McSWIGGAN, O. A. (1978). Adenovirus type 21 keratoconjunctivitis. *Brit. J. Ophthal.*, **62**, 836–837.

DAROUGAR, S., QUINLAN, M. P., GIBSON, J. A., JONES, B. R. and McSWIGGAN, O. A. (1977). Epidemic keratoconjunctivitis and chronic papillary conjunctivitis in London due to adenovirus type 19. *Brit. J. Ophthal.*, **61**, 76–85.

DAVIDSON, S. I. (1964). Epidemic keratoconjunctivitis. *Brit. J. Ophthal.*, **48**, 573–580.

DAWSON, C. R., HANNA, L. and TOGNI, B. (1972). Adenovirus type 8 infections in the U.S.A. IV. *Arch. Ophthal.*, **87**, 258–268.

DAWSON, C. R., HANNA, L., WOOD, T. R. and DESPAIN, R. (1970). Adenovirus type 8 keratoconjunctivitis in the United States. III. *Amer. J. Ophthal.*, **69**, 473–480.

DEJONG, J. C., WIGAND, R., WADELL, G., KELLER, D., MUZERIE, C. J., WERMEMBOL, A. G. and SCHAAP, G. J. (1981). Adenovirus 37: identification and characterisation of a medically important new adenovirus type of sub-group D. *J. Med. Virol.*, **7**, 105–118.

DESMYTER, J., DEJONG, J. C., SLATERUS, K. W. and VERLAECT, H. (1974). Keratoconjunctivitis caused by adenovirus type 19. *Brit. Med. J.*, **4**, 406.

DUDGEON, J., BHARGARA, S. K. and ROSS, C. A. C. (1969). Treatment of adenovirus infection of the eye with 5-iodo-2'-deoxyuridine. *Brit. J. Ophthal.* **53**, 530–533.

FOX, J. P., HALL, C. E. and COONEY, M. K. (1977). Observations of adenovirus infections. *The Seattle Virus Watch.* **VII**, 105, 362–386.

FUCHS, E. (1889). Keratitis puctata superficialis. *Wien. Klin. Wschr.* **2**, 837.

GIGLIOTTI, F., WILLIAMS, W. T., HAYDEN, F. G., HENDLEY, J. O., BENJAMIN, J., DICKENS, M., GLEASON, C., PERRIELLO, V. C. and WOOD, J. (1981). Etiology of acute conjunctivitis in children. *J. Pediatrics*, **98**, 531–536.

GOLDEN, B., McKEEN, A. P. and COPPEL, S. P. (1971). Epidemic keratoconjunctivitis: a new approach. *Trans. Amer. Acad. Ophthal. Otolaryng.*, **75**, 1216.

HARA, J., ISHIBASHI, T., FUJIMOTO, F., DANJYO, S., KINEKAWA, Y. O. and MAEDA, A. (1980). Adenovirus type 10 keratoconjunctivitis with increased intraocular pressure. *Amer. J. Ophthal.*, **90**, 481–484.

HARNETT, G. B. and NEWNHAM, W. A. (1981). Isolation of adenovirus type 19 from male and female genital tracts. *Brit. J. Vener. Dis.*, **57**, 55–57.

HIERHOLZER, J. C. and RODRIGUEZ, F. H. (1981). Antigenically intermediate human adenovirus strain associated conjunctivitis. *J. Clin. Microbiol.*, **13**, 395–397.

HILLEMAN, M. R. and WERNER, J. H. (1954). Recovery of a new agent from patients with acute respiratory illness. *Proc. Soc. Exp. Biol. (N.Y.)*, **85**, 183.

HOGAN, M. J. and CRAWFORD, J. W. (1942). Epidemic keratonconjunctivitis. *Amer. J. Ophthal.*, **25**, 1059–1078.

HUEBNER, R. J. and ROWE, W. P. (1957). Adenovirus as etiological agents in conjunctivitis and keratoconjunctivitis. *Amer. J. Ophthal.*, **43**, 20–25.

IRVING, L., KENNET, M., LEWIS, F., BIRCH, C. and DONALDSON, A. (1981). Adenovirus eye infections in an Australian city 1972–1979. *J. Hyg. (Lond.)*, **86**, 95–103.

JAWETZ, E. (1962). Adenovirus type 8 and the story of epidemic keratoconjunctivitis. *Trans. Ophthal. Soc. U.K.*, **82**, 613–619.

JAWETZ, E., KIMURA, S. J., HANNA, L., COLEMAN, V. R., THYGESON, P. and NICHOLAS, A. (1955). Studies on the etiology of epidemic keratoconjunctivitis. *Amer. J. Ophthal.*, **40**, 200–209.

JAWETZ, E., THYGESON, P., HANNA, L., NICHOLAS, A. and KIMURA, S. J. (1956). Antibodies to APC virus type 8 in epidemic keratoconjunctivitis. *Proc. Soc. Exp. Biol. (N.Y.)*, **92**, 91–95.

JONES, B. R. (1958). The clinical features of viral keratitis and a concept of their pathogenesis. *Proc. Roy. Soc. Med.*, **51**, 13–20.

JONES, B. R. (1962). Adenovirus infection of the eye in London. *Trans. Ophthal. Soc. U.K.*, **88**, 621–640.

KIERNAN, J. P., SCHANZLIN, D. J. and LEVEILLE, A. S. (1981). Stevens-Johnson syndrome associated with adenovirus conjunctivitis. *Amer. J. Ophthal.*, **92**, 543–545.

LAIBSON, P. R. (1975). Adenoviral keratoconjunctivitis. *Int. Ophthal. Clin.*, **15**, 187–201.

LAIBSON, P. R., DHRIRI, S., OCONER, J. and ORTILAN, G. (1970). Corneal infiltrates in epidemic keratoconjunctivitis. *Arch. Ophthal.*, **84**, 36–40.

LAIBSON, P. R., ORTILAN, G. and DUPRE-STRACHAN, S. (1968). Community and hospital outbreak of E.K.C. *Arch. Ophthal.*, **80**, 467–473.

LEVANDOWSKI, R. A. and RUBENIS, M. (1981). Nosocomial conjunctivitis caused by Adenovirus type 4. *J. Infect. Dis.*, **143**, 28–31.

LOCATCHER-KHORAZO, D. and SEEGAL, B. C. (1972*a,b*). *Microbiology of the Eye*. (*a*) p. 281, (*b*) p. 287. St. Louis: Mosby.

LUND, O. E. and STEFANI, F. H. (1978). Corneal histology after E.K.C. *Arch. Ophthal.*, **96**, 2085–2088.

O'DAY, D. M., GUYER, B., HIERHOLZER, J. C., ROSING, K. J., and SCHAFFNER, W. (1976). Clinical and laboratory evaluation of epidemic keratoconjunctivitis due to adeno-virus types 8 and 19. *Amer. J. Ophthal.*, **81**, 207–215.

ORMSY, H. L. and AITCHISON, W. S. (1955). The role of the swimming pool in the transmission of pharyngoconjunctival fever. *Canad. Med. Ass. J.*, **73**, 864–866.

PAVAN-LANGSTON, D. and DOHLMAN, C. (1972). A double blind clinical study of adenine arabinoside therapy of viral keratoconjunctivitis. *Amer. J. Ophthal.*, **74**, 81–88.

PERIERA, H. G. (1972). Persistent infection by adenoviruses. *J. Clin. Path.*, **25**, Suppl. 6, 39–42.

PETTIT, T. H. and HOLLAND, G. N. (1979). Chronic keratoconjunctivitis associated with ocular adenovirus infection. *Amer. J. Ophthal.*, **61**, 73–75.

ROSEN, L. (1960). A hemagglutination inhibition technique for typing adenoviruses. *Amer. J. Hyg.*, **71**, 120–128.

ROWE, W. P., HUEBNER, R. J., GILMORE, L. K., PARROTT, R. H. and WARD, R. D. (1953). Isolation of a cytopathogenic agent from human adenoids undergoing spontaneous degeneration in tissue culture. *Proc. Soc. Exp. Biol. (N.Y.)*, **84**, 570.

SCHAAP, G. J. P., DEJONG, J. C., VAN BIJSTEWELD, O. P. and BEEKHUIS, W. H. (1979). A new intermediate adenovirus type causing conjunctivitis. *Arch. Ophthal.*, **97**, 2336–2338.

SCHWARTZ, H. S., YAMASHIROYA, H. and WINKLER, J. (1979). Development of adenoviral induced corneal lesions in cyclophosphamide treated animals. *ARVO Abstract*, **12**, 24.

SWANZY, H. (1915). *Diseases of the Eye*, p. 144. London: Lewis.

THYGESON, P. (1957). Office and dispensary transmission of epidemic keratoconjunctivitis. *Amer. J. Ophthal.*, **43**, 98–101.

TULLO, A. B. (1980). Clinical and epidemiological features of adenovirus keratoconjunctivitis. *Trans. Ophthal. Soc. U.K.*, **100**, 263–267.

TULLO, A. B. (1981). Shipyard eye. *Brit. Med. J.*, **283**, 1056.

TULLO, A. B. and HIGGINS, P. G. (1979). An outbreak of adenovirus keratoconjunctivitis in Bristol. *Brit. J. Ophthal.*, **63**, 621–626.

TULLO, A. B. and HIGGINS, P. G. (1980). An outbreak of adenovirus type 4 conjunctivitis. *Brit. J. Ophthal.*, **64**, 489–493.

WADELL, G. (1979). Classification of human adenoviruses by SDS-polyacrylanide gel electrophoresis of structural polypeptides. *Intervirology*, **11**, 47–57.

WADELL, G. and DEJONG, J. C. (1980). Restriction endonucleases in identification of a genome type of adenovirus 19 associated with keratoconjunctivitis. *Infection & Immunity.*, **27**, 292–296.

WADELL, G. and VARSANYI, T. M. (1978). Demonstration of three different subtypes of adenovirus type 7 by DNA restriction site mapping. *Infection & Immunity.*, **21**, 238–246.

ZOGRAFOS, L. (1977). La Keratoconjucivitie de l'adenovirus type 10. *Ophthalmologica (Basel)*, **174**, 61–64.

ZWEIGHAFT, R. M., HIERHOLZER, J. C. and BRYAN, J. A. (1977). Epidemic keratoconjunctivitis at a Vietnamese refugee camp in Florida. *Amer. J. Epidem.*, **106**, 399–407.

CHAPTER ELEVEN

Acute Haemorrhagic Conjunctivitis

PETER G. HIGGINS

THE enteroviruses, together with the rhinoviruses, are the two most important groups of human picornaviruses. The enteroviruses have been subdivided into the polioviruses (3 types), Coxsackieviruses type A (24 types), Coxsackieviruses type B (6 types) and the echoviruses (33 types). When it became apparent that these divisions were not absolute it was decided in 1969 that all new enteroviruses would be called simply *enterovirus*, and four serotypes have been recognised to date (enterovirus types 68 to 71).

The enteroviruses are small, approximately 27 nm in diameter, non-enveloped viruses containing single-stranded RNA. They are relatively stable and can remain viable for days at room temperature, and for months at 4°C. They are, however, inactivated by heat and free chlorine but are resistant to acid, lipid solvents, proteolytic enzymes and many common disinfectants such as phenols, alcohol and quaternary ammonium compounds.

The natural habitat of the enteroviruses is the gut and they spread by the faecal-oral route. Most infections are subclinical, especially in children, although they can give rise to a wide range of clinical illness. Many enteroviruses can cause aseptic meningitis, 'summer flu', sore throat and respiratory infections, any of which may be accompanied by a rash. Other illnesses result from infections with a limited number of enteroviruses: Bornholm disease and infections of the heart (Coxsackieviruses type B), hand, foot and mouth disease (mainly Coxsackieviruses type A, especially type A16), herpangina (Coxsackieviruses type A), and acute haemorrhagic conjunctivitis are examples.

Infections with enteroviruses have a seasonal distribution in temperate climates, being most common in summer and autumn. The prevalence of any one serotype varies in a cyclical fashion, giving rise to epidemics separated by periods of reduced activity during which the proportion of susceptibles increases and permits subsequent infections to progress to an epidemic. This pattern was typified by poliomyelitis in developed countries before the introduction of vaccine.

It is only in the last decade that enteroviruses have been shown to contribute significantly to the aetiology of acute conjunctivitis. Two apparently new enteroviruses, enterovirus type 70 and another which ultimately proved to be a prime variant of the already recognised Coxsackievirus type A24, gave rise to widespread epidemics of conjunctivitis in Africa and Asia in the early 1970s and again, in 1981, to the current extensive outbreaks in the Americas. The ocular diseases caused by the two viruses were very similar and when they occurred in the same area, either at the same time or consecutively, observers were unable to distinguish between them on clinical grounds. Characteristically the infection had a very short incubation period, affected both eyes, caused swelling of the eyelids and chemosis, was associated with pain and a serous discharge and resolved, without sequelae, in a week to ten days. The subconjunctival haemorrhages which give the disease its name were present in virtually all cases in the original outbreak but were less evident in some of the subsequent epidemics. The major epidemics have occurred in the developing countries in the tropics, and only small outbreaks have been reported from a limited number of countries in the temperate zone.

The disease was first recognised as a clinical entity in Ghana in 1969. Over thirteen and a half thousand cases were seen in the clinic in Accra between June and October, of which almost nine thousand presented in August. Although no causal agent was isolated, a viral aetiology was suspected from the clinical features of the cases studied. However, they differed from those associated with epidemic adenovirus keratoconjunctivitis, and the name 'epidemic haemorrhagic conjunctivitis' was suggested (Chatterjee et al., 1970). From Ghana the epidemic spread along the west coast reaching Lagos in Nigeria by October of the same year, where the local populace preferred to call the condition 'Apollo 11 disease' (Parrott, 1971) for it was prevalent at the time of the Apollo 11 landing on the moon. Morocco was affected by the end of 1970 (Bourdieu, 1973) and Tunisia the following year (Whitcher et al., 1976).

In the latter half of 1970 epidemics of the disease were occurring in Indonesia (Kono et al., 1972) and it is possible that the condition had been present the previous year (Kono, 1975). As in Africa, the disease spread widely, reaching Singapore (Yin-Murphy, 1972) and Hong Kong in 1970, and proceeding, via Malaysia and Thailand (Dumavibhat et al., 1973) to the Indian sub-continent by 1971 (Roy et al., 1972). It was in India that the possibility of neurological complications following acute haemorrhagic conjunctivitis (AHC) was first recognised (Bharucha and Mondkar, 1972). In 1971 the disease had also reached Taiwan (Tai et al., 1974) and Japan (Kono et al., 1972; Mitsui et al., 1972) and the first European outbreaks were observed (Jones, 1972; Schaap, 1974).

The virus most commonly isolated from these outbreaks was the enterovirus type 70 but others were associated with the Coxsackievirus type A24. Indeed, the latter virus was the first to be isolated, being found in a high proportion of patients' samples during the 1970 Singapore epidemic (Yin-Murphy, 1972).

Coxsackievirus type A24, alone or together with enterovirus type 70, has also been shown to be the cause of other epidemics of AHC, in Hong Kong in 1970 (Mirkovic et al., 1974), in Bangkok in 1975 (Thongcharoen and Wasi, 1978), Vellore in 1975 (Christopher et al., 1977), Bangladesh in 1975 (Yin-Murphy, 1976), Brunei in 1975 (Yin-Murphy, Lim and Ho, 1976) and Sri Lanka in 1975 (Higgins and Chapman, 1977).

In many of these countries epidemics of AHC occurred annually or slightly less frequently for several years and were shown to be caused by one or other of these two enteroviruses (Dawson et al., 1974; Hung et al., 1976; Metselaar et al., 1976; Yin-Murphy et al., 1976; Thongcharoen and Wasi, 1978; Kawamoto, 1979). Thereafter, the incidence fell and few epidemics were reported between 1975 and 1980 although sporadic cases were observed during this period (Yin-Murphy, 1980; Wadia et al., 1981; John et al., 1981).

Evidence of renewed activity came in the report of an outbreak of AHC caused by Coxsackievirus type A24 in Madras in the latter half of 1979 (WHO Wkly. Epidem. Rec., 1980a) and of another outbreak, this time in Kenya, in early 1980 when the infecting agent was enterovirus type 70 (WHO Wkly. Epidem. Rec., 1980b). Further cases of AHC in Madras at the end of 1980 (Thakur, 1981) were followed in mid-1981 by outbreaks in other parts of India and Pakistan (Katiyar et al., 1981; Wadia et al., 1981; WHO Wkly. Epidem. Rec., 1981a, b) and also in Africa, in Nigeria (WHO Wkly. Epidem. Rec., 1981a) and in Zäire (Desmyter et al., 1981).

The first report of cases in the Americas came from central and northern countries of South America, and AHC then spread through the Caribbean (WHO Wkly. Epidem. Rec., 1981a and c) to reach Florida in September 1981 (WHO Wkly. Epidem. Rec., 1981d). In a number of the epidemics the causal agent was shown to be enterovirus 70 (Kono et al., 1981; WHO Wkly. Epidem. Rec., 1981b and c).

Clinical Features

Although no aetiological agent was isolated from the original outbreak in Ghana the clinical features of the disease were sufficiently distinct for it to be recognised as a new form of conjunctivitis. The most outstanding sign of that outbreak was the presence of subconjunctival haemorrhages which varied in size but were present in every case (Plate IIIb). In subsequent epidemics haemorrhages have not been such a constant feature and have been observed in as few as 28 per cent of cases in Japan with enterovirus type 70 infections (Minami et al., 1976) and 6 per cent of ocular infections with Coxsackievirus type A24 in Singapore (Yin-Murphy et al., 1976). Furthermore, subconjunctival haemorrhages may occur with other infections, notably those with adenovirus type 4 (Muzzi et al., 1975; Tullo and Higgins, 1980) and also with adenovirus type 11 which has been reported as responsible, along with enterovirus type 70, for mixed epidemics of AHC (Tai et al., 1974; Yin-Murphy et al., 1976; Arnow et al., 1977). Although subconjunctival haemorrhage is an important sign in AHC, it is by no means diagnostic. Haemorrhages may occur into the skin of the lids (Figure 11.1). A follicular conjunctivitis may be associated (Figure 11.2).

In all the outbreaks the majority of infections have been bilateral. This may

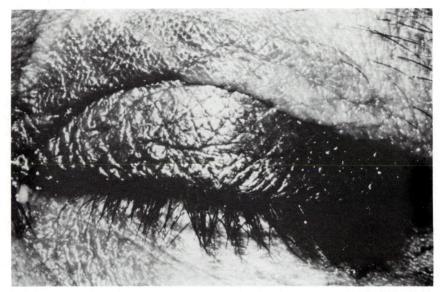

Figure 11.1. Haemorrhage into the skin of the upper lid in acute haemorrhagic conjunctivitis. (Courtesy, Dr. Penny A. Asbell.)

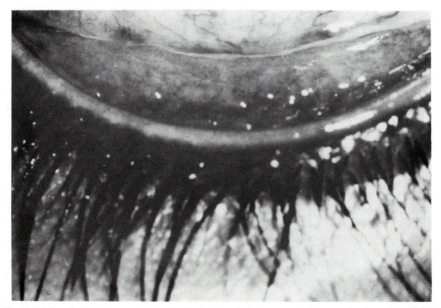

Figure 11.2. Follicles appearing in the lower tarsal plate in acute haemorrhagic conjunctivitis. (Courtesy, Dr. Penny A. Asbell.)

be present at the onset of the illness or it may result from infection passing from one eye to the other, which usually occurs early in the disease. The incubation period is short, being less than 24 hours, and has been confirmed for both viruses following accidental infection of laboratory staff (Sasagawa *et al.*, 1976; Langford *et al.*, 1979) and hospital cross-infection (Dawson *et al.*, 1974).

The earliest symptoms are pain, foreign-body sensation and lachrymation with congestion of the conjunctiva. The lids are markedly swollen, commonly there is a follicular conjunctivitis, and chemosis has frequently been reported. Corneal involvement is limited to a superficial epithelial keratitis and significant stromal opacities do not occur (Chatterjee *et al.*, 1970; Parrott, 1971; Pramanik, 1971; Jones, 1972; Kono *et al.*, 1972; Mitsui *et al.*, 1972; Roy *et al.*, 1972; Dumavibhat *et al.*, 1973; Golden and Smit, 1974; Likar *et al.*, 1975; Minami *et al.*, 1976; Whitcher *et al.*, 1976; Yin-Murphy *et al.*, 1976; Arnow *et al.*, 1977; Christopher *et al.*, 1977).

Other findings are more variable but do not appear to depend on the type of the infecting enterovirus. In some instances it has been noted that a high proportion of the patients have a lymphadenopathy of the pre-auricular lymph nodes (Chatterjee *et al.*, 1970; Mitsui *et al.*, 1972; Roy *et al.*, 1972; Likar *et al.*, 1975; Minami *et al.*, 1976; Whitcher *et al.*, 1976; Yin-Murphy *et al.*, 1976) while in other epidemics this has been a rare occurrence (Parrott, 1971; Pramanik, 1971; Dumavibhat *et al.*, 1973). Similarly, the incidence of respiratory and constitutional symptoms have varied from outbreak to outbreak (Parrott, 1971; Pramanik, 1971; Minami *et al.*, 1976; Whitcher *et al.*, 1976; Yin-Murphy, *et al.*, 1976).

AHC is a clinical entity which can be distinguished from other forms of conjunctivitis on clinical grounds on many occasions, but can also be mimicked by certain adenovirus infections of the eye. It should also be stressed that it is not possible on clinical, or even epidemiological grounds, to distinguish between AHC caused by enterovirus type 70 and that caused by Coxsackievirus type A24.

The presentation of AHC may be impressive but the condition, in all but a very few cases, is benign, with complete resolution occurring in one or two weeks, and with no sequelae.

Very rarely, cases of radiculomyelitis follow AHC caused by enterovirus 70 after an interval ranging from a few days to eight weeks but commonly being two or three weeks. The onset is frequently preceded by a prodromal illness of malaise and fever which gives way to root pain and paraesthesia which may persist for up to two weeks. Muscle weakness or a flaccid paralysis quickly follows. The lower limbs are more commonly affected than the upper and the brunt of the disease falls on the proximal rather than the distal portion of the limb. When the upper limbs are involved there is often a history of injections into, or excessive use of, the limb immediately prior to onset of paralysis. The clinical picture is one closely resembling poliomyelitis, with asymmetrical flaccid paralysis and loss of reflexes. Progress is also similar, with a proportion recovering to be able to walk unaided. The commonest residual disability is difficulty in rising from the squatting position, but a proportion of patients remain paraplegic. During the acute phase there is a cellular response in the

CSF, mainly lymphocytic, which is present for a few days but the accompanying increase in CSF protein persists for weeks (Wadia *et al.*, 1973; Kono *et al.*, 1974; Hung *et al.*, 1976; Kono *et al.*, 1976; Phuapradit *et al.*, 1976; Kono *et al.*, 1977).

During the 1981 epidemic of AHC in India, neurological complications were again observed. (Wadia *et al.*, 1981; Mondkar, 1981; Katiyar *et al.*, 1981; Thakur, 1981). Not only has there been an increase in the number of polio-like illnesses accompanying the conjunctivitis, but also cases of single or multiple cranial-nerve palsies, especially of the VIIth nerve, have been reported. These cranial-nerve lesions occur alone or with paralysis of limbs, but their onset appears to follow the conjunctivitis more rapidly than does the polio-like illness involving the limbs.

Epidemiology

Much of the epidemiology of AHC becomes apparent when one considers the origin and geographical spread of the infecting agents, their mode of transmission and the incidence of infection at various age levels.

There is no incontrovertible evidence for determining the geographical origin of AHC caused by infections with either virus. What is known is that in the year 1969–70 two foci of AHC appeared in the world, one in Africa and another in Asia. The infecting agent in both centres was probably enterovirus 70, while Coxsackievirus type A24 was isolated in Singapore in 1970. It has been suggested (Kono, 1975) that Moslem pilgrims may have played a part in establishing these two foci but there is little evidence to support such a theory. However, any form of pilgrimage which brings closely together subjects from widely separated regions to which they subsequently return, offers an excellent opportunity for the spread and dissemination of any infectious agent.

It is quite amazing that not one, but two, enteroviruses should, within such a short period of time, emerge as major causes of acute conjunctivitis. Kono (1975) postulates that enterovirus type 70 may represent the 'humanisation' of an animal enterovirus facilitated by the close contact between animals and babies which may occur in parts of Africa. Such a possibility cannot be excluded but, intuitively, an explanation that would also account for the adaptation of Coxsackievirus A24 to the eye would be preferred. If the responsible factor were to reside in host resistance or mode of transmission of the agents, it would not even be necessary to propose the appearance of a new enterovirus but merely the manifestation of the presence of an already existing enterovirus which had not previously caused symptoms.

For whatever reason these two viruses should commence to cause ocular disease, there is no doubt that the two foci of infections were in such areas that spread could occur with great ease. Poor hygiene resulting from poverty, ignorance or custom, together with overcrowding, facilitates case-to-case transmission, and under these conditions AHC gave rise to epidemics of un-paralleled size in recent times. It is estimated that over a million cases occurred in Calcutta between May and July 1971 (Kono, 1975) and half a million cases in Bombay between March and September of that year (Wadia *et al.*, 1973). Further evidence of the size of these epidemics is provided by the fact that the local population ascribed names to the disease such as 'Apollo 11 disease' and

'Joy Bangla' (Pramanik, 1971). The effect of overcrowding and poor hygiene can be judged by comparing the incidence of disease in various socio-economic groups during an outbreak. In Nigeria 24 per cent of labourers were clinically affected but only 6 per cent of the Nigerian managerial staff and 2 per cent of the expatriate managerial staff suffered (Parrott, 1971). Similarly, 43 per cent of Vietnamese refugees developed AHC, mainly on the crowded evacuation vessels, but only 1 per cent of the Americans attending them contracted the disease (Arnow et al., 1977).

The initial epidemics of AHC spread throughout Africa and Asia, and epidemics of similar proportions have recently affected South America, the Caribbean and Southern U.S.A. However, only limited outbreaks have been recorded in certain European countries and none in Australasia. In Europe, and commonly in Japan, the spread of the disease has been restricted to household contacts or has occurred as nosocomial outbreaks centred on ophthalmic units, in the same way as adenovirus epidemic keratoconjunctivitis spreads in those countries with high standards of hygiene (Jones, 1972; Mitsui et al., 1972; Schaap, 1974; Likar et al., 1975; Minami et al., 1976). A similar pattern can be expected among the more prosperous areas of the USA, but widespread infections, as seen in South America and the Caribbean would be forecast for the poorer sections of this country.

There is no doubt that the spread of both viruses can be accomplished by transfer of the ocular discharge. With Coxsackievirus A24 there are other possibilities for the virus can be recovered from the eye for only the first two days of symptoms but it is readily isolated from the throat and faeces for very much longer, at least 20 days (Langford et al., 1979). Enterovirus 70 is seldom isolated from the faeces (Sasagawa et al., 1976) although this has been accomplished on occasions (Mirkovic et al., 1973; Kono et al., 1977).

The spread of AHC viruses is similar to that of adenovirus type 8, with natural epidemics being replaced by hospital-based outbreaks in those areas where the standard of hygiene of the general community has been raised. Similarly, with both adenovirus type 8 and enterovirus type 70 infections, the conjunctival element of the clinical picture is often lacking in younger members of the population (Kono, 1975; Hung et al., 1976; Minami et al., 1976). Very few people had antibody to enterovirus 70 before 1969 so it would be expected that the introduction of a new virus would lead to disease which would affect all age groups equally. This might be modified by the standard of hygiene exhibited by individuals, with the result that young children would be expected to have a somewhat higher incidence of AHC than adults. In fact the converse proved to be true, with a lower incidence of AHC in children under 15 years of age than in adults. However, serological estimation of infection following outbreaks of AHC showed that children did in fact have the highest incidence of infection, but only a small proportion of them presented with ocular manifestations (Mathur et al., 1977). It is characteristic of enterovirus infections that a higher proportion of infections are subclinical in children than in adults.

In the developed countries the incidence of AHC is, again, greatest in adults and even in the aged, but this can be attributed, in part at least, to the iatrogenic nature of the disease in these countries, where the age of those attending ophthalmic centres is likely to be greater than the national average.

It is not easy to estimate the incidence with which neurological symptoms complicate AHC. It is believed that approximately 500,000 cases of AHC occurred in Bombay in 1971 and 19 cases of radiculomyelitis were observed (Wadia et al., 1973). If this is the true incidence, or if the proportion of 1 in 10,000 (Hung and Kono, 1979) is accepted, it is not surprising that few other areas have reported this type of complication. Many of the outbreaks, including all those in Europe and Japan, would be expected to yield less than one case of radiculomyelitis per outbreak. However, in addition to the 19 cases described as occurring in Bombay, 26 cases were reported from Thailand (Kono et al., 1977), 33 from Taiwan (Hung et al., 1976), and 8 from Senegal (Kono et al., 1976). There may be some doubt as to the authenticity of a few of the cases which failed to give a history of AHC and also did not possess antibodies to enterovirus type 70 in their convalescent sera, but the majority do appear to be related to AHC and in most instances the possibility of poliovirus infection had been considered and excluded.

The age range of the patients with radiculomyelitis reflected that of those suffering from AHC, with no case of neurological complication in children under 15 years of age. The sex distribution of AHC was generally equal, but in Taiwan there was a male preponderance of 3:1 (Hung et al., 1976). Of the 86 cases of radiculomyelitis recorded in the literature, 61 are males, but this is heavily influenced by the Taiwan figures which show the same sex distribution as in AHC in that country.

The manner of presentation of the neurological complications of AHC differed in the 1981 epidemic in India, with a proportion of the cases showing cranial-nerve lesions. This was not the only contrast with the previous 1971 epidemic, for there was also an apparent increase in the incidence of these complications; 94 such cases had been reported from five centres in three regions of the country by the end of 1981 (Wadia et al., 1981; Katiyar et al., 1981; Thakur, 1981; Mondkar, 1981; John et al., 1981).

Diagnosis

The diagnosis of AHC can often be made on clinico-epidemiological grounds. Infection will commonly be part of an epidemic and it can be differentiated from adenovirus epidemic keratoconjunctivitis by the absence of subepithelial lesions of the cornea. The presence of subconjunctival haemorrhages may well be helpful, but on occasions, when caused by adenoviruses, they will be misleading. It is therefore desirable if not essential to have virological confirmation of the clinical diagnosis. This can be achieved either by isolating the virus or by producing serological evidence of infection with one of the two known causal enteroviruses.

The isolation of Coxsackievirus A24 is simple, as it will readily grow in a number of continuous cell lines. However, it is important that eye swabs are collected early in the illness as infectious virus disappears from the ocular discharge within 2 days of the onset of symptoms, by which time the tears possess neutralising activity (Langford et al., 1979). Enterovirus 70 is a much more fastidious virus, requiring such conditions as blind passage in human embryo kidney cultures, and some strains have been isolated only after

PLATE III

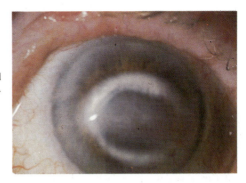

(a) Severe rebound zoster keratitis in a patient treated for six months with topical corticosteroid for minor corneal opacities.

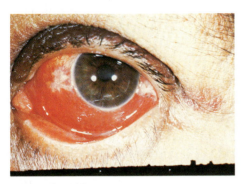

(b) Subconjunctival haemorrhages in acute haemorrhagic conjunctivitis.

(c) 'Tomato sauce' and 'ketchup' appearance seen in patients with active retinitis due to generalised cytomegalovirus infection. (Courtesy, Mr John Scott.)

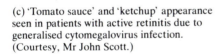

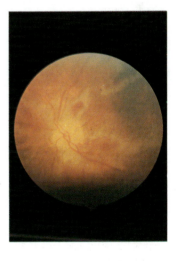

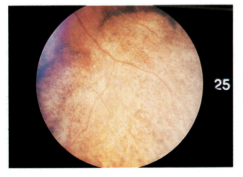

25

(d) Retinal pigment epithelial atrophy in a patient with an immunodeficiency and a history of generalised cytomegalic inclusion disease. (Courtesy, Mr Paul Mills.)

adaptation in human embryo conjunctival organ cultures (Higgins and Scott, 1973). Whatever method has been used to culture, the virus isolation rates have seldom reached the efficiency achieved for the isolation of Coxsackievirus A24. Numerous enterovirus-like particles have been seen by electron-microscopy of negatively stained conjunctival scrapings taken within 2 days of the onset of symptoms with enterovirus 70 conjunctivitis (Mitsui *et al.*, 1972).

Paired sera, one collected early in the illness and a second during the convalescent phase, can be used to demonstrate the presence of a rise in antibody to one of the two enteroviruses. Such a rise would establish that the illness and the infection were concurrent.

The diagnosis of enterovirus 70 radiculomyopathy is less easy to achieve. Virus could not be isolated from conjunctiva, throat, faeces, CSF, blood or urine of the cases in Bombay (Wadia *et al.*, 1973) nor from the CSF of 10 cases in Thailand, but one strain was isolated from 7 stool samples from these patients (Kono *et al.*, 1977). It was argued that if virus spread from the eye to the CNS the necessary viraemia would prove a greater stimulus than local disease, with the result that cases of radiculomyelitis would have higher convalescent antibody titres to enterovirus 70 than those with just AHC. On the basis of an early survey it was suggested that a neutralising antibody titre of 1/16 or greater was diagnostic of radiculomyelitis (Kono *et al.*, 1974; Green *et al.*, 1975). However, it was later shown that there was no significant difference between mean titres to enterovirus 70 in those with AHC and those with AHC and neurological complications (Kono *et al.*, 1977). Some would attach considerable significance to the fact that 2 patients with radiculomyopathy showed a rise of antibody titre despite the acute serum being taken after the onset of neurological signs (Kono *et al.*, 1977). Others might prefer to think of this as slower antibody production in these individuals. The antibody response to enterovirus 70 AHC can be poor, as demonstrated by two laboratory infections which occurred in Japan (Sasagawa *et al.*, 1976). More satisfactory evidence for the causal role of enterovirus 70 in the neurological complications of AHC has come from recent studies of cerebral spinal fluid (CSF) antibody. Kono and his colleagues (1981) demonstrated the presence of antibody to enterovirus 70 in the CSF of six out of eight patients with AHC and paralysis. Even more convincing were the results obtained by studying five patients with AHC and polio-like illness in Vellore (John *et al.*, 1981). Convalescent serum and CSF were obtained simultaneously from each patient, and all had raised serum antibody titres to enterovirus 70. Four patients also had CSF antibody and the ratio of serum to CSF antibody titres excluded the possibility of transfer of antibody across the blood-brain barrier. The fifth patient, whose CSF antibody titre was less than 1/4, was subsequently shown to have an intramedullary glioma. This technique can now be used to determine whether enterovirus 70 can produce paralysis in patients without an associated conjunctivitis. A rise in antibody titre between samples of CSF taken in the acute and convalescent phases of the illness would be conclusive.

Poliomyelitis is still prevalent in the areas where cases of radiculomyelitis have occurred but has been convincingly excluded as a cause of paralysis in a number of instances (Kono *et al.*, 1977).

Investigational and Experimental Virology

The viruses isolated from the early epidemics of AHC were readily recognised as enteroviruses, and a number of independent investigators proceeded to demonstrate that the viruses possessed all the characteristics necessary for inclusion within this group (Kono et al., 1972; Yin-Murphy, 1972; Kapsenberg, 1973; Higgins et al., 1974; Nejmi et al., 1974; Tai, 1974; Yamazaki et al., 1974; Jayavusu et al., 1975; Roy et al., 1975). Difficulties were encountered when none of the strains could be neutralised by antisera to any of the known enteroviruses. During the course of characterising the isolates it became apparent that some were pathogenic for suckling mice and others were not (Higgins et al., 1974) i.e. some behaved as a Coxsackievirus and others as an echovirus. It was also shown that these two groups were serologically distinct (Yin-Murphy and Lim, 1972; Yin-Murphy, 1973a,b,c; Higgins et al., 1974) although at that time all of the isolates in each group were closely related to each other antigenically. Eventually the 'echotype' virus was determined to be a new virus, enterovirus type 70 (Mirkovic et al., 1973) while the 'Coxsackie-like' virus was shown to be a prime variant of the established Coxsackievirus type A24 (Mirkovic et al., 1974).

By using plaque size and kinetic neutralisation tests it was shown that four of the early enterovirus 70 isolates could be subdivided into three groups (Esposito et al., 1974). A later study of 12 strains of enterovirus 70, 10 of which had been isolated in Japan between 1971 and 1976, showed that 1971 and some 1972 isolates resembled the prototype, other strains isolated in 1972 and those in 1973 were intermediate and strains isolated from 1974 to 1976 were prime variants (Kawamoto, 1979). Antigenic variation of this type is common among the enteroviruses. The causal role of both enteroviruses in AHC was easy to establish because of the high frequency with which virus was isolated from cases, and the rise in neutralising antibody to the infecting virus which occurred in patients over the course of the illness. Final proof for both viruses was provided by accidental laboratory infections which gave rise to AHC from which the virus could be recovered (Sasagawa et al., 1976; Langford et al., 1979).

Coxsackievirus A24 was recognised long before the epidemics of AHC occurred and therefore some people would have pre-existing antibody in their sera, but enterovirus 70 was a new virus and sera collected before the pandemic would not be expected to possess any antibody to this particular virus. Sera collected in Lucknow before 1971 failed to neutralise enterovirus 70 (Mathur et al., 1977) and only 0·3 per cent of sera collected between 1970 and 1974 from people living in eastern and south-eastern U.S.A. contained neutralising antibody to any of 3 or 4 strains of enterovirus 70 (Hierholzer et al., 1975). However, about 5 per cent of pre-epidemic sera collected in Ghana and Indonesia contained antibody at a titre of 1/8 or greater (Kono et al., 1975). If this reaction is specific it would indicate a limited presence of the virus prior to the emergence of AHC.

The inability to isolate enterovirus 70 from the CSF of cases of radiculo-myelitis made it difficult to prove this virus was the aetiological agent. The great majority of cases were preceded by AHC so that the isolation of virus from other sites and the demonstration of a rise in serum antibody could be as well related to one illness as the other. However, the presence of antibody to enterovirus 70 in high titre in the CSF of patients with neurological complications of AHC (Kono et al., 1981; John et al., 1981) confirms enterovirus 70 as the causal agent. Furthermore, there is some supportive experimental evidence as this virus will produce paralysis when inoculated into the CNS of the monkey, but only when large amounts are used (Kono et al., 1973). Interestingly enough, virus was not recovered from the CNS of these animals but an antibody response was obtained. The same authors reported the production of ocular discharge and haemorrhage in one of four monkeys following conjunctival inoculation. Again, virus was not recovered from the eye. Workers in Thailand have produced fever and conjunctivitis in rabbits and monkeys with enterovirus 70 by the same route but no haemorrhages were observed (Jayavusu et al., 1975). One of three monkeys developed muscle weakness after the conjunctivitis had resolved. Kono and his colleagues (1973) liken the neurovirulence of enterovirus 70 to that of polio vaccine which is compatible with the relatively small number of cases of neurological complication compared to the enormous number of cases of AHC.

The author has observed conjunctivitis in mice inoculated, not with enterovirus 70 but with the prime variant of Coxsackievirus A24. This virus is less pathogenic for suckling mice than most of the lower numbered serotypes so that many of the litter survive infection and only a proportion develop paralysis. However, ocular lesions were observed in approximately 3 per cent of mice which survived 30 days. The onset varied between 24 and 30 days after subcutaneous inoculation and, in those mice which were not sacrificed, persisted for 10 days before recovery was complete. In the white mice used, the most striking sign was the swelling of the eyelids which results in complete closure of the palpebral fissure. Evidence of discharge was also seen, but the lesions did not appear to be troublesome to the affected mice. Conjunctivitis, which in one instance was bilateral, occurred only in those mice already affected by paralysis. Virus was not recovered from eye swabs nor from the eye and conjunctiva when used as organ cultures. Bacterial cultures were sterile or yielded a scanty growth of non-pathogens.

The inoculation of virus into the conjunctival sac of mice three to four weeks old failed to produce conjunctivitis in the following 30 days, irrespective of whether or not they had been inoculated subcutaneously with the virus when 24–48 hours old. These findings suggest that neither replication of the virus in the conjunctiva nor previous sensitisation of the conjunctiva by systemic infection is the cause of the conjunctivitis seen in mice. The mechanism by which conjunctivitis does occur in mice and other animals would appear to be different from that in man and be more closely related to that responsible for paralysis in humans and monkeys.

Prevention and Treatment

The great similarity which exists between the epidemiology of epidemic keratoconjunctivitis and AHC would indicate that those measures which have proved effective in limiting the spread of type 8 adenovirus would be equally efficient in curtailing epidemics of AHC. For this reason it has been advocated that great attention should be paid to the washing of hands between examining patients and the adequate sterilisation of instruments (Dawson *et al.*, 1974). Such procedures should rapidly halt those outbreaks based on ophthalmic units as seen in Japan and Europe. The community epidemics have all occurred in areas where overcrowding is common and hygiene poor, and it is only by changing these conditions that epidemics of this nature can be prevented.

It has been suggested that attention should be given to developing a vaccine to protect against the neurological complications of enterovirus 70 infections (Wadia *et al.*, 1981). However, it should be remembered that the need for such a vaccine will be greatest in those regions where poliomyelitis still exists. No greater, and possibly less, success can be expected in respect of any enterovirus 70 vaccine programme.

There is disagreement as to whether enterovirus 70 grows better at 33°C than 37°C (Miyamura *et al.*, 1974; Tokuda *et al.*, 1973; Miyamura *et al.*, 1976) but all accept that the virus grows less well at temperatures above 37°C. It has been postulated that this property of the virus be utilised in treatment (Stanton *et al.*, 1977). Under certain conditions both enterovirus 70 and Coxsackievirus A24 are poor inducers of interferon but are sensitive to it, and the suggestion has been made that the application of interferon to the conjunctival sac could be a simple and effective method of treatment of AHC (Stanton *et al.*, 1977). As both eyes are commonly involved a controlled study could easily be performed and it is hoped that advantage will be taken of the current epidemic in the Americas to answer this question. Until interferon is readily available and its efficacy proved there is no specific treatment for this self-limiting condition.

Outlook

The massive epidemics which occurred in the early seventies in Asia and Africa are now affecting the Americas and recurring small epidemics can be expected in the latter region for the next few years. Thereafter it is very probable that the occurrence of sporadic cases and sub-clinical infections in children will lead to a similar situation to that seen with other enteroviruses. During periods of minimal activity by these two enteroviruses the number of those who are not immune will increase to allow minor epidemics every few years but they are unlikely to reach the proportions of those seen initially when virtually the whole population was susceptible. It is to be hoped that the standard of living will be raised in those areas which have suffered the maximal impact of the epidemics so that, even if the pool of susceptibles does increase, both viruses will experience greater difficulty in passing from one host to another and so reduce the size of any potential outbreak.

REFERENCES

ARNOW, P. M., HIERHOLZER, J. C., HIGBEE, J. and HARRIS, D. H. (1977). Acute hemorrhagic conjunctivitis. A mixed outbreak among Vietnamese refugees on Guam. *Amer. J. Epidem.*, **105**, 68–74.

BHARUCHA, E. P. and MONDKAR, V. P. (1972). Neurological complications of a new conjunctivitis. *Lancet*, **2**, 970.

Bourdieu, J. P. (1973). A propos de l'épidémie de conjonctivite observée au Maroc en 1971. *Maroc Med.*, **53**, 45–60.

Chatterjee, S., Quarcoopome, C. O. and Apenteng, A. (1970). Unusual type of epidemic conjunctivitis in Ghana. *Brit. J. Ophthal.*, **54**, 628–30.

Christopher, S., John, T. J., Charles, B. and Roy, S. (1977). Coxsackie A24 variant EH27/70 and enterovirus type 70 in an epidemic of acute haemorrhagic conjunctivitis—a preliminary report. *Indian J. Med. Res.*, **65**, 593–5.

Dawson, C. R., Whitcher, J. P. and Schmidt, N. J. (1974). Editorial: Acute hemorrhagic conjunctivitis. *J. Amer. Med. Ass.*, **230**, 727–8.

Desmyter, J., Colaert, J., Maertens, K. and Muyumbe, T. (1981). Enterovirus 70 haemorrhagic conjunctivitis in Zäire, 1981 versus 1972. *Lancet*, **2**, 1054–5.

Dumavibhat, P., Panpatana, P., Wasi, C., Jatikavanij, V., Sarasombath, S. and Thongcharoen, P. (1973). An outbreak of acute haemorrhagic conjunctivitis in Thailand. *J. Med. Ass. Thailand*, **56**, 267–272.

Esposito, J. J., Hierholzer, J. C., Obijeski, J. F. and Hatch, M. H. (1974). Characterization of four virus isolates obtained during acute haemorrhagic conjunctivitis outbreaks. *Microbiology*, **11**, 215–27.

Golden, B. and Smit, P. (1974). Epidemic haemorrhagic conjunctivitis. *S. Afr. Med. J.*, **48**, 619.

Green, I. J., Hung, T. P. and Sung, S. M. (1975). Neurologic complications with elevated antibody titre after acute hemorrhagic conjunctivitis. *Amer. J. Ophthal.*, **80**, 832–4.

Hierholzer, J. C., Hillard, K. A. and Esposito, J. J. (1975). Serosurvey for 'acute hemorrhagic conjunctivitis' virus (enterovirus 70) antibodies in the south-eastern United States, with review of the literature and some epidemiologic implications. *Amer. J. Epidem.*, **102**, 533–44.

Higgins, P. G. and Chapman, T. E. D. (1977). Coxsackie A24 and acute haemorrhagic conjunctivitis in Sri Lanka. *Lancet*, **1**, 361.

Higgins, P. G. and Scott, R. J. D. (1973). The isolation of enteroviruses from cases of acute conjunctivitis. *J. Clin. Path.*, **26**, 706–11.

Higgins, P. G., Scott, R. J., Davies, Patricia M. and Gamble, D. R. (1974). A comparative study of viruses associated with acute haemorrhagic conjunctivitis. *J. Clin. Path.*, **27**, 292–6.

Hung, T. P. and Kono, R. (1979). Neurological complications of acute haemorrhagic conjunctivitis (A polio-like syndrome in adults). In *Handbook of Clinical Neurology*, Vol. 38, pp. 595–623. Eds. P. J. Vinken, G. W. Bruyn and H. L. Klawans. Amsterdam: North Holland.

Hung, T. P., Sung, S. M., Liang, H. C., Landsborough, D. and Green, I. J. (1976). Radioculomyelitis following acute haemorrhagic conjunctivitis. *Brain*, **99**, 771–90.

Jayavusu, C., Santiswatdinont, P., Srimarut, S. and Sangkawibha, N. (1975). Characterization of a virus associated with epidemic conjunctivitis in Thailand. *Biken's J.*, **18**, 249–55.

John, J. J., Christopher, S. and Abraham, J. (1981). Neurological manifestations of acute haemorrhagic conjunctivitis due to enterovirus 70. *Lancet*, **2**, 1283–4.

Jones, B. R. (1972). Epidemic haemorrhagic conjunctivitis in London, 1971: A conjunctival picornavirus infection. *Trans. Ophthal. Soc. U.K.*, **92**, 625–7.

Kapsenberg, J. G. (1973). Virus isolatie bij enn plaatselijke epidemie van haemorrhagische conjunctivitis in Veenedaal. *Ber. Rijks Inst. Volksgezond. Utrecht*, **33**, 160–1.

Katiyar, B. C., Misra, S., Singh, R. B. and Singh, A. K. (1981). Neurological syndromes after acute epidemic conjunctivitis. *Lancet*, **2**, 866–7.

Kawamoto, H. (1979). Antigenic analysis of acute haemorrhagic conjunctivitis viruses (enterovirus type 70). *Microbiol. Immunol.*, **23**, 859–66.

KONO, R. (1975). Apollo 11 disease or acute haemorrhagic conjunctivitis: A pandemic of a new enterovirus infection of the eyes. *Amer. J. Epidem.*, **101**, 383–390.

KONO, R., MIYAMURA, K., OGINO, T., WADIA, N. H., WADIA, P. N., KATRAK, S. M. and MISRA, V. P. (1981). Antibody titres to enterovirus type 70 in the 1981 Indian epidemic of acute haemorrhagic conjunctivitis. *Lancet*, **2**, 924–5.

KONO, R., MIYAMURA, K., TAJIRI, E., ROBIN, Y. and GIRARD, P. (1976). Serological studies of radiculomyelitis occurring during the outbreak of acute haemorrhagic conjunctivitis in Senegal in 1970. *Jap. J. Med. Sci. Biol.*, **29**, 91–4.

KONO, R., MIYAMURA, K., TAJIRI, E., SASAGAWA, A., PHUAPRADIT, P., ROONGWITHU, N., VEJJAJIVA, A., JAYAVASU, C., THONGCHAROEN, P., WASI, C. and RODPRASSERT, P. (1977). Virological and serological studies of neurological complications of acute haemorrhagic conjunctivitis in Thailand. *J. Infect. Dis.*, **135**, 706–13.

KONO, R., MIYAMURA, K., TAJIRI, E., SHIGA, S., SASAGAWA, A., IRANI, P. F., KATRAK, S. M. and WADIA, N. H. (1974). Neurologic complications associated with acute haemorrhagic conjunctivitis virus infection and its serologic confirmation. *J. Infect. Dis.*, **129**, 590–3.

KONO, R., SASAGAWA, A., ISHII, K., SUGIURA, S., OCHI, M., MATSUMIYA, H., UCHIDA, Y., KAMEYAMA, K., KANEKO, M. and SAKURAI, N. (1972). Pandemic of a new type of conjunctivitis. *Lancet*, **1**, 1191–4.

KONO, R., SASAGAWA, A., MIYAMURA, K. and TAJIRI, E. (1975). Serologic characterization and sero-epidemiologic studies on acute hemorrhagic conjunctivitis (AHC) virus. *Amer. J. Epidem.*, **101**, 444–57.

KONO, R., UCHIDA, N., SASAGAWA, A., AKAO, Y., KODAMA, H., MUKOYAMA, J. and FUJIWARA, T. (1973). Neurovirulence of acute haemorrhagic conjunctivitis virus in monkeys. *Lancet*, **1**, 61–3.

LANGFORD, M. P., STANTON, G. J., BARBER, J. C. and BARON, S. (1979). Early-appearing antiviral activity in human tears during a case of picornavirus epidemic conjunctivitis. *J. Infect. Dis.*, **139**, 653–8.

LIKAR, M., TALANYI-PFEIFER, L. and MARIN, J. (1975). An outbreak of acute haemorrhagic conjunctivitis in Yugoslavia in 1973. *Path. et Microbiol.*, **42**, 29–35.

MATHUR, A., SHARMA, B. and CHATURVEDI, U. C. (1977). The investigation of a recurrence of an AHC virus epidemic at Lucknow: a serosurvey for AHC virus antibodies before and after the epidemic. *J. Hyg. (Lond.)*, **79**, 219–24.

METSELAAR, D., AWAN, A. M. and ENSERING, H. L. (1976). Acute haemorrhagic conjunctivitis and enterovirus 70 in Kenya. *Trop. Geogr. Med.*, **28**, 131–6.

MINAMI, K., KONNO, K., HONMA, M., MIZUNO, H. and FUJIMURA, S. (1976). An epidemic of acute haemorrhagic conjunctivitis in Sendai area, 1973–4. *Tohoku J. Exp. Med.*, **120**, 329–37.

MIRKOVIC, R. R., KONO, R., YIN-MURPHY, M., SOHIER, R., SCHMIDT, N. J. and MELNICK, J. L. (1973). Enterovirus type 70: the etiologic agent of pandemic acute hemorrhagic conjunctivitis. *Bull. Wld. Hlth. Org.*, **49**, 341–46.

MIRKOVIC, R. R., SCHMIDT, NATHALIE, J., YIN-MURPHY, M. and MELNICK, J. L. (1974). Enterovirus etiology of the 1970 Singapore epidemic of acute conjunctivitis. *Intervirology*, **4**, 119–27.

MITSUI, Y., KAJIMA, M., MATSUMARA, K. and SHIOTA, H. (1972). Haemorrhagic conjunctivitis, a new type of epidemic viral keratoconjunctivitis. *Jap. J. Ophthal.*, **16**, 33–40.

MIYAMURA, K., SASAGAWA, A., TAJIRI, E. and KONO, R. (1976). Growth characteristics of acute haemorrhagic conjunctivitis (AHC) virus in monkey kidney cells. II. Temperature sensitivity of the isolates obtained at various epidemic areas. *Intervirology*, **7**, 192–200.

MIYAMURA, K., YAMAZAKI, S., TAJIRI, E. and KONO, R. (1974). Growth characteristics of acute haemorrhagic conjunctivitis (AHC) virus in monkey kidney cells. I. Effect of temperature on viral growth. *Intervirology*, **4**, 279–86.

MONDKAR, V. P. (1981). Cranial nerve paralyses associated with acute haemorrhagic conjunctivitis. *Lancet*, **2**, 584.

MUZZI, A., ROCCHI, G., LUMBROSO, B., TOSATO, G. and BARBIERI, F. (1975). Acute haemorrhagic conjunctivitis during an epidemic outbreak of adenovirus type 4 infection. *Lancet*, **2**, 822–3.

NEJMI, S., GAUDIN, O. G., CHOMEL, J. J., BAAJ, A., SOHIER, R. and BOSSHARD, S. (1974). Isolation of a virus responsible for an outbreak of acute haemorrhagic conjunctivitis in Morocco. *J. Hyg. (Lond.)*, **72**, 181–3.

PARROTT, W. F. (1971). An epidemic called Apollo. An outbreak of conjunctivitis in Nigeria. *Practitioner*, **206**, 253–5.

PHUAPRADIT, PRIDA, ROONGWITHU, N., LIMSUKON, P., BOONGIRD, P. and VEJJAJIVA, ATHASIT (1976). Radioculomyelitis complicating acute haemorrhagic conjunctivitis. *J. Neurol. Sci.*, **27**, 117–22.

PRAMANIK, D. D. (1971). Joy Bangla. An epidemic of conjunctivitis in India. *Practitioner*, **207**, 805–6.

ROY, I. S., ROY, S. N. and AHMED, E. (1972). Epidemic acute conjunctivitis. *Brit. J. Ophthal.*, **56**, 501–3.

ROY, I., SARKAR, J. K., CHAKRAVARTY, M. S., MUKHERJEE, K. K., MUKHERJEE, M. K., CHAKRAVARTY, S. K., ROY, I. S., MITRA, B. K. and SEN, G. C. (1975). Virological studies on the epidemic of conjunctivitis in Calcutta. *Indian J. Med. Res.*, **63**, 27–30.

SASAGAWA, A., KONO, R. and KONNO, K. (1976). Laboratory acquired infection of the eye with AHC virus. *Japan J. Med. Sci. Biol.*, **29**, 95–7.

SCHAAP, G. J. P. (1974). Acute haemorrhagic conjunctivitis in Rotterdam—July 1971. (Personal communication.)

STANTON, G. J., LANGFORD, M. P. and BARON, S. (1977). Effect of interferon, elevated temperature and cell type on replication of acute hemorrhagic conjunctivitis viruses. *Infection & Immunity*, **18**, 370–6.

TAI, F. U. (1974). Characterisation of viruses isolated in Taiwan during 1971 outbreaks of acute haemorrhagic conjunctivitis. *Chin. J. Microbiol.*, **7**, 179.

TAI, F. U., LIN, H. M., CHU, S., WEI, H. Y. and HIERHOLZER, J. C. (1974). A new form of acute conjunctivitis epidemic in Taiwan. A simultaneous outbreak of adenovirus type 11 and 'acute haemorrhagic conjunctivitis' virus infections. *Chin. J. Microbiol.*, **7**, 79–88.

THAKUR, L. C. (1981). Cranial nerve paralyses associated with acute haemorrhagic conjunctivitis. *Lancet*, **2**, 584.

THONGCHAROEN, P. and WASI, C. (1978). Picornavirus haemorrhagic conjunctivitis in Thailand 1971–5. *Abst. IV Int. Cong. Virol, The Hague*, 650.

TOKUDA, M., IMAI, J., MATSUO, Y., KOMODA, H. and TAKAHASHI, H. (1973). Studies on acute haemorrhagic conjunctivitis virus. *Ann. Res. Inst. Virus Res. Kyoto Univ.*, **16**, 15–24.

TULLO, A. B. and HIGGINS, P. G. (1980). An outbreak of adenovirus type 4 conjunctivitis. *Brit. J. Ophthal.*, **64**, 489–93.

WADIA, N. H., IRANI, P. F. and KATRAK, S. M. (1973). Lumbosacral radiculomyelitis associated with pandemic acute haemorrhagic conjunctivitis. *Lancet*, **1**, 350–2.

WADIA, N. H., WADIA, P. N., KATRAK, S. M. and MISRA, V. P. (1981). Neurological manifestations of acute haemorrhagic conjunctivitis. *Lancet*, **2**, 528–9.

WHITCHER, J. P., SCHMIDT, NATHALIE, J., MABROUK, R., MESSADI, M., DAGHFOUS, T., HOSHIWARA, I. and DAWSON, C. R. (1976). Acute haemorrhagic conjunctivitis in Tunisia. *Arch. Ophthal.*, **94**, 51–55.

WHO Weekly Epidemiological Record (1980*a*). Epidemic haemorrhagic conjunctivitis. **55**, 149.

WHO Weekly Epidemiological Record (1980*b*). Acute haemorrhagic conjunctivitis. **55**, 175.

WHO Weekly Epidemiological Record (1981*a*). Acute haemorrhagic conjunctivitis. **56**, 293–4.

WHO Weekly Epidemiological Record (1981*b*). Enterovirus 70 surveillance. Acute haemorrhagic conjunctivitis. **56**, 254.

WHO Weekly Epidemiological Record (1981*c*). Acute haemorrhagic conjunctivitis. **56**, 346.

WHO Weekly Epidemiological Record (1981*d*). Acute haemorrhagic conjunctivitis in the American region. **56**, 311.

WHO Weekly Epidemiological Record (1981*e*). Acute haemorrhagic conjunctivitis. **56**, 325–6.

YAMAZAKI, S., NATORI, K. and KONO, R. (1974). Purification and biophysical properties of acute haemorrhagic conjunctivitis virus. *J. Virol.*, **14**, 1357–60.

YIN-MURPHY, M. (1972). An epidemic of picornavirus conjunctivitis in Singapore. *S.E. Asian J. Trop. Med. Pub. Hlth.*, **3**, 303–9.

YIN-MURPHY, M. (1973*a*). The picornaviruses of acute haemorrhagic conjunctivitis: a comparative study. *S.E. Asian J. Trop. Med. Pub. Hlth.*, **4**, 305–10.

YIN-MURPHY, M. (1973*b*). The picornaviruses of epidemic conjunctivitis. *S.E. Asian J. Trop. Med. Pub. Hlth.*, **4**, 11–14.

YIN-MURPHY, M. (1973*c*). Viruses of acute haemorrhagic conjunctivitis. *Lancet*, **1**, 545–6.

YIN-MURPHY, M. (1976). Simple tests for the diagnosis of picornavirus epidemic conjunctivitis (acute haemorrhagic conjunctivitis). *Bull. Wld. Hlth. Org.*, **54**, 675–679.

YIN-MURPHY, M. (1980). Personal communication.

YIN-MURPHY, M. and LIM, K. H. (1972). Picornavirus epidemic conjunctivitis in Singapore. *Lancet*, **2**, 857–8.

YIN-MURPHY, M., LIM, K. H. and HO, Y. M. (1976). A Coxsackie type A24 epidemic of acute conjunctivitis. *S.E. Asian J. Trop. Med. Pub. Hlth.*, **7**, 1–5.

CHAPTER TWELVE

Viral Infections of the Fetus and Newborn

Introduction

A major unsolved problem in medicine today concerns the large number of children born each year with congenital malformations. Often it is the essential organs of the body such as the central nervous system and cardiovascular system which are affected. Little is known about the causation of congenital malformations despite the remarkable advances which have occurred in medical science in the last decade. The causes can be classified as environmental, in that they may be directly attributed to an infection or ionising radiation, or genetic, due to chromosomal anomalies and mutant gene effects, or mixed genetic and environmental, which may indeed account for the majority of congenital malformations. A number of viruses have been incriminated as a cause of prenatal disease leading to fetal damage and spontaneous abortion, stillbirth, congenital defects or other forms of damage. However, the association between maternal virus disease and congenital infection is ill-defined. Viruses may produce long-term effects on the individual which have not yet been realised. Where disease is produced immediately after birth the relationship appears to be clear. It is becoming apparent that not all infectious agents, especially viruses, behave in a conventional way in regard to stimulating immune responses and causing disease processes.

Although a great deal of work has been carried out on the induction of malformation in developing chick embryos and certain mammalian species, the relevance of this work to human malformation is difficult to interpret because of the differences in the structure and function of the placenta between species. There is therefore difficulty in the extrapolation of data from one species to another. There is no animal model for the study of the pathogenesis of rubella infection and its effect on the fetus, and it is true that the essential observations have come from detailed human studies. However, there are a number of models which test the vertical transmission of disease by viruses. The Bittner agent of mice is associated with a high incidence of mammary carcinoma in certain strains of mice. The animal leukaemia virus may infect the ovum directly and can be passed to the offspring, with the onset of disease several months after birth. Human cytomegalovirus may be passed to the newborn child with the mother's milk. Baby hamsters can develop hydrocephalus and aqueductal stenosis in this way as a result of secondary congenital mumps infection, and it is possible or feasible that a similar phenomenon may occur in man.

The criteria for establishing a causal relationship between a maternal infection and congenital defects or fetal damage have been suggested by Hanshaw and Dudgeon (1978). The clinical criteria are based on each infection inducing a syndrome with a repetitive pattern of clinical disease. Epidemiological features should indicate that the same manifestations are observed with the same agent following maternal illness in different countries. Virological evidence should show persistence of the infective agent in fetal tissues, and the induction of a chronic infective state after birth. Immunological evidence should reveal persistence of an antibody in the child after the normal decline of maternal antibody, and the presence of antibody in the IgM fraction. However, these criteria cannot be satisfied in all situations. Although clear-cut evidence exists in the case of maternal rubella and CMV infection, the evidence in mumps, measles, poliomyelitis, chickenpox and hepatitis is less well established. Thus, several large-scale prospective studies were carried out to examine the effect of these infections, and it was concluded that the overall evidence was not convincing. However, mumps virus has been incriminated as a cause of congenital defects more often than any virus other than rubella, although proof is still lacking. Ylinen and Jarvinen (1953) in Finland found a 22 per cent incidence of malformation in children whose mothers had parotitis in the first trimester, compared with 10 per cent in the second or third trimesters. In the Manson report (1960) there was an excess number of deaths occurring in infants in the second year of life from a variety of causes following maternal influenza between the 13th and 28th weeks of pregnancy. Smallpox vaccine definitely can cause fetal death and damage, particularly after primary vaccination. The evidence for this is substantial and justifies the recommendation that live vaccines are contra-indicated in pregnancy. Live attenuated rubella vaccines administered inadvertently during pregnancy have been known to affect the fetus, and in one case, structural damage to the lens of the eye has been reported (Modlin et al., 1975). Fetal abnormalities may be more frequent in mothers who have acquired Epstein-Barr virus infections during pregnancy (Icart and Didier, 1981), or the BK polyomavirus (Gibson et al., 1981).

Recently the development of advanced laboratory techniques has resulted in recognition of a broad spectrum of disease and a more frequent occurrence of herpetic infection in the neonate. The ocular manifestations of neonatal infection consists of conjunctivitis, keratitis, chorioretinitis, optic neuritis, cataract, uveitis, and microphthalmia, which occur in about 10 per cent of neonates with dissemination of the HSV infection and in 33 per cent of those with localised infection. Type 2 HSV is the major cause of neonatal disease, and the only agent which has been found in herpetic chorioretinitis. Brick *et al.* (1981) have investigated the effect of subacute cutaneous inoculation of HSV 2 in New Zealand white rabbits shortly after birth. Within 24 hours a cutaneous lesion was induced, and foci of infection occurred in many other organs, including the eye, by the third day and thereafter. Death of the animals occurred on the fifth day with infection of the central nervous system. HSV 2 was isolated from mononuclear and plasma cells of peripheral blood, indicating the possible role of both elements in dissemination of the virus. Forty per cent of animals developed ocular lesions consisting of retinal folds with or without degenerative changes. Iritis and choroiditis also developed in some eyes. Infectious virus could be isolated from 33 per cent of the eyes by days 4 and 5. The authors considered that the newborn rabbit may serve as a suitable experimental model for the study of herpes-simplex-induced chorioretinitis in the human newborn.

The human fetus responds immunologically to virtually all known intra-uterine and perinatal infections. Measurement of humoral immune responses plays an important role in the laboratory diagnosis of these infections. A feature of intra-uterine infection is that many of the agents may persist for varying time intervals. Thus the infection may last throughout fetal life, but it can extend to several weeks after birth, and in some instances it may persist for years. Defence mechanisms in the fetus are non-specific or specific. Non-specific mechanisms operate in the early stages of infection and do not depend upon specific recognition. Specific mechanisms, which are initiated by the lymphoid system, respond to a particular infectious agent or antigen. Fetal and neonatal immunity must take into account the transfer of antibody and immune cells from the mother before birth, and the consumption of antibody and other protective substances in colostrum and milk after birth (Table 12.1).

The importance of T-lymphocytes in recovery from viral infections has

TABLE 12.1

IMMUNE DEFENCE MECHANISMS IN THE FETUS AND NEWBORN

Non-specific

Skin
Mucous membrane
Breast milk (lysozyme, complement, lactoferrin,
    immunocompetent cells)
Antibody (passive transfer across the placental membranes)
Amnionic fluid (IgG, lysozyme, transferrin)
Covering fetal membranes (lost following rupture)
The placental barrier (infection may occur in CMV, HSV,
    vaccinia and varicella infection in the mother)
Production of interferon by the placenta
Phagocytosis (polymorphonuclear, monocytic)
The complement system

Specific

Humoral
Cell-mediated

already been described, and a defect in cell-mediated immunity has been postulated as a cause for the persistence of chronic infection in several of the intra-uterine viral infections, especially rubella and CMV infections. Suppression of cell-mediated immune reactions have not however been demonstrated conclusively in either of these infections (Denman, 1982). The major difficulty in the investigation has been the lack of suitable antigen. Fucillo *et al.* (1974) using chromium-release lymphocytotoxicity micro-assay systems to examine cell-mediated immunity in congenital rubella found evidence of a defective response. Similarly, in a study of congenital CMV, the reactivity of lymphocytes in mixed lymphocyte cultures was found to be diminished in children with symptomatic disease, but not in those with asymptomatic infections (Emodi *et al.*, 1973). Investigations of immune function in congenital rubella have sought to prove a hypothesis that virus persistence is associated with a defect in host defence mechanisms due to the development of a tolerant state, or an active immunosuppressive effect of the virus. However, this has not been clearly demonstrated and the whole question remains as yet unanswered.

CONGENITAL CYTOMEGALOVIRUS INFECTION

When the cytomegalovirus comes into contact with the unborn infant the infection may be contained by several of the defence mechanisms of the fetus, or there may be disease which ranges from subtle abnormality not detectable at birth to severe generalised disease which is apparent at birth or shortly after. The latter form of disease has been more fully documented than the former associated with mild manifestations. The importance of congenital CMV infection as a medical problem is related to the long-term development of infants, there being at least 10 infected infants who do not have clinical abnormality for every single infant born with overt signs of cytomegalic inclusion disease (CID). It was the impression that CMV infection was associated with severe illness in the newborn in a high proportion of cases, and that it carried a high probability of death or marked damage to the central nervous system. Since laboratory procedures for identification became available, it has been shown that CMV can indeed produce devastating disease in the newborn, but also that congenital infection, although relatively common, is usually inapparent at a clinical level and that it has a benign course which can be recognised if laboratory studies are performed. Many individuals develop antibody following unrecognised infection acquired during childhood or young adulthood. A small proportion of normal individuals may have a form of infectious mononucleosis or possibly symptoms of a respiratory illness with CMV infection. Clinical disease is more likely to be evident in those who are immunologically deficient because of neoplastic disease or are undergoing treatment with immunosuppressants. Following infection, virus excretion occurs intermittently in the face of high levels of circulating antibody. Dissemination probably occurs by close contact with an excreter, or spread may occur through the placenta or via blood transfusions.

Biological Characteristic of the Virus

CMV is morphologically indistinguishable from varicella zoster, herpes simplex, and other members of the herpesvirus family. Tissue culture may demonstrate a large proportion of forms which are incompletely endowed with nucleic acid. These empty or partially empty forms are non-infectious, and indicate that the synthesis of virus *in vitro* is defective. Human strains replicate to form complete virus only in human culture tissue. As in the case of varicella zoster, human fibroblasts infected with CMV are associated with contraction and rounding of cells, and the development of intranuclear and intracyto-plasmic inclusions, cellular enlargement, and the eventual formation of foci of altered cells which may fuse into giant forms. The virus is mostly cell associated although supernatants from tissues culture may contain large amounts of infectious virus. The viral agent is labile to low pH, fat solvents and temperature. Preservation is achieved by rapid freezing and storage at $-60°C$. Inactivation occurs at $-20°C$ more rapidly than at $4°C$ making ordinary refrigerator temperatures more acceptable for short-term storage.

The virus is best isolated by direct inoculation of fresh material into cultures of human fibroblasts. There is a certain amount of evidence that different strains of CMV exist, but there is little to suggest that the different syndromes caused by CMV are related to these strain differences. CMV can produce latent infections similar to the other herpesviruses which may reactivate under various conditions.

Laboratory Diagnosis

Isolation of the virus can be carried out usually from the pharynx, the buffy coat of peripheral blood, breast milk, urine, stools, tears, cervix and semen. Human fibroblast cultures should be inoculated and observed for six to eight weeks for the appearance of foci of swollen cells with intranuclear inclusions.

Serologically, complement fixation tests using a single strain of CMV antigen are used to detect antibody. It is unclear whether infection with one strain of virus precludes infection with another. An indirect haemagglutination method has been developed for the serological diagnosis. This test is more sensitive than complement fixation. It reflects the presence of antibody in IgG and IgM subclasses, whereas complement-fixing antibody affects principally IgG. Neutralisation, platelet aggregation, and fluorescent antibody techniques have also been used, but are somewhat laborious and variable in their results. As with rubella infection, the identification of CMV-specific antibody is important in the diagnosis of recent infection. It has been measured with the use of an indirect fluorescent antibody technique.

Intra-uterine Infections and Congenital Abnormality

Epidemiology—Cytomegalovirus causes intra-uterine infection in $0.7–18.0$ per cent of newborn babies. Several follow-up studies have shown a high frequency of at least mild developmental disorders of the central nervous system among congenitally infected infants (Starr *et al.*, 1970; Melish and Hanshaw, 1973). Some congenital infections are symptomless and at birth only a few congenitally infected babies show typical severe cytomegalic inclusion disease, with hepatosplenomegaly, thrombocytopenia, seizures and chorio-retinitis (Hanshaw, 1971). Infections may also occur in the first months of life, when it is called perinatal. CMV has been isolated frequently from the urine towards the end of pregnancy, and it has been suggested that cervical virus may be responsible for perinatal infection. Such infection is asymptomatic, and like congenital CMV infection it leads to the excretion of virus which may persist in the presence of humoral antibody for several months (Alford *et al.*, 1973; Numazaki *et al.*, 1970).

CMV infection as betokened by excretion of the virus in the urine is common within the population, and is frequent during pregnancy (Hurley and de Louvois, 1980). It is found in the urine of 2–3 per cent of pregnant women. However, primary infection is uncommon and it is thought to be about 1 in 200 women who become seropositive during pregnancy. The incidence of reported infections in England and Wales between 1976–1978 was of the order of 3·4 per 100,000 live births, and the incidence of severe disseminated cytomegalic inclusion disease approximates towards 1 in 100,000 live births. It is therefore easy to comprehend why there is little information concerning ocular disease in babies with recognised disease.

Infection with CMV in the appropriate species produces characteristic histopathological changes, including greatly enlarged (cytomegalic) cells containing intranuclear and cytoplasmic inclusions. The inclusions were formerly called salivary-gland viruses because they were frequently found in these glands in children and lower animals during routine histological examinations (Farber and Wolbach, 1932).

Cytomegalic inclusion disease describes a clinical syndrome with widespread involvement in newborn infants and which may have a fatal outcome (Birdsong *et al.*, 1956; Medearis, 1964). More recently, CMV infections have been recorded in children and adults with malignant disorders of the haemopoietic system (Bodey *et al.*, 1965; Cangir and Sullivan, 1966; Gottman and Beatty, 1962; Peace, 1958), in people with debilitating disease (Fisher and Davis, 1958; Nash *et al.*, 1970; Symmers, 1960; Wong and Warner, 1962; Wyatt *et al.*, 1951), and in patients with primary or secondary immunodeficiency disorders (Hill *et al.*, 1964; Kanich and Craighead, 1966).

Originally the diagnosis of CMV infections was made on postmortem tissue examined by histology, but in 1950 Wyatt *et al.* suggested that a diagnosis could be aided by finding characteristic cells in the urine. In 1956 the virus was isolated from salivary gland and renal tissue (Smith, 1956), while virus was later found in adenoid and liver tissue, and in urine (Rowe *et al.*, 1956; Weller *et al.*, 1957). Epidemiological studies using diagnostic serological techniques suggest that there is a high incidence of subclinical infection, such that a positive serological test does not necessarily indicate that there is a causal relationship between the disease under investigation and the implied presence of CMV.

Although the clinical manifestations of the disease vary, there is a recognisable syndrome complex in congenital and acquired infections. *In utero* infection may result in death of the fetus or a syndrome which includes jaundice, prematurity, hepatosplenomegaly, thrombocytopenia, purpura, pneumonitis, and damage to the central nervous system, with microcephaly, mental and motor retardation, calcification around the ventricles, chorioretinitis, and optic atrophy. Infection *in utero* is therefore not necessarily fatal, some children surviving with deficits in the central nervous system, while the infection remains in others (Birnbaum *et al.*, 1969). In the acquired form, clinical disease is not always apparent. Postmortem studies in infants more than 3 months of age dying of other causes showed evidence of CMV infections in the salivary glands in between 8 and 32 per cent (Seifert and Oehme, 1957), possibly largely due to postnatal infections. Acquired infection in children may produce subacute or chronic hepatitis, interstitial pneumonitis, or acquired haemolytic anaemia (Table 12.2). A syndrome similar to infectious mononucleosis has been described as occurring in children or adults following blood transfusion (Kääriäinen *et al.*, 1966*b*), where there is a concomitant rise of serum CMV antibody level (Kääriäinen *et al.*, 1966*a*).

TABLE 12.2

SYNDROMES IN CHILDREN AND ADULTS
FOLLOWING INFECTION BY CMV

Neonatal infections
   Congenital
   Acquired
Infections in children and adults
   Mononucleosis
   Hepatitis
   CMV infection following transfusion
   CMV infection following organ transplant
   CMV infection following malignant disease
   Encephalitis ⎫
   Guillain-Barré syndrome ⎬ possible relationship
   Ulcerative colitis ⎭

Pathogenesis—The various forms of CMV infection carry different consequences which is probably related to the level of the immune responses following the infection. Congenital infection may be associated with significant residual damage to the central nervous system, whereas acquired infection is often not associated with any long-term disability, even when it occurs in the newborn. Primary infection of the mother during the first three months of gestation is associated with a high probability of infection in the newborn; whether such infection is associated with birth defects remains unclear. Recurrent CMV infection during pregnancy is unlikely to result in the delivery of an infected baby.

Based on the available information concerning the relation between primary infection in the first trimester of pregnancy and the production of genetic abnormality, certain speculations can be made. During primary infection, a maternal viraemia would be expected, and under certain conditions virus in small quantities may cross the placenta to initiate foci of replication in fetal tissues. Maternal IgG crosses the placenta to interact with CMV which proliferates in the fetal host. The eventual manifestations of fetal disease must depend upon the relative amounts of virus and antibody. In the majority of instances where the amount of antibody is adequate, little virus-induced disease can occur, but where virus is in excess, with inadequate immune response, then it would be expected that disease would be induced in the fetus. However, cell-mediated immunity responses would be reduced or absent, which would allow proliferation of virus inside the cell, while antibody would exert its influence on extracellular virus only. Thus as long as live virus is not allowed to enter the cell, it seems likely that intra-uterine infection with CMV will be largely contained.

Immune response—Antibody to CMV is produced following CMV infection, and appears to persist throughout life. The primary response is highly specific. There is no cross-reactivity with other members of the herpesvirus group using complement fixation tests. Specific IgM antibody can be detected in neonates and elevated IgM can be found in the cord blood which indicates possible intra-uterine CMV infection (Reynolds *et al.*, 1974).

T-cells play a role in recovery from CMV infections as shown by studies in nude mice which succumb to experimental infection with sublethal dosages of CMV (Olding *et al.*, 1975; Starr, 1976). Studies in mothers and infants with congenital infection due to CMV demonstrated reduced CMI using ^{51}Cr release assay. It was considered there was a specific impairment in CMI to CMV in the mothers of infected infants, and similar observations were made in patients with persistent CMV infections (Rola-Pleszcsynski *et al.*, 1977).

Ocular disease in CMV infection—The first report of ocular involvement in congenital cytomegalic inclusion disease appeared in 1947 (Kalfayan) following which reports were infrequent (Christensen *et al.*, 1957; Dvorak-Theobald, 1959; Gottman and Beatty, 1962; Manshot and Daaman, 1962; Miklos and Orban, 1964; Smith, Zimmerman and Harley, 1966; Frenke *et al.*, 1980). Inclusion-bearing cells were reported by Christensen *et al.* (1957) in the retina and choroid of an infant.

Cytomegalic Inclusion Disease Uveitis

Burns (1959) cites a case of proven generalised cytomegalic inclusion disease in whom an agent was isolated from the anterior chamber that produced inclusions in tissue culture similar to those previously isolated in the urine. It was felt that the evidence was such that it supported a diagnosis of cytomegalic inclusion disease uveitis. An illness occurred in a premature infant aged 5 weeks with hepatosplenomegaly, periventricular cerebral calcification and anaemia. Later there was fever, vomiting, petechiae, thrombocytopenia and leucocytosis. By six months, hydrocephalus and mental retardation were apparent. At 110 days of age, the right cornea was clear. The anterior chamber showed a flare, but no cells. An acute and a healed area of choroiditis was noted with perivascular exudation around a superotemporal vessel. In the opposite eye there was a healed pigmented lesion on the nasal side. The ocular condition subsequently deteriorated with progressive uveitis. Eventually the right cornea became cloudy, the iris vascularised and the uveitis persisted. There were subsequent improvements and recrudescences of inflammation. A final examination showed optic atrophy and a pebbled appearance in the retina of each eye.

The ocular abnormalities which have been found in congenital cytomegalovirus inclusion disease are chorioretinitis, strabismus and optic atrophy. Microphthalmia, cataract, retinal necrosis and calcification, together with optic disc and anterior chamber malformation have been described in association with generalised congenital disease. However, Hanshaw and Dudgeon (1978) stated that the presence of an unusual abnormality such as microphthalmia and cataract is evidence that the disease process is probably not due to CMV. The chorioretinitis is considered to be similar to that caused by *Toxoplasma gondii*, where central retinal lesions can be produced. Cerebral calcification may occur in areas around the ventricles in the subependymal region. Such appearances are characteristic of severe congenital cytomegalovirus encephalitis occurring early in pregnancy. Microcephaly is associated with calcium deposition, obstruction of the fourth ventricle and, rarely, hydrocephalus. In patients with cerebral calcification, chorioretinitis, optic atrophy and strabismus may be found.

Immunisation—If convincing evidence can be obtained supporting the impression that primary CMV infection, rather than a recurrence of it, during pregnancy, results in fetal infection, clinical illness and eventual residual damage, then there is a good basis for considering the use of a vaccine. However, vaccination does not necessarily mean that lasting protection would be achieved, there being rare reports of CMV infection in consecutive pregnancies. A cause for concern is the malignant potential of the herpesviruses. This potential has been implicated particularly in lower animals; thus, irradiated CMV has been shown to cause transformation *in vitro* in hamster cells (Albrecht and Rapp, 1973). Killed vaccine is unlikely to be easy to achieve because the virus probably does not multiply to a high enough titre to make this practicable. Thus, effective vaccine would depend on the use of live virus (Elek and Stern, 1974). Preliminary results using a vaccine preparation demonstrate that mild local signs develop at the site of injection in 50 per cent of subjects, and in two subjects an adenopathy developed. No subjects developed disturbance in liver function or excreted virus in throat secretions or urine. Live vaccine has been found to stimulate antibody without inducing significant side-effects. Whether the antibody which has been induced will persist and prevent subsequent infection *in utero* is at present unknown. The role of cell-mediated immunity in response to natural, as compared to vaccine, virus, and its role in protection against viral reactivation or protection have not been reported. Further work is required on the nature of these fundamental immune reactions in the maternal immune system, and their influence on protection against viral invasion of the fetus.

RUBELLA VIRUS

Biological Characteristics

Rubella is an RNA virus which is sensitive to a variety of chemical agents, including ether, and is inactivated at a pH below 6·8 and above 8·1, and by ultraviolet irradiation. Unstable at room temperature, it is best preserved at −60°C or below. Sections of infected tissue-culture cells examined by electron-microscopy show virus particles which are spherical, measuring 50 to 70 nm in diameter, with 30 nm electron-dense cores. Virions can be seen to be budding into intracellular vesicles or directly from the marginal membrane. Released virus is covered with projections which can cause these particles to haem-agglutinate certain fowl red blood cells. The rubella nucleocapsid core contains a single strand of infectious RNA, which is unstable and has therefore created difficulties in the study of its structure. The virion has been reported to contain three to eight structural proteins, the major ones being two glycoproteins and a non-glycosylated core protein. Taxonomically the position of the rubella virus is with the togaviruses, because it is an RNA virus with an envelope. It is apparent that there is one antigenic type and that there is no cross-reactivity with alpha viruses or other members of the togavirus group. Nevertheless, there are differences in the biological behaviour of different strains, including the capacity to induce interferon *in vitro* and transmissibility to rabbit fetuses.

The virus was cultured in 1962 for the first time in the United States. This was a breakthrough in that it made possible an accurate dilineation of the clinical epidemiology of the disease, and it also made it possible to determine the behaviour of the virus in population groups. It also provided an opportunity for the development of vaccines for the control and prevention of congenital rubella. The PHV strain of live attenuated rubella vaccine was developed by Meyer *et al.* (1966) and the Cendehill strain was developed shortly thereafter by Prinzie *et al.* (1969). Plotkin (1969) developed a strain which was used in several European countries at about the same time. Vaccines have now been used for some 10 years and their impact on the rubella problem is now being clearly defined as beneficial.

Laboratory Methods

Most rubella diagnosis is done by serological tests because virus isolation is either not practicable or is too slow to help in the treatment of a clinical problem. In the investigation of infants with suspected congenital infection or abnormality, virus may be excreted for some months. Virus has been isolated from cataracts and infected brain tissues up to 12 years after birth (Cremer *et al.*, 1975). A proportion of babies are normal at birth but may excrete the virus for a short time. Although virus may be isolated from a number of sites, a throat swab in transport medium is convenient.

Rubella propagates in several cell cultures and lines. Primary cell cultures, such as African green or Patas monkey kidney and continuous Vero culture systems, are suitable. However, the virus does not produce a cytopathic effect by virus growth, but it can be detected by interference with the growth of a subsequently added indicator virus, e.g. Echo 11, or passage into further cell lines such as RK13, BHK21, SIRC in which rubella cytopathic effect can be detected.

There are a number of serological methods available for the measurement of antibodies. The most widely used is haemagglutination inhibition, and less frequently, complement fixation. Other techniques include neutralisation immunodiffusion, indirect fluorescence, platelet aggregation and haemadsorption inhibition tests. The test to be selected depends on the nature of the clinical situation and the purpose for which the test is being done. In diagnosis and survey work haemagglutination inhibition is suitable. The titres of 90 per cent of antibody-positive sera fall between 1:16 and 1:256. As in most viral infections neutralising antibodies to rubella virus are considered to be the most closely correlated with immunity. However, there is a close correlation between haemagglutination inhibition and neutralisation and so the former technique has become standard. Rubella-specific IgM antibody is present transiently following primary infection and its estimation is therefore a method of detecting recent or current experience of the virus. The test is useful when rubella antibody is present in newborn infants with congenital disease, as it distinguishes between passively transferred maternal antibody, and fetally produced antibody. Since IgM cannot be transferred across the placenta, it therefore represents a positive immune response which has occurred in the fetus in response to rubella infection contracted *in utero*.

Epidemiology—The peak years of reported rubella cases occurred in 1935, 1943 and 1974 in the United States. In the United Kingdom epidemics occurred between 1940 and 1943 and from 1962 to 1964. Sizeable epidemics therefore occur approximately every 6–9 years with major ones occurring at 30-year intervals. However there is a regular occurrence of cases each year associated with the periodic epidemics. Serological surveys have shown an 85 per cent immunity level. The epidemiological feature which is puzzling is how to explain the extensive outbreaks which occur after long periods of time. It is difficult to comprehend why a particular epidemic should gather force, and result in the production of serious consequences in a community, as happened in 1964. Although no significant antigenic differences between strains have been documented, viruses may alter biological characteristics and eventually present an enhanced capacity to spread. At the same time host factors may also be involved, the periodic severe recurrences probably being a reflection of a gradual increase in the number of susceptible persons in the population, which facilitates the spread of the virus through the community.

Geographically rubella is worldwide in its distribution. In certain countries, however, epidemics occur between which there appears not to be a low level of background infection. Thus there are differences between the incidences of seropositive individuals in different countries, which cannot be explained. In Taiwan and Barbados it has been noticed that the incidence of antibody in the newborn is low between epidemics. Indeed, the epidemiology of rubella on islands is different from that in large continents. Thus, some countries have endemic rubella for many years, while others suffer epidemics which are not set against a background of endemic disease. The largest number of cases regularly appear in the larger countries in March, April and May. It is a disease which primarily affects school children, with a peak incidence in the 5- to 9-year age group.

Systemic manifestations of rubella—The disease we know as rubella was first described in the German literature in the mid-eighteenth century, and was first mentioned in the English literature in 1814. The term *rubella* was introduced in 1886 but the disease is still commonly known as 'German measles'. The clinical manifestations are mild and so the disease did not provoke much comment. It was not until Gregg's important observations in 1941 that there was a resurgence of interest.

Rubella is a seasonal disease, occurring most often in the spring, while epidemics occur approximately every 7 years. It is worldwide in its distribution, and when endemic it occurs most often in young children, especially males. The incubation period is 8 days, and lymphadenopathy develops prior to other manifestations. The posterior auricular and occipital nodes are usually involved. There may be a generalised proliferation with enlargement of the nodes, which are large and firm. In the prodromal period there may be catarrhal inflammation of the upper respiratory tract associated with fever, malaise, muscular aches and headaches.

The rash appears 12 to 20 days after exposure, the average time of development being 16 days. Subclinical disease patterns may occur without the appearance of the typical rash. The exanthem is macular papular on the skin of the face and chest, abdomen, thighs and upper extremities. It may last for 1 to 4 days and is preceded by a transient blush of the face and trunk. Fever may occur, but it is low grade and associated with the rash. Complications are rare and may include encephalitis without demyelinisation. In the uncommon fatal case, necrotising vasculitis has been reported. Thrombocytopenic purpura occurs fairly often, but a mild arthritis, rheumatoid in nature, is probably the most common complication. The small and medium-sized joints are involved and symptoms may persist for one week. The disease may be accompanied by a mild leucopenia in the early stages, with a relative lymphocytosis in the latter stages. In the presence of the typical clinical features, the diagnosis does not present a clinician with undue difficulty, but on occasions there may be confusion with the following disease entities: modified rubeola, roseola infantum, erythema infectiosum and mild scarlet fever, infectious mono-nucleosis, delayed serum rashes, drug reactions and erythema multiforme.

The Congenital Syndrome

In 1941 Sir Norman Gregg, an Australian ophthalmologist working in Sydney, published his paper entitled 'Congenital cataract following German measles in the mother', in which he established that many children referred to him with congenital cataract had been *in utero* during an extensive outbreak of rubella. These findings were confirmed by other research workers, who reported that the children were on many occasions also deaf. In addition, there was good evidence that they also suffered from cardiac lesions. During the years following these important associations, prospective enquiries were carried out; the starting point was the mother with a rubella-like illness during pregnancy, the babies subsequently being examined for congenital abnormalities. These studies suggested that the incidence of abnormality was lower than had previously been suggested when infection was acquired during the first trimester of pregnancy, but if it was contracted within the first month, the defects were shown to be frequently severe and multiple, occurring in up to 60 per cent of newborn infants. The defects then declined to an incidence of 5 per cent at the 13th–16th weeks, which remains approximately double the incidence of major congenital abnormality in the population at large.

Fetal damage may result from at least two mechanisms: the virus may cause chromosomal damage and induce infected cells to divide more slowly, as a result of which infants are born smaller than healthy infants (Figure 12.1), or chronic rubella infection may cause endothelial cell damage and thrombosis in

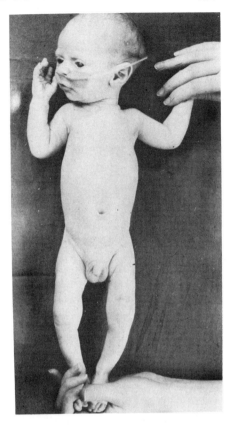

Figure 12.1. Newborn baby with congenital rubella syndrome, with low birth weight. There was a rash, ventriculoseptal defect, hepatosplenomegaly, typical bony changes and congenital glaucoma. (Courtesy, Mr. David Taylor.)

small fetal blood vessels, leading to tissue necrosis which may produce further damage and malformed organs. The retardation in the rate of growth of cells, if it occurs during the critical period of organogenesis (i.e. before the 8th week of pregnancy), may induce multiple congenital defects.

There may be a high fetal wastage from spontaneous and therapeutic abortion. Congenital rubella is also associated with a high spontaneous neonatal mortality rate which varies from 10 per cent to 30 per cent. Babies with severe congenital heart disease have a particularly high neonatal mortality rate. At birth the characteristic features of congenitally acquired rubella include multisystem disease, persistent virus excretion and an active rubella-specific immune response. Transient lesions include thrombocytopenic purpura, hepatosplenomegaly, and areas of radiotranslucency at the ends of long bones which may last for days or weeks but are not followed by development of permanent sequelae. Since virus replication continues after birth, congenitally acquired rubella is not a static disease, and lesions which are not apparent at birth but which are detected during follow-up are described as developmental defects. It is therefore important to keep in mind that such defects, because they occur after birth, do not exclude infections with rubella virus from the range of aetiological factors.

Clinical Features of the Congenital Rubella Syndrome

The varieties of fetal damage which occur depend on the stage of pregnancy in which rubella involved the embryo. The severity of damage may present a spectrum varying from mild auditory disease to the presentation of multisystem or organ abnormalities. It is noteworthy that rubella contracted in the fifth month of pregnancy or later is unlikely to produce signs of disease in the offspring. The serious effects occur where infection occurs in the mother during the first two months of gestation (Roy and Deutsch, 1966). The lesions produced include thrombocytopenic purpura, hepatomegaly, and spleno-megaly. It is in the early part of gestation that the disease is most likely to produce disease of the special senses such as defects in hearing and ocular defects. The ocular defects can occur in association with cardiomyopathy, which probably results from infection at a crucial time in the organogenesis of the heart and eye (Boniuk, 1972).

The systemic effects are possibly related to the decreased rate of multiplication of cells in organs where the virus is able to replicate (Table 12.3). The decreased rate of intra-uterine growth may continue postnatally with a failure to thrive. There may be prematurity by weight, and mental and physical developmental retardation which can persist into early childhood. The virus may persist in the tissues such as the lens (Menser et al., 1967), which can be a further complication in management. In many organs the virus persists with a minimum of apparent clinical effects. Focal areas of necrotic cardiac and skeletal muscle have been reported following pathological examination of infected infants (Spiro, 1966), together with interstitial pneumonitis and focal hyalinisation of the glomeruli, without significant inflammatory responses in these lesions (Korones et al., 1965). Radiological changes occur in the distal, femoral and proximal tibial metaphyses, where the trabecular pattern is altered with the appearance of small linear areas of radiolucency and increased bone density (Rudolf et al., 1965). The pathological features include abnormal bone deposition, primarily in the laying down and calcification of osteoid.

TABLE 12.3

CONGENITAL RUBELLA SYNDROME: SYSTEMIC ABNORMALITIES

General	Failure to grow and thrive
Cardiovascular system	Patent ductus arteriosus, atrial septal defects, tetralogy of Fallot, peripheral pulmonary stenosis, Wolff-Parkinson-White syndrome, transposition of great vessels
Gastro-intestinal system	Cleft palate, oesophageal atresia, pancreatic insufficiency, hepatomegaly, splenomegaly
Central nervous system	Encephalomyelocele, myelocele, meningocele, microcephaly, delayed functional development, mental retardation
Skeletal system	Alteration of trabecular appearance in proximal tibial and distal femoral metaphyses ('celery stalk' appearance), skull with bulging fontanelles
Blood	Thrombocytopenic purpura, pancytopenia
Special senses	Ocular defects, auditory defects.

Ocular Abnormalities

The ophthalmologist may be one of the key persons in the team of paediatricians who can help in reaching a presumptive diagnosis in the congenital rubella syndrome (Table 12.4). Congenital cataracts, or cataracts appearing and progressing after birth are one of the most helpful findings.

TABLE 12.4

CONGENITAL RUBELLA SYNDROME: OCULAR DEFECTS

Ocular abnormality	Clinical appearance	Treatment
Iris hypoplasia	Poor development of stroma and dilator; iris transilluminates	Nil
Cataract	Congenital—or appears after birth	Aspiration with single-stage procedure. Use maximal postoperative dilatation
Microphthalmos	Cornea 8–10 mm diameter	Nil
Retinopathy	Widespread mottling or blotchy pigment deposits usually of greatest density at macula. Fluorescein angiography reveals pigment epithelial defect	Nil
Strabismus	Usually convergent, secondary or paralytic	Treat primary lesion prior to squint
Glaucoma	Symptoms and signs of buphthalmos, associated with cataract or corneal opacity occasionally	Platelet count should be performed before surgery to prevent hyphaema

Embryopathic cataracts appear in the offspring owing to the transplacental transmission of an infection from the mother usually acquired during the first three months of pregnancy (Figure 12.2). Thus, congenital cataracts have followed viral infections in the early months of pregnancy in measles, poliomyelitis, and influenza (Lefebvre and Merlen, 1948), herpes zoster (Duehr, 1955) and epidemic parotitis (di Ferdinando, 1952; Agarwal and Raizada, 1954).

Rubella is the commonest maternal infection to produce such a lesion. The cataracts may be associated not infrequently with widespread abnormalities elsewhere. In a group of 50 patients born after the 1940–1 epidemic and examined by Hertzberg (1968), there were 10 patients who had had cataract surgery. In 60 per cent cataract occurred in the presence of other congenital abnormalities of the eye, including secondary retinal pigmentary degeneration, atrophy of the iris, mesodermal dysgenesis, corneal opacities, congenital glaucoma, strabismus or nystagmus and microphthalmos.

The cataract may be bilateral, may be nuclear, atypical or total, and may progress after birth to complete opacification which may become shrunken and fibrotic (Ehrlich, 1948). Rarely, an infant is born with clear lenses, the opacities occurring after some months (Menser et al., 1966).

Histology shows destruction of the posterior epithelial cells, which occurs about one month after maternal infection has presented (Figure 12.3 and 12.4).

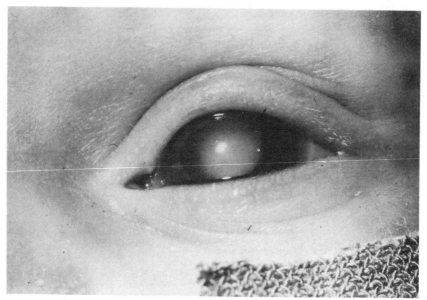

Figure 12.2.   Rubella cataract associated with buphthalmos in a newborn infant. (Courtesy, Mr. David Taylor.)

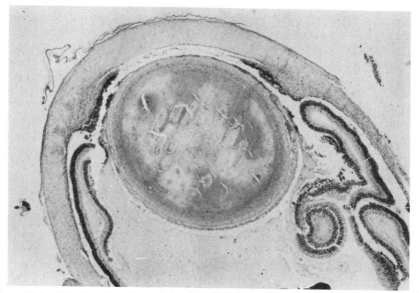

Figure 12.3.   Histological section of rubella cataract showing abnormalities in the posterior epithelial cells (×24). (Courtesy, Professor Alec Garner.)

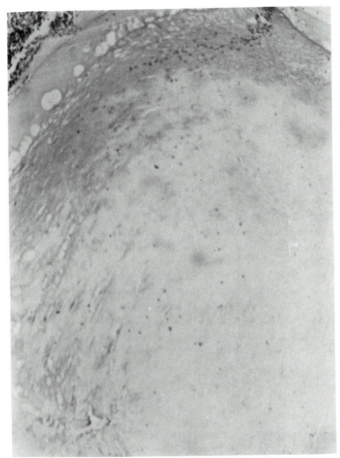

Figure 12.4.   Histological section of a rubella cataract showing abnormality of the posterior epithelial cells (×82). (Courtesy, Professor Alec Garner.)

The subcapsular and equatorial cells may remain relatively unaffected at first, but may later degenerate and suffer complete destruction. The persistence of the virus in the tissues probably accounts for the change and further development of the cataract after birth, when the virus has often been recovered (Cotlier *et al.*, 1966; Hambridge *et al.*, 1966; Reid and Murphy, 1966; Murphy *et al.*, 1967). Virus has been isolated from the developing lens fibres of experimentally infected rats (Bohigian *et al.*, 1968).

In addition to cataract, other features include a variable degree of microphthalmia, corneal changes, glaucoma, retinopathy and strabismus. Microphthalmia is usually not severe, but is a common feature. Iris hypoplasia has been considered to be a further sign which results in poor dilatation following the use of mydriatic prior to cataract surgery. It has been noticed that irides in suspect rubella infants are often peculiar in colour and consistency, and transillumination may be of help in reaching a diagnosis in certain instances. Deficits in the pigment epithelium may be demonstrable by this technique.

Various ocular autostimulation phenomena have been reported in the congenital rubella syndrome; these include the child pressing on the eyes to produce phosphenes, passing the hand before the eye with the least degree of cataract formation, and head wagging while fixing the eyes on a bright light (Roy, 1967). However, these kinds of phenomena are not unique to the rubella syndrome and probably represent a response in the child to an early visual deficit, which may occur in other conditions where rubella infection plays no causal role.

Glaucoma

In a series of 15 patients with infantile glaucoma studied by Boniuk (1972), there were 7 patients with the congenital rubella syndrome with bilateral glaucoma, 2 of whom had central corneal rings. In more than 200 patients studied in the Rubella Clinic at Texas Children's Hospital, the incidence of glaucoma was less than 3 per cent (Boniuk, 1972). The glaucoma was associated with deafness, cerebral palsy and cataracts, and was encountered following cataract surgery. Pathological studies revealed incomplete cleavage of the chamber angle and focal areas of necrosis near the ciliary processes. It would seem appropriate that patients with congenital glaucoma should have laboratory investigations to exclude the congenital rubella syndrome. In treating certain patients with glaucoma, care should be taken in excluding thrombocytopenia prior to surgery, in order to avoid the risk of operative or postoperative hyphaema.

Rubella Retinopathy

In his initial report before the Ophthalmological Society of Australia, Gregg failed to mention that *in utero* exposure to rubella could result in a retinopathy. The initial observation is attributed to Mitchell, an Australian physician quoted by Gregg in a discussion at the Australian Ophthalmological Society in 1946. Rubella retinitis is now recognised as one of the three most frequent ocular abnormalities in the newborn with congenital rubella. The exact incidence varies according to various series considerably (Alfano, 1966; Hamilton *et al.*, 1948; Hertzberg, 1969; Marks, 1947; Morlet, 1949; Roy *et al.*, 1966). The retinitis may be the only indication of congenital rubella, or it may occur in conjunction with any of the known ocular or systemic stigmata.

The appearance of the retina is typical in most cases and the literature has been well summarised by Krill (1972): widespread pigment deposits with their greatest density apparent at the macula, with on occasions isolated macular pigmentary reactions, or sometimes peripheral pigmentary reactions. The deposits may be uni-ocular or binocular and may be restricted to one or more sectors of the eyes. Commonly, both eyes are involved. The pigment has been described as blotchy, forming clumps at the macula, and at times large, flat, black deposits of irregular outline.

There may be loss of the foveal reflex, and there may be a dust-like stippling of the retinal periphery. Pallor of the optic nerve has been reported in some cases, but the retinal vessels remain normal (Hamilton *et al.*, 1948; Long and Danielson, 1945). The retinitis causes little or no visual deficit, the visual acuity and visual fields, dark adaptation, colour vision and electroretinography remaining normal or near normal in patients with no other ocular complication of rubella (Babel and Dieterle, 1960, Francois, 1963; Hertzberg, 1968).

Pathological studies have been carried out on eyes with rubella retinitis, and confirm that the changes are limited to the pigment epithelium and are characterised by focal areas of increased and decreased pigmentation, together with atrophic changes (Krill *et al.*, 1968). The changes may affect the macula or the equator. No other abnormalities have been recorded in the rest of the retina or the choroid. Fluorescein studies reflect the diffuse abnormality of the pigment epithelium, demonstrating pigment epithelial deficits throughout the posterior pole and the mid-periphery.

The observation of a pigmentary retinopathy in newborns or infants should arouse some suspicion of rubella as an aetiological agent, even if there is no history of it in the first trimester of pregnancy. The association of cataracts or microphthalmia with the retinopathy suggest rubella. Deafness and certain systemic abnormalities such as cardiac disease also suggest rubella as an aetiological agent.

The differential diagnosis includes congenital tapetoretinal degeneration, which was originally described by Leber (1867) as amaurosis congenita. Such children may also suffer from cataracts and also rarely from keratoconus. There is severe visual impairment resulting from the retinal abnormality. A minimal response is obtained in the ERG, which thereby easily distinguishes it from congenital rubella. Rarely, other viral infections, when contracted during the first trimester of pregnancy, are thought to cause ocular abnormalities in the newborn infant on occasions, and to produce similar retinal changes as in rubella. These infections include morbilli, varicella (LaForet and Lynch, 1947; LaPlane *et al.*, 1950) and influenza (Mann, 1957). Radiation (Francois and Haustate-Gosset, 1962) has also been considered as a factor in the aetiology of pigmentary retinopathy in newborns which has little effect on retinal function. Pigmentation may also be a prominent feature in congenital toxoplasmosis and cytomegalic inclusion disease, although the pigmentation in these two conditions is usually markedly different from that following maternal rubella.

Krill (1972) has stressed the benign nature of rubella retinopathy, and reported on the fluorescein angiogram in adolescents or young adults with typical retinal changes (Figure 12.5). The changes, although affecting the pigmentary epithelium, produce little effect on electrodiagnostic investigations or on retinal function. Irreversible loss of visual function occurs in the presence of other congenital ocular abnormalities in rubella, such as cataract or glaucoma. Microphthalmic eyes probably have abnormal retinal development and always have poor vision.

In 1978, Deutman and Grizzard reported their fluorescein angiographic changes in three cases with presumed rubella retinopathy who also suffered from congenital deafness. Unilateral subretinal neovascularisation, haemor-

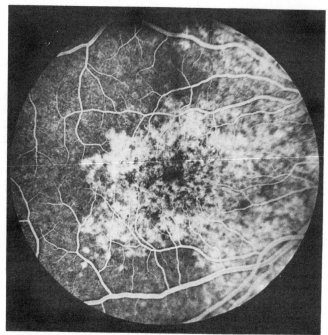

Figure 12.5. Fluorescein angiogram of presumed rubella retinopathy in a young adult with a history of the congenital rubella syndrome. There is a patchy disturbance of the pigment epithelium, particularly marked around the posterior pole. (Courtesy, Dr. C. McCulloch.)

rhage and scarring were demonstrable. These retinal changes occurred at the macula and resulted in considerable reduction in the visual acuity. It was considered that the alterations in the retinal pigment epithelium probably predisposes rubella infants to develop choroidal neovascularisation later in life. However, the diagnosis of rubella syndrome was based on clinical criteria, such as the characteristic appearance of the fundus, congenital deafness, a negative family history of ocular disease or deafness, and good vision without nystagmus. In one of the three patients, there was a subnormal ERG with equal rod and cone dysfunction.

Electroretinograms were performed in 28 patients with ocular signs of the post-rubeola syndrome by Obenour (1972). In every case in which rubella retinopathy alone was present (30 eyes), the ERG was normal, except for two borderline cases. Seven abnormal ERGs were obtained from patients whose eyes were severely affected by other anormalities, including microphthalmia, secondary cataracts and nystagmus.

Preventive Measures

The severity of congenital rubella defects is clearly a prime indication for the use of preventive measures. Before the introduction of rubella vaccination in the United Kingdom the total number of reported cases of congenital rubella defects was approximately 250 per annum. Theoretically, congenital rubella can be prevented by immunisation, either passively or actively, like other forms of infectious disease, but there is an important difference in the approach to the prevention of congenital defects by immunisation procedures. The object is to protect the fetus rather than just the parent, and this is best achieved by immunising women before they reach childbearing age, thus bridging the gaps in immune protection left by nature. In this way the number of susceptible women at risk of contracting the disease in pregnancy can be reduced.

The vaccination policy in the United Kingdom, and in any European country, recommends selective immunisation. Thus, all girls between the ages of 11 and 14 years are offered the vaccine without pretesting for their rubella-immune status. Vaccination is offered to adult women, and groups at risk of disease such as teachers, doctors, nurses and nursery staff, who have been shown to be susceptible as a result of negative serology, but who are not pregnant, nor likely to become so for at least three months after vaccination. In contrast, in the United States, mass vaccination for all children of both sexes aged 1 year to puberty is recommended. In addition, vaccination is recommended for adolescent and adult females provided that their immune status is known prior to vaccination.

Rubella prevention—It is too early to say which of the two vaccination policies is correct. However, there is enough evidence to show that serious epidemics of rubella are diminishing, and that the number of babies born with the congenital rubella syndrome is considerably reduced, whatever the vaccination policy used.

The cases of congenital rubella confirmed or suspected in England, Scotland and Wales fell from a level of 60 reported cases in 1970 to 47 reported cases in 1979, and three reported cases in 1980. During this decade, there have been 625 reported cases overall (*British Medical Journal*, 1981). Analysis of 83 children born after May 1978 showed that 56 had proved defects, 7 had suspected defects, and the remaining 20 were apparently normal though they had laboratory evidence of prenatal infection. In the first group, cataract, deafness, congenital heart disease and microcephaly were the common defects. Pneumonitis was diagnosed in five children. Of children with proven defects, 9 died. Of the 83 cases, 27 had cataract and 7 had other ocular defects. Congenital heart disease occurred in 30 babies and microcephaly in 20. Twenty-one had sensorineural deafness, and there were 29 additional suspect cases. In 1980 there was little rubella in England and Wales. There was an epidemic of rubella in the period 1978–79.

Treatment of Congenital Cataract

Congenital cataract, although one of the more unfortunate effects of the congenital rubella syndrome, is a reversible complication and allows of eventual rehabilitation. Although a two-stage process of lens removal was investigated by Yanoff et al. (1968), it was noted that there was a high incidence of phthisis bulbi. This contrasted impressively with the good results obtained in their surgical treatment of congenital cataracts of other types (Scheie et al., 1967). It was thought that the lack of success was related to the persistence of the virus in the tissues and therefore the authors recommended that the surgery should be delayed to a later stage in the development of the child. Boniuk and Boniuk (1972) felt that there is no correlation between rubella viral persistence and the serious complications following cataract surgery, unless multiple procedures are carried out. They recommend that as much lens matter as possible should be removed as a primary procedure. It was not felt that there is an indication for delay, and in a number of centres the operation is carried out at the earliest opportunity in order to ensure the development of the best possible vision. Aspiration of the lens is an operation which has had considerable success when all possible lens material is removed in one procedure. It is also important that maximal dilatation of the pupil should be achieved following the surgery, to prevent the production of dense posterior synechiae. More recently it has been the practice to remove congenital cataracts using lensectomy through a limbal incision with removal of the anterior vitreous. Since it has been found that in extremely early cataract extraction in the newborn, extracapsular methods result in a prolific regeneration of the posterior capsule, leaving a fibrotic cyclitic membrane with adherence of the pupil margin to it, it has been considered that lensectomy and anterior vitrectomy carries a better prognosis for the ultimate vision which can be regained for the child (Taylor, personal communication). It nevertheless remains to be seen whether these techniques which remove the lens *in toto*, and therefore ensure that there is no diaphragm between the anterior and posterior segments, will result in maintained vision in the long term.

Rubella in Animals

The use of experimental animal models for rubella infection is now of theoretical interest only, owing to the progress that has been made in elucidating the epidemiology of rubella infection in humans, and the development of an effective vaccine. Animal experiments show that the lens is a favourite target organ for the virus by virtue of its isolation and encapsulation. Where virus particles replicate inside the lens is not clear, and whether the lens capsule prevents the egress of the virus outwardly has not been ascertained. In the developing lens there is continuous DNA synthesis which would be expected to afford an excellent opportunity for the virus to survive and replicate. It has been suggested that the RNA-rubella virus may compete with the amino acids or nucleotides normally incorporated into the lens DNA or the ribosomal cytoplasmic RNA. According to Boniuk and Zimmerman (1967), the basophilic chromatin-like material found in the nucleus of the human rubella-infected lens represents damaged DNA or retained virus. Electron-microscopy of rubella-infected rat lenses substantiates the destructive effects of virus in the production of nuclear DNA (Cotlier *et al.*, 1968). Inhibition of the rate of mitosis in cells may be brought about by the virus (Plotkin and Vaheri, 1967). In addition, the persistence of the virus in the lens may be contributed to by the high protein content of the latter. Weller and Neva (1962) reported that low titres of infective virus may persist for several days in media with high protein concentrations, whereas the virus becomes inactivated at 37° in 2 per cent fetal calf serum.

Studies have been performed to investigate the possible causes of uveitis seen postoperative to the congenital rubella syndrome. Jacoby (1972) reported that intravitreal injection of rubella stimulated the production of rubella serum antibody, and almost half of the group of animals tested showed a spontaneous delayed intra-ocular response, particularly where systemic antibody reached high titres. If rubella virus were introduced as a subsequent injection, with or without lens protein, there was an intense and prolonged immediate reaction in all animals. However, the presence of lens protein in the injection did not seem to alter the magnitude of the inflammatory response, indicating that the lens material itself cannot be considered responsible for the severe inflammatory reaction found postoperatively in the newborn. Where a purified suspension of virus was introduced into the vitreous in the absence of culture medium, the primary ocular response was not very marked, although the secondary response was considerably enhanced.

It is possible therefore to consider the cataract removal as a sensitising episode, where the intralenticular virus is released into the vitreous cavity, with, in addition to the production of a systemic immune response, a localised sensitisation of the ocular tissues such that more than one intra-ocular procedure may well lead to a severe immunological inflammatory reaction. Thus Zimmerman and Silverstein (1961) have demonstrated that the inflammatory reaction in ocular tissues following intravitreal injection of antigen have the appearances characteristic of those of a typical delayed hypersensitivity reaction, with plasma-cell infiltration of the iris and the ciliary body. It is possible that the plasma cells seed the eye and remain capable of proliferating and differentiating, and producing antibody at the site should antigen reappear. Silverstein (1963) demonstrated that competent cells responsible for hypersensitivity uveitis develop extra-ocularly and invade intra-ocular tissue, where they remain indefinitely capable of responding to intra-ocular antigenic stimulation whenever the specific antigen is introduced.

The severe immunological responses inducing postoperative uveitis and even phthisis bulbi in the human may have a similar mechanism in their production. The animal experiments seem to confirm the thesis that lens removal in the congenital rubella syndrome should be carried out as a complete primary procedure and not as a two-stage operation.

Varicella Zoster

Maternal varicella was first recognised as a cause of congenital anomalies by Laforet and Lynch (1947) who described an underdeveloped infant with cerebral cortical atrophy, cicatricial skin lesions over the left lower extremity, undescended testicles, defective development of the toes of the right foot, and bilateral optic atrophy, with a peculiar darkish pigmentation of the retina, bilateral nystagmus and a questionable pupillary reaction to light stimulation. Chorioretinitis has been documented by McKendry and Bailey (1973) and Charles et al. (1977). There was also histological evidence of lens involvement noted by the same authorities and also by Srabstein et al. (1974). Cotlier (1978) reported a case of unilateral congenital cataract secondary to maternal varicella in a 16-month-old infant who underwent successful cataract surgery. However, although there was a significant titre of specific antibody in the infant, no virus was cultured from the aspirated lens material. A wide spectrum of lesions is present in congenital varicella, which range from early death (Laforet and Lynch, 1947) to central nervous system involvement with cerebral or cerebellar atrophy (McKendry and Bailey, 1973; Charles *et al.*, 1977). The severity of the congenital syndrome depends upon the time in gestation at which the infection occurs. Infections in the mother occurring before the twelfth week of pregnancy were associated with multiple systemic lesions, while conversely, isolated involvement of the eye resulted from maternal infection during the fourth month of gestation in the patients of Charles *et al.* (1977) and of Cotlier (1978).

REFERENCES

AGARWAL, L. P. and RAIZADA, L. N. (1954). Congenital membranous cataract, dentigerous cysts and multiple fibrolipomata. *Brit. J. Ophthal.*, **38**, 383.

ALBRECHT, T. and RAPP, F. (1973). Malignant transformation of hamster embryo fibroblasts following exposure to ultraviolet-irritated human cytomegalovirus. *Virology*, **55**, 53–61.

ALFANO, J. E. (1966). Ocular aspects of the maternal rubella syndrome. *Trans. Amer. Acad. Ophthal. Otolaryng.*, **70**, 235–66.

ALFORD, C. A., REYNOLDS, D. W., STAGNO, S., HOSTRY, T. S. and TILLER, M. (1975). Diagnosis of chronic perinatal infections. *Amer. J. Dis. Child.*, **129**, 455–63.

BABEL, J. and DIETERLE, P. (1960). Cataracte apparemment héréditaire d'origine embryopathique confin. *Confin. Neurol.*, **20**, 122–4.

BIRDSONG, M., SMITH, D. E., MITCHELL, F. N. and COREY, J. H. (1956). Generalised cytomegalic inclusion disease in newborn infants. *J. Amer. Med. Ass.*, **162**, 1305–1308.

BIRNBAUM, G., LYNCH, J. I., MARGILETH, A. M., LONERGAN, W. M. and SEVER, J. L. (1969). Cytomegalovirus infections in newborn infants. *J. Pediat.*, **75**, 789–95.

BODEY, G. P., WERTLAKE, P. T., DOUGLAS, G. and LEVIN, R. H. (1965). Cytomegalic inclusion disease in patients with acute leukaemia. *Ann. Intern. Med.*, **62**, 899–906.

BOHIGIAN, G. M., FOX, J. and COTLIER, E. (1968). Immunofluorescent localisation of rubella virus in lens, retina and heart of congenital rubella-infected rats. *Amer. J. Ophthal.*, **65**, 196–201.

BONIUK, M. and ZIMMERMAN, L. E. (1967). Ocular pathology in the rubella syndrome. *Arch. Ophthal.*, **77**, 455–73.

BONIUK, V. (1972). Systemic and ocular manifestations of the rubella syndrome. In: *Rubella and Other Intraocular Viral Diseases in Infancy*, pp. 67–76. Ed. M. Boniuk. International Ophthalmology Clinics, Vol. 12. Boston: Little, Brown & Co.

BONIUK, V. and BONIUK, M. (1972). The incidence of phthisis bulbi as a complication of cataract surgery in the congenital rubella syndrome. In: *Rubella and Other Intraocular Viral Diseases in Infancy*. Ed. M. Boniuk. International Ophthalmology Clinics, Vol. 12. Boston: Little, Brown & Co.

BRICK, D. C., OH, J. O. and SICHERT, S. E. (1981). Ocular lesions associated with dissemination of type 2 herpes simplex virus from skin infections in newborn rabbits. *Invest. Ophthal. Vis. Sci.*, **21**, 681–8.

British Medical Journal (1981). Epidemiology Report. National congenital rubella surveillance programme. **282**, 324.

BURNS, R. P. (1959). Cytomegalic inclusion disease uveitis. *Arch. Ophthal.*, **61**, 376–87.

CANGIR, A. and SULLIVAN, M. (1966). The occurrence of cytomegalic infections in childhood leukaemia. *J. Amer. Med. Ass.*, **195**, 616–22.

CHARLES, N. C., BENNETT, T. W. and MARGOLIS, S. (1977). Ocular pathology of congenital varicella syndrome. *Arch. Ophthal.*, **95**, 2034–7.

CHRISTENSEN, L., BEEMAN, H. W. and ALLEN, A. (1957). Cytomegalic inclusion disease. *Arch. Ophthal.*, **57**, 90–99.

COTLIER, E. (1978). Congenital varicella cataract. *Amer. J. Ophthal.*, **86**, 627–9.

COTLIER, E., FOX, J., BOHIGIAN, G., BEATY, C. and DUPRE, A. (1968). Pathogenic effects of rubella virus in embryos and newborn rats. *Nature*, **217**, 38–40.

COTLIER, E., FOX, J. and SMITH, M. (1966). Rubella virus in the cataractous lens of congenital rubella syndrome. *Amer. J. Ophthal.*, **62**, 233–5.

CREMER, N. E., OSHIRO, L. S., WEIL, M. L., LENNETTE, E. H., ITABASHI, H. H. and CARNAY, L. (1975). Isolation of rubella virus from brain in chronic progressive panencephalitis. *J. Gen. Virol.*, **29**, 143–53.

DENMAN, A. M. (1982). Pregnancy and immunological disorders. *Brit. Med. J.*, **284**, 999.

DEUTMAN, A. F. and GRIZZARD, W. S. (1978). Rubella retinopathy and subretinal neovascularisation. *Amer. J. Ophthal.*, **85**, 82–7.

DI FERDINANDO, R. Malformazioni congenite da embriopatia rubeolica e parotitica. *Boll. Oculist.*, **31**, 427–441.

DUEHR, P. A. (1955). Herpes zoster as cause of congenital cataract. *Amer. J. Ophthal.*, **39**, 157–161.

DVORAK-THEOBALD, G. (1959). Cytomegalic inclusion disease: Report of a case. *Amer. J. Ophthal.*, **47**, 52–62.

EHRLICH, L. H. (1948). Spontaneous absorption of congenital cataract following maternal rubella. *Arch. Ophthal.*, **39**, 205–209.

ELEK, S. and STERN, H. (1974). Development of a vaccine against mental retardation caused by cytomegalovirus infection *in utero*. *Lancet*, **1**, 1–5.

EMODI, G., MIGGIANO, A. OLAFSSON, A. and JUST, M. (1973). Studies of cellular immunity in congenital cytomegalovirus infection. *Acta Paediat. Scand.* (Suppl.), **236**, 43–44.

FARBER, S. and WOLBACH, S. B. (1932). Intranuclear and cytoplasmic inclusions ('protozoan-like bodies') in salivary glands and other organs of infants. *Amer. J. Path.*, **8**, 123–36.

FISHER, E. R. and DAVIS, E. (1958). Cytomegalic inclusion disease in the adult. *New Engl. J. Med.*, **258**, 1036–40.

FRANCOIS, J. (1963). Etiology of congenital cataracts. *Vie Med.*, **43**, 1327–48.

FRANCOIS, J. and HAUSTATE-GOSSET (1962). Cataracte juvenile chez deux jurnelles univitellines. *J. Genet. Hum.*, **12**, 154–67.

FRENKE, L. D., KEYS, M. P., HEFFEREN, S. J., ROLA-PLESZCZYNSKI, M. and BELLANTI, J. A. (1980). Unusual eye abnormalities associated with congenital cytomegalovirus infection. *Pediatrics*, **66**, 763–6.

FUCILLO, D. A., STEELE, R. W., HENSEN, S. A., VINCENT, M. M., HARDY, J. M. and BELLANTI, J. A. (1974). Impaired cellular immunity to rubella virus in congenital rubella. *Infection and Immunity*, **9**, 81–4.

GIBSON, P. E., FIELD, A. M., GARDNER, S. D. and COLEMAN, D. V. (1981). Occurrence of IgM antibodies against BK and JC polyomaviruses during pregnancy. *J. Clin. Path.*, **34**, 674–9.

GOTTMAN, A. W. and BEATTY, E. C. (1962). Cytomegalic inclusion disease in children with leukaemia or lymphosarcoma. *Amer. J. Dis. Child.*, **104**, 180–4.

GREGG, N. M. (1941). Congenital cataract following German measles in the mother. *Trans. Ophthal. Soc. Aust.*, **3**, 35–46.

GREGG, N. M. (1946). Further observations on congenital defects in infants following maternal rubella. *Trans. Ophthal. Soc. Aust.*, **4**, 119–131.

HAMILTON, J. B. (1942). Eye disease found in Australian 8-year survey. *Med. J. Aust.*, **1**, 45–47.

HAMILTON, J. B. *et al.* (1948). Rubella retinitis in Tasmania. *Trans. Ophthal. Soc. Aust.*, **8**, 114.

HAMRIDGE, K. W., SHAFFER, D., and MARSHALL, W. C. *et al.* (1966). Congenital rubella: report of two cases with generalised infection. *Brit. Med. J.*, **1**, 650–2.

HANSHAW, J. B. (1971). Congenital cytomegalovirus infection: a fifteen-year perspective. *J. Infect. Dis.*, **123**, 555–61.

HANSHAW, J. B. and DUDGEON, J. A. (1978). Viral diseases of the fetus and newborn. Introduction. *Maj. Probl. Clin. Pediat.*, **17**, 1–9.

HERTZBERG, R. (1968). Twenty-five year follow up of ocular defects in congenital rubella. *Amer. J. Ophthal.*, **66**, 269–71.

HERTZBERG, R. (1969). Ocular defects in congenital rubella. *Med. J. Aust.*, **1**, 594–5.

HILL, R. B., JR., ROWLANDS, D. T., JR. and RIFKIND, D. (1964). Infectious pulmonary disease in patients receiving immunosuppressive therapy for organ transplantation. *New Engl. J. Med.*, **271**, 1021–7.

HURLEY, R. and DE LOUVOIS, J. (1980). Serious infections in obstetric and neonatal practice. *J. Roy. Soc. Med.*, **73**, 770.

ICART, J. and DIDIER, J. (1981). Infections due to Epstein-Barr virus during pregnancy. *J. Infect. Dis.*, **143**, 499.

JACOBY, R. M. (1972). Intravitreal challenge of rabbit eyes with live rubella virus and homologous lens protein. In: *Rubella and Other Intraocular Viral Diseases in Infancy*, p. 147 (International Ophthalmology Clinics, Vol. 12). Ed. M. Boniuk. Boston: Little Brown & Co.

KÄÄRIÄINEN, L., KLEMOLA, E. and PALOHEIMO, J. (1966*a*). Rise of cytomegalovirus antibodies in infectious mononucleosis-like syndrome after transfusion. *Brit. Med. J.*, **1**, 1270–2.

KÄÄRIÄINEN, L., PALOHEIMO, J. and KLEMOLA, E. (1966*b*). Cytomegalovirus mononucleosis. Isolation of the virus and demonstration of subclinical infections after fresh blood transfusion in connection with open heart surgery. *Ann. Med. Exp. Fenn.*, **44**, 297–301.

KANICH, R. E. and CRAIGHEAD, J. E. (1966). Cytomegalovirus infection and cytomegalic inclusion disease in renal homotransplant recipient. *Amer. J. Med.*, **40**, 874–82.

KORONES, S. B., AINGER, L. E. and MONIF, G. R. (1965). Congenital rubella syndrome: New clinical aspects with recovery of virus from infected infants. *J. Pediat.*, **67**, 166–81.

KRILL, A. E. (1972). Retinopathy secondary to rubella. In: *Rubella and Other Intraocular Viral Diseases in Infancy*, p. 89 (International Ophthalmology Clinics, Vol. 12). Ed. M. Boniuk. Boston: Little Brown & Co.

KRILL, A. E., NEWELL, F. W. and CHISHTI, M. I. (1968). Fluorescein studies in diseases affecting the retinal pigment epithelium. *Amer. J. Ophthal.*, **66**, 470–84.

LAFORET, E. G. and LYNCH, C. L. (1947). Multiple congenital defects following maternal varicella. *New Engl. J. Med.*, **236**, 534–537.

LAPLANE, R., BREGEAT, P. and OSSOPORSKI, B. (1950). Un cas d'embryopathie consécutif d'une varicelle maternelle. *Arch. Franç. Pédiat.*, **7**, 530.

LEBER, T. (1867). Ueber retinitis pigmentosa und angerboren amaurose. *Albrecht v. Graefes Arch. Klin. Exp. Ophthal.*, **15**, 1.

LEFEBVRE, G. and MERLEN, J. (1948). La plase de la rubeole et des autres facteurs infectieux on toxiques survenus en cours de gestatin dans la genese des malformations et dystrophies congenitalis. *Ann. Pédiat.*, **171**, 266–276.

LONG, J. C. and DANIELSON, R. W. (1945). Cataract and other congenital defects in infants following rubella in the mother. *Arch. Ophthal.*, **34**, 24–27.

McKENDRY, J. B. and BAILEY, J. D. (1973). Congenital varicella associated with multiple defects. *Canad. Med. Assoc. J.*, **108**, 66–8.

MANN, I. (1957). *Development Abnormalities of the Eye*, 2nd edit. Philadelphia: Lippincott.

MANSHOT, W. A. and DAAMAN, C. B. (1962). Case of cytomegalic inclusion disease with ocular involvement. *Ophthalmologica*, **143**, 137–40.

MANSON, M. M., LOGAN, W. P. D. and LOY, R. M. (1960). *Rubella and other virus infections during pregnancy*. Rep. Publ. Hlth. Med. Subj. No. 101. London: HMSO.

MARKS, E. D. (1947). Pigmentary abnormalities in children congenitally deaf following maternal German measles. *Brit. J. Ophthal.*, **31**, 119.

MEDEARIS, D. N., JR. (1964). Observations concerning human cytomegalovirus infection and disease. *Bull. Johns Hopk. Hosp.*, **114**, 181–211.

MELISH, M. E. and HANSHAW, J. B. (1973). Congenital cytomegalovirus infection. Developmental progress of infants detected by routine screening. *Amer. J. Dis. Child.*, **126**, 190–4.

MENSER, M. A., HARLEY, J. D. and J. D. HERTZBERG, R. *et al.* (1967). Persistency of virus in lens for three years after prenatal rubella. *Lancet*, **2**, 387–8.

MENSER, M. A., HARLEY, J. D., HOUSEGO, G. J. and MURPHY, A. M. (1966). Possible clinical factors in the postnatal development of rubella cataracts. *Lancet*, **2**, 771.

MEYER, H. M., PARKMAN, P. D. and PANOS, T. C. (1966). Attenuated rubella virus: Production of an experimental live virus vaccine and clinical trial. *New Engl. J. Med.*, **275**, 575–80.

MIKLOS, G. and ORBAN, T. (1964). Ophthalmic lesion due to cytomegalic inclusion disease. *Ophthalmologica*, **148**, 98.

MODLIN, J. F., BRANDLING-BENNETT, A. D., WITTE, J. F., CAMPBELL, C. C. and MYERS, J. D. (1975). A review of 5 years experience with rubella vaccine in the United States. *Pediatrics*, **55**, 20–9.

MORLET, C. (1949). Rubella retinitis in Western Australia. *Trans. Ophthal. Soc. Aust.*, **9**, 212.

MURPHY, A. M., REID, R. R., POLLARD, I. *et al.* (1967). Rubella cataracts: further clinical and virologic observations. *Amer. J. Ophthal.*, **64**, 1109–19.

NASH, G., MORRIS, J. A., FOLEY, F. D. and PRUETT, G. A. (1970). Disseminated cytomegalic inclusion disease in a burned adult. *J. Amer. Med. Ass.*, **214**, 587–8.

NUMAZAKI, Y., YANO, M., MORIZUKA, T., TAKAI, S. and ISHIDA, M. (1970). Primary infection with human cytomegalovirus: Virus isolation from healthy infants and pregnant women. *Amer. J. Epidemiol.*, **91**, 410–17.

OBENOUR, L. C. (1972). The electroretinogram in rubella retinopathy. In: *Rubella and Other Intraocular Viral Diseases in Infancy*, p. 105. (International Ophthalmology Clinics, Vol. 12). Ed. M. Boniuk. Boston: Little, Brown & Co.

OLDING, L. B., JENSEN, F. C. and OLDSTONE, M. B. (1975). A pathogenesis of cytomegalovirus infection. 1. Activation of virus from bone marrow derived lymphocytes by *in vitro* allogenic reaction. *J. Exp. Med.*, **141**, 561–72.

PEACE, R. J. (1958). Cytomegalic inclusion disease in adults: A complication of neoplastic disease of the hemopoietic and reticulohistiocytic systems. *Amer. J. Med.*, **24**, 48.

PLOTKIN, S. A., FARQUHAR, J. D. and KATZ, M. *et al.* (1969). Attenuation of R.A. 27/3 rubella virus in WI-38 human diploid cells. *Amer. J. Dis. Child.*, **118**, 178–85.

PLOTKIN, S. A. and VAHERI, A. (1967). Human fibroblasts infected with rubella virus produce a growth inhibitor. *Science*, **156**, 659–661.

PRINZIE, A., HUYGELEN, C., GOLD, J., FARQUHAR, J. and McKEE, J. (1969). Experimental live attenuated rubella virus vaccine: clinical evaluation of Cendehill strain. *Amer. J. Dis. Child.*, **118**, 172–177.

REID, R. R. and MURPHY, A. M. (1966). Isolation of rubella virus from congenital cataracts removed at operation. *Med. J. Aust.*, **1**, 540–2.

REYNOLDS, D. W., STAGNO, S., STUBBS, K. G., DAHLE, A. J., LIVINGSTONE, M. M., SAXON, S. S. and ALFORD, C. A. (1974). Inapparent congenital cytomegalovirus infection with elevated cord IgM levels. Causal relation with auditory and mental deficiency. *New Engl. J. Med.*, **290**, 291–6.

ROLA-PLESZCSYNSKI, M., FRENKEL, L. D., FUCILLO, D. A., HENSEN, S. A., VINCENT, M. M., REYNOLDS, D. W., STAGNO, S. and BELLANTI, J. A. (1977). Specific impairment of cell-mediated immunity in mothers of infants with congenital infection due to cytomegalovirus. *J. Infect. Dis.*, **135**, 386–91.

ROWE, W. P., HARTLEY, J. W., WATERMAN, S., TURNER, H. F. and HUEBNER, R. J. (1956). Cytopathogenic agent resembling human salivary gland virus recovered from tissue cultures of human adenoids. *Proc. Soc. Exp. Biol. (N.Y.)*, **92**, 418–24.

ROY, F. H. (1967). Ocular autostimulation. *Amer. J. Ophthal.*, **63**, 1776–7.

ROY, F. H. and DEUTSCH, A. R. (1966). The congenital rubella syndrome. Ocular pathogenesis and related embryology. *Amer. J. Ophthal.*, **62**, 236–8.

ROY, F. E., HIATT, R. L. and KORONES, S. E. *et al.* (1966). Ocular manifestation of congenital rubella syndrome: Recovery of virus from affected infants. *Arch. Ophthal.*, **75**, 601–7.

RUDOLPH, A. J., SINGLETON, E. B. and ROSENBERG, H. S. *et al.* (1965). Osseous manifestations of the congenital rubella syndrome. *Amer. J. Dis. Child.*, **110**, 428–33.

SCHEIE, H. G., SCHAFFER, D. B., PLOTKIN, S. A. and KERTESZ, E. D. (1967). Congenital rubella cataracts: surgical results and virus recovery from intraocular tissue. *Arch. Ophthal.*, **77**, 440–4.

SEIFERT, G. and OEHME, J. (1957). *Pathologie und Klinik der cytomegalie.* Leipzig: Thieme.

SILVERSTEIN, A. M. (1963). The effect of x-irradiation on the development of immunologic uveitis. *Invest. Ophthal.*, **2**, 58–62.

SMITH, M. E., ZIMMERMAN, L. E. and HARLEY, R. D. (1966). Ocular involvement in congenital cytomegalic inclusion disease. *Arch. Ophthal.*, **76**, 696–9.

SMITH, M. G. (1956). Propagation in tissue cultures of a cytopathogenic virus from human salivary gland virus (S.G.V.) disease. *Proc. Soc. Exp. Biol. (N.Y.)*, **92**, 424–30.

SPIRO, A. J. (1966). Skeletal muscle lesions in the congenital rubella syndrome. *Amer. J. Dis. Child.*, **112**, 427–428.

SRABSTEIN, J. C., MORRIS, N. and LARKE, R. P. *et al.* (1974). Is there a congenital varicella syndrome? *J. Pediat.*, **84**, 239–43.

STARR, J. G., BART, R. D. and GOLD, E. (1970). Inapparent congenital cytomegalovirus infection: clinical and epidemiological characteristics in early infancy. *New Engl. J. Med.*, **282**, 1075–8.

STARR, S. E. (1976). Murine cytomegalovirus in nude mice. *Clin. Res.*, **24**, 69.

SYMMERS, W. S. C. (1960). Generalised cytomegalic inclusion body disease associated with pneumocystic pneumonia in adults: Report of three cases, with Wegener's granulomatosis, thrombotic purpura and Hodgkin's disease as predisposing conditions. *J. Clin. Path.*, **13**, 1–21.

WELLER, T. H., MACAULEY, J. C., CRAIG, J. M. and WIRTH, P. (1957). Isolation of intranuclear inclusion producing agents from infants with illness resembling cytomegalic inclusion disease. *Proc. Soc. Exp. Biol. (N.Y.)*, **94**, 4–12.

WELLER, T. H. and NEVA, F. A. (1962). Propagation in tissue culture of cytopathic agents from patients with rubella-like illness. *Proc. Soc. Exp. Biol. (N.Y.)*, **111**, 215–25.

WONG, T. W. and WARNER, N. E. (1962). Cytomegalic inclusion disease in adults: report of 14 cases. *Arch. Path.*, **74**, 403–22.

WYATT, J. P., HEMSATH, F. A. and SOASH, M. D. (1951). Disseminated cytomegalic inclusion disease in an adult with primary refractory anemia or transfusional siderosis: Report of a case. *Amer. J. Clin. Path.*, **21**, 50–55.

WYATT, J. P., SAXTON, J., LEE, R. S. and PINKERTON, H. J. (1950). Generalised cytomegalic inclusion disease. *J. Pediat.*, **36**, 271–294.

YANOFF, M., SCHAFFER, D. B. and SCHEIE, H. C. (1968). Rubella ocular syndrome: clinical significance of viral and pathological studies. *Trans. Amer. Acad. Ophthal. Otolaryng.*, **72**, 896–902.

YLINEN, O. and JARVINEN, P. A. (1953). Parotitis in pregnancy. *Acta Obstet. Gynec. Scand.*, **32**, 121–132.

ZIMMERMAN, L. E. and SILVERSTEIN, A. M. (1961). In: *Immunopathology of Uveitis.* Eds. E. Maumenee and A. M. Silverstein. Baltimore: Williams and Wilkins.

CHAPTER THIRTEEN

Other Virus Diseases of the Eye

THIS chapter deals with virus infections of the eye which are less well known, and often of less significance to the patient. However, it is anticipated that in the future virus-related disease of the eye will emerge in the form of immune complex disease. Circulating immune complexes are known to be associated with various phenomena in the eye such as uveitis, which may follow a minor systemic viral disease. In the following chapter those viruses which are known to cause infections of the external eye or the retina will be described.

THE CYTOMEGALOVIRUS

The conditions caused by cytomegalovirus (CMV) are associated with large inclusion-bearing cells in tissue sections. CMV has been recognised as a cause of human disease and a general problem in many populations throughout the world. It has a major impact in causing congenital infections, generally as a result of primary infection occurring early in pregnancy, and has already been discussed (Chapter 12).

The mode of transmission in the majority of cases is not clearly known. However the CMV is considered to be highly contagious. It can be recovered from saliva, urine and serum of infected individuals. One mode of transmission is via blood products, particularly fresh whole blood. The primary disease in normal individuals varies in severity; the majority of those infected hardly experience a distinctive syndrome. Clinically recognised disease may last from one to several weeks and on occasions months. Patients develop fever, malaise, hepatosplenomegaly and lymphocytosis, with the appearance of atypical lymphocytes. There is a lymphadenopathy in some individuals.

An increased incidence in severity of infection may occur in many groups of patients who have undergone immunosuppression. Those with rheumatological disease or those receiving cytotoxic therapy for underlying malignancies, and also organ transplant recipients, suffer severe infections with CMV. Patients with malignancies have an increased shedding of CMV with evidence of severe infection, these patients presenting either with pneumonia or with disseminated infection with the involvement of many organs. Bone-marrow transplant patients can also suffer from these infections. CMV may be transferred in renal tissue to seronegative individuals, who undergo a primary syndrome typical of CMV mononucleosis.

Infectious mononucleosis is characterised by an atypical lymphocytosis which is principally of T-cell origin. Epstein-Barr virus is the major cause of the disease and the pathogenesis of this infection has been well studied. Similar T-cell responses are seen in the rarer CMV mononucleosis. Patients with CMV-induced infectious mononucleosis have increased numbers of immunoglobulin-producing cells. The non-specific activation of this immunoglobulin synthesis has been investigated in EBV and CMV mononucleosis (Haswell Elkins *et al.*, 1983). It has become evident that CMV may be capable of inducing non-specific polyclonal immunoglobulin synthesis, although it does not appear to be as potent an inducer as EBV.

Diagnosis

Many techniques exist. Antibody can be measured using the complement fixation test, but sensitive tests such as fluorescent antibody staining, indirect haemagglutination and enzyme-linked immuno-absorbent assay may replace complement fixation. Virus isolation is performed on diploid tissue culture cells, generally using the urine as the most likely positive material.

Cell-mediated immunity can be assessed by using lymphocyte transformation techniques. Patients who have been immunosuppressed show limited transformation levels.

Cytomegalic Inclusion Disease in the Adult Patient

Infection with the CMV may take a number of different forms in its systemic manifestations (Table 12.2, p. 293). There are a number of reports of involvement of the eye, usually in the form of retinitis. The ocular manifestations usually occur in debilitated or immunosuppressed patients and in those undergoing cytotoxic therapeutic regimes for blood dyscrasias or metastatic tumours. In particular it has been seen in patients who have undergone renal transplantation (Mills, 1977). The clinical appearance is one of granular, yellow-white areas of retinal necrosis, haemorrhages and vascular sheathing with attenuation (de Venecia *et al.*, 1971; Egbert *et al.*, 1980; Plate (IIIc). Chumbley *et al.* (1975) described cytomegalovirus retino-uveitis with hypopyon in a renal transplant recipient. Biiateral cytomegalovirus panuveitis was described in a previously healthy young woman receiving immunosuppressive doses of systemic corticosteroid. There may be dense vitreous opacities associated with granulomatous panuveitis, not necessarily accompanied by retinitis. The virus may be isolated from the saliva, cervix and the eye (Berger *et al.*, 1979). The most serious complication of retino-uveitis is retinal detachment. The detachment is initially exudative, and may become complicated by a rhegmatogenous component. Broughton *et al* (1978) described bilateral retinal detachments which developed in a renal allograft patient several months after the onset of cytomegalic retinitis. Laser photocoagulation was used to limit the posterior extent of one detachment until the detachment was surgically repaired. Many cases have now been reported (Pollard *et al.*, 1981). The retinal lesions generally present as an exudative retinitis which is often located in a perivascular area. It later becomes haemorrhagic. There is little evidence of vitreous involvement, which enables one to distinguish it from other forms of retinitis, particularly toxoplasmosis. In many cases the retinitis progresses to blindness. Haemorrhagic areas may develop and the areas of retinal inflammation may become confluent, with the eventual appearance of retinal pigment atrophy (Plate III*d* and Figure 13.1).

Pathology

Large inclusion-bearing cells were originally found in the kidney, lung or liver of infants who had died from various causes. It was noted that there was a similarity between the appearance of the inclusion-containing cells, which were called 'cytomegalia', and the intranuclear inclusions seen in skin lesions caused by herpesviruses. Infection of a cell is accompanied by contraction and rounding of the membrane, followed by the development of intranuclear and intracytoplasmic inclusions. These cells enlarge and eventually form foci of altered cells, some of which may fuse to produce giant cells (Figure 13.2). Histological studies demonstrate degeneration and necrosis in the retina with little extension of an inflammatory response into the vitreous. The major site of infection is thought to be the retina. Those found in the nucleus are known as the Cowdry A type which demonstrate a so-called 'owl eye' appearance with a halo in paraffin-embedded sections. The formation of a halo cannot be seen in epoxy-resin-embedded sections. Electron-microscopy demonstrates CMV particles of differing developmental stages in intranuclear inclusions. These have been described as empty capsids, capsids with electron-lucent cores, and capsids with electron-dense cores, based on the different stages of development. In addition, capsids with bar-like structures and particles similar to perichromatin-like granules have been described. Taylor *et al.* (1981) found evidence of CMV following retinal biopsy. Figure 13.3 demonstrates typical inclusion bodies in retinal tissue taken postmortem where it can be seen that there are cytomegaolovirus-like particles shown by subsequent electron microscopy (Figure 13.4). The retinal necrosis is thought to be caused by occlusion of retinal vessels. This might be caused by CMV infection of the vascular endothelial cells. Masuyama *et al.* (1981) were not able to demonstrate this; however, retinal arterioles occluded with proliferating smooth muscle cells originating from the vascular wall were found. This might explain the necrotic aspect of the clinical picture. In this study cytomegalic cells were demonstrated in the iris, ciliary body and choroid.

Epidemiology

Cytomegalovirus infection varies in incidence from one transplantation centre to another (Fine *et al.* 1972; Coulson *et al.*, 1974; Simmons *et al.*, 1974; Fiala *et al.*, 1975; Ho *et al.*, 1975). In some units CMV infection occurred in 96 per cent of renal transplant subjects (Fiala *et al.*, 1975; Fiala *et al.*, 1976), the morbidity being in the order of 60 per cent, most subjects suffering a febrile syndrome with arthralgia, while 15 per cent had viral pneumonitis, 15 per cent had viral hepatitis and 4 per cent had retinitis. The factors which influence the

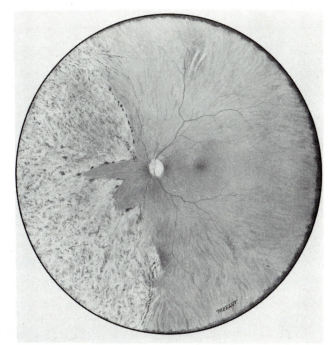

Figure 13.1. Retinal drawing of the distribution of atrophy of the pigmentary epithelium following cytomegalic inclusion disease in an immunodeficient patient.

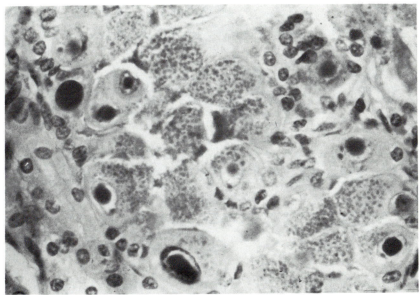

Figure 13.2. Renal tissue demonstrating cytoplasmic and nuclear inclusion bodies in an immunodeficient patient, postmortem.

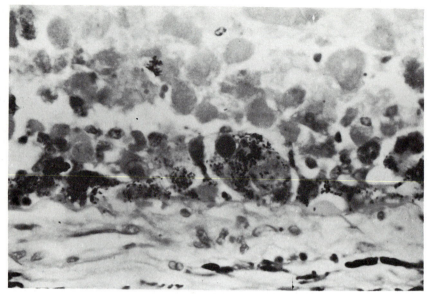

Figure 13.3. Postmortem tissue showing inclusion bodies. The patient had the classical retinal changes associated with CMV retinitis. (Courtesy, Mr. John Scott.)

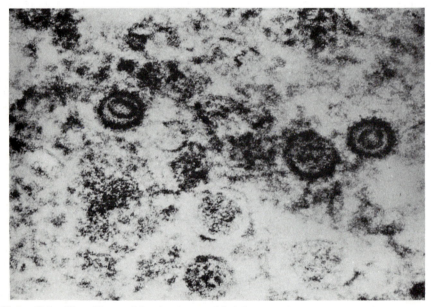

Figure 13.4. Virus-like particles demonstrated by electron-microscopy in retinal tissue taken postmortem from an immunosuppressed patient. (Courtesy, Mr. John Scott.)

clinical course of transplant recipients have been poorly understood, and to help to elicit some of the factors which might be involved in the induction to retinal disease, the time-course, intensity and leucocyte-site in cytomegalovirus viraemia were investigated (Fiala *et al.*, 1977). In 61 transplant patients, five patients had chronic viraemia which lasted more than six months, two of these developed typical cytomegalovirus retinitis and a severe fungal infection after viraemia which lasted 11 months. Retinitis did not develop in 22 patients in whom the viraemia was of short duration. The infectious cytomegalovirus was largely associated with polymorphonuclear leucocytes, while in one patient with terminal illness the virus was associated with monocytes during a granulocytic response which accompanied the infection. Monocytes may serve as a second line of defence against cytomegalovirus when there is a depletion of neutrophils. These cells may not only help in the destruction of cytomegalovirus, but may also disseminate the virus to various target organs such as the liver, spleen, kidney and eye. Cytomegalic retinitis probably results from intensive and chronic cytomegalovirus viraemia, and it is important that the leucocyte deficit which accompanies the disease should be identified, so that appropriate action may be taken to avoid the more serious consequences such as occur with overwhelming infections.

Porter and his associates (1972) estimated the incidence of retinitis following cytomegalovirus infection in renal transplants to be 5 per cent, but Astle and Ellis (1974) reported on incidence of only 1·3 per cent.

Treatment

In a trial of therapy in a group of immunosuppressed patients using adenine arabinoside intravenously (Pollard *et al.*, 1980 and 1981) several patients with progressive retinitis demonstrated apparent improvement in the eye lesions following such treatment. However, when the immunosuppressive therapy was reduced in other patients there was also a therapeutic response. Measurement of virus shedding provided a parameter of effectiveness during antiviral therapy. The dosages of the antiviral required to alter the course of CMV retinitis were higher than those required in other herpesvirus infections and were associated with haematological and gastro-intestinal side-effects. There is evidence of spontaneous resolution in a number of patients. Careful ophthalmological examination may allow early diagnosis and management in patients who have undergone major transplant surgery.

The Epstein-Barr Virus

An unusual malignant lymphoma occurring in African children was first described by Burkitt in 1958; it was restricted to hot and wet areas below an altitude of 4,500 feet. Burkitt reasoned that the distribution corresponded to a mosquito belt and considered that the cancer might be caused by a mosquito-borne virus. Following an intensive search for virus in lymphomas and in cultured cell lines derived from them, Epstein and Barr identified a herpesvirus which is now known as the Epstein-Barr virus. The EB virus genome is integrated with that of the cells of the African lymphoma and has also been identified in nasopharyngeal carcinomas in peoples of Southern Chinese extraction. In 1964 Epstein and his colleagues recovered a herpesvirus from cultured tumour cells. The Epstein-Barr virus (EBV) is integrated into the chromosomes of all lines of EB tumour cells, some of which yield active virus spontaneously, while others can be activated to yield particles by chemical treatment. EBV was found to be the aetiological agent of infectious mono-nucleosis (Niederman *et al.*, 1968).

The virus is a distinctive member of the herpes group. EBV appears very similar to other herpesviruses on EM. Two laboratory strains are recognised. Virus has been cultivated in suspensions of primate lymphocytes which may yield small amounts of extracellular virus. The capacity for persistence and latency of EBV in a non-productive form creates a situation where later reactivation under conditions of immunosuppression such as in malaria, and therepeutic immunosuppression may be possible. The African Burkitt lymph-oma and nasopharyngeal carcinoma may be expressions of reactivation. The EBV is capable of transforming uninfected primate lymphocytes and inducing in them the potential for unlimited proliferation, which is now known as immortalisation.

The prevalence of antibody to EBV has been determined on a wide scale. In developing and tropical countries, most children have been infected by the age of six years. The disease is unlikely to be clinically recognisable in such countries. In Western communities the percentage of children who have been infected under the age of six years amounts to about 50 per cent. If a delay in exposure to the virus occurs and infection is initiated between the ages of 15 and 25 years it may emerge as a significant clinical entity as infectious mononucleosis. Typically, it may present in the young adult as fever, pharyng-itis, lymphadenitis and splenomegaly, with disturbed liver function and characteristic atypical large lymphocytes in the peripheral blood. It may be insidious in onset with malaise and lethargy. High, fluctuating fever, chills, and headaches may be a later manifestation. Enlargement of the posterior cervical lymph glands is usual, and axillary and other glands are also frequently involved. Neurological complications occasionally occur, particularly the Guillain-Barré syndrome, Bell's palsy, meningo-encephalitis and transverse myelitis.

Ocular Manifestations

There may be a direct involvement of the eye or its adnexa with a conjunctivitis associated with hyperaemia and a follicular response in the tarsal plates, with associated white spots which are possible focal collections of inflammatory cells. A granulomatous mass may sometimes appear which is associated with a pre-auricular adenopathy. Subconjunctival haemorrhages may be associated. Rarely, a membranous conjunctivitis can occur. Keratitis is rare. It may be sectorial or take the form of initial superficial punctate erosions in the epithelium, and stromal disease may develop in the underlying region. Palpebral and periorbital oedema together with dacryo-adenitis and dacryocystitis, episcleritis, uveitis, optic neuritis, retinal oedema and haem-orrhages have all been reported. Palsies of the extra-ocular muscles, together with nystagmus and conjugate deviations of gaze have been recorded. Conjunctivitis is thought to be the most common ocular manifestation. There may be mild unilateral or bilateral conjunctival injection, or an extensive follicular or membranous conjunctivitis. These changes may either precede or follow the manifestations of the generalised disease. The conjunctivitis may be a reflection of the lymphoproliferative nature of the infection. Perivascular lymphoid infiltrates with necrosis were reported by Meisler *et al*. (1981).

Pox Viridae

The pox viruses are the largest and most complex of all viruses. The pox viridae are divided into six genera on the basis of antigenic and morphological differences. Several pox viruses may cause infection in the human, including smallpox (variola), molluscum contagiosum (Figure 13.5), cowpox, milker's nodes and orf. Most diseases are associated with pustular skin lesions, which may be localised or part of a generalised rash.

Smallpox itself has been eradicated as a result of the WHO smallpox campaign. Surveillance so far suggests that the virus of smallpox no longer exists anywhere on earth, and therefore a discussion of the ocular effects is no longer necessary (Table 13.1). However, it must be kept in mind that following the control of smallpox in West Africa, further cases of pox disease appeared in man in 1970 in the absence of any known smallpox disease in the community. The isolated virus was identified as monkey pox virus. Cases of human monkey pox infection have been recognised, and several have died. Of further concern is the recovery of virus strains indistinguishable from variola virus from two

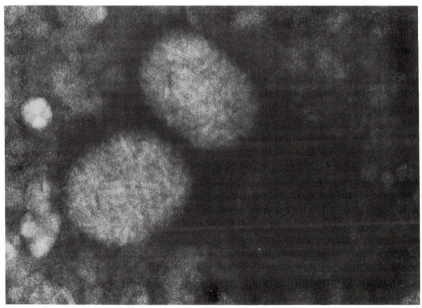

Figure 13.5.   Electronmicrograph of the causal agent of molluscum contagiosum. Most of the pox viruses are morphologically indistinguishable from each other (× 140,000).

TABLE 13.1

OCULAR MANIFESTATIONS OF VARIOLA

Catarrhal conjunctivitis
Haemorrhagic conjunctivitis
Phlyctens or pustules on conjunctiva
Ulceration of bulbar conjunctiva with membrane
    formation
Subsequent corneal ulceration when phlyctenular
    lesions situated at the limbus
Disciform keratitis
Hypopyon ulcers (secondary microbial agents)
Dense corneal scarring
Phthisis bulbi

normal monkey kidney cell lines taken from cynomolgus monkeys from Malaysia (Gispen and Brand-Saathof, 1972), and the recovery of a single strain from kidney cells from a chimpanzee caught in Zaire (Marennikova *et al.*, 1972). Thus, the infectious agent can be found in other primates although it has not yet been ascertained that any human variola case has originated in monkey disease. Isolates such as this which are obtained in the absence of known human smallpox indicates that there is a need for careful study of primates and other mammalian populations before finally declaring that global eradication has been accomplished.

The pox viruses are large enough to be seen under a light microscope, using critical illumination. The structure of the virion of vaccinia and smallpox appear to be identical. There is no nucleocapsid conforming to either of the two types of symmetry found in other viruses, and hence it is sometimes called a complex variant. There is an outer membrane of tubular shaped lipoprotein subunits arranged irregularly to enclose a dumb-bell-shaped core and two lateral bodies of an unknown nature. The core contains viral DNA together with protein but the exact arrangements are not yet determined. The nucleic acid is double-stranded DNA with a molecular weight of 160 million daltons. The core proteins include a transcriptase and several other enzymes. The lipoprotein of the membrane is synthesised *de novo* and not derived by budding from cellular membranes. As would be expected from its multiplicity of polypeptides, the virion contains numerous antigens, which can be recognised by gel diffusion systems. There is extensive cross-neutralisation between viruses belonging to the same genus but none between viruses of different genera.

VACCINIA

With the eradication of smallpox the indications for vaccination have now largely disappeared. Nevertheless, in certain parts of the world it remains a statutory requirement which implies that ocular disease due to vaccination, although rare, could remain a possibility. Most of the cases which have been reported are not due to auto-inoculation, although this may occur, but are due to contamination after contact with a vaccination vesicle of another person. The clinical picture varies considerably and is dependent upon the patient's previous experience of the infective organism. In patients without immunity an alarming condition may occur, while in the presence of good immunity a blepharoconjunctivitis alone may present. In non-immune individuals redness and swelling of the lids appears after three days, and the eyes may become completely closed. This situation may mimic the appearance of orbital cellulitis. A non-follicular, purulent conjunctivitis may occur, but on occasions a pseudomembranous conjunctivitis involving the palpebral conjunctiva may coexist.

The corneal complications are serious at times, and have been recorded in 30 per cent of cases. They range between a punctate superficial keratitis and a chronic disciform keratitis. At its onset there is a granular opacification with swelling of the epithelial cells which necrose and form small clumps of opacification. With EM the cells can shown to contain virus. Beneath the epithelial disease opacities develop within the stroma (Figure 13.6). These may resemble the lesions seen in adenoviral conjunctivitis. They may persist for many months or years. Ulcers have also been recorded which may have a prolonged course and cause severe pain. Eventually, involvement of the stroma may supervene with collagen melting in association. Disciform keratitis may also occur as a delayed phenomenon. Both superficial and deep vascularisation may be associated. A kerato-uveitis can also result. As in herpes simplex disease it seems likely that the epithelial lesion is due to viral proliferation in

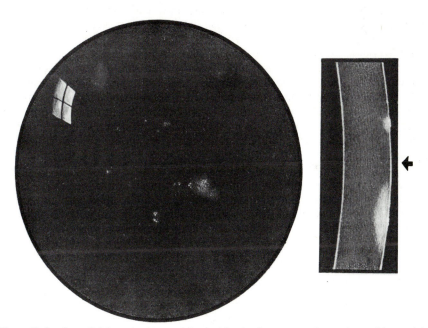

Figure 13.6. Superficial punctate stromal opacities in the cornea of a patient with vaccinial keratitis. (Courtesy, Professor Barrie Jones.)

this layer, while the stromal involvement is due to immunological processes, directed against further spread of the virus, which simultaneously operate to induce tissue damage and loss of corneal transparency.

Treatment

At the epithelial stage it has been shown, in animal models of vaccinia keratitis, that the vaccinial agent can be effectively treated with antivirals which act against other DNA viruses (Shiota *et al.*, 1981). Thus, a series of experiments showed that IDU, F_3T and Ara AMP were effective in reducing the severity of the keratitis. Adenine arabinoside and hypoxanthine arabinoside were highly effective and were superior to trifluorothymidine and idoxuridine, which themselves were more effective than controls.

MOLLUSCUM CONTAGIOSUM

Molluscum contagiosum is a specifically human disease, characterised by discrete nodules 2–5 mm in diameter, limited to the epidermis and occurring in most parts of the body. Lesions are white in colour, painless and umbilicated. At the top of each lesion there can be seen a small white core. Cells within the nodule are hypertrophied and contain large hyaline acidophillic cytoplasmic masses called molluscum bodies (Figure 13.7). These consist of a spongy matrix divided into cavities in each of which are clustered masses of virus particles which have the same general structure as those of the vaccinia virus. Incubation varies between 14 and 50 days. Attempts to transmit infection to experimental animals have failed. It is probably transmitted through minor abrasions, and exposure in specific environments such as swimming pools.

Ocular Disease

Molluscum may grow on the lid margins in positions where the lesions can be difficult to identify, amongst the lashes, or at the inner canthus (Figure 13.8). A secondary conjunctivitis may be produced which is persistent and associated with a follicular reaction in the fornices and on the tarsal plates (Plate IV*a*). In severe cases corneal complications can occur, with punctate epithelial keratitis and occasionally a filamentary keratitis. Vascularisation may be associated. It has been considered that the conjunctival reaction results from the influence of toxic products released from the main focus of disease. It appears just as likely that the infectious agent enters the conjunctival sac to induce a local immune response.

Treatment

The tumours can be excised with a sharp, pointed knife, or the contents of the molluscum can be evacuated with a small curette and placed on a slide for examination for inclusion bodies. Removal results in rapid improvement in symptoms and regressions of conjunctival and corneal disease.

PAPOVAVIRUSES

The papovaviruses are small, non-enveloped icosahedral viruses which

PLATE IV

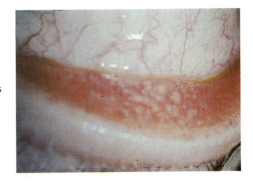

(a) Follicular conjunctivitis affecting the lower tarsal plate and fornix in a patient with a molluscum body amongst the lashes of the upper lid.

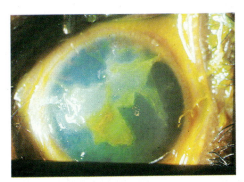

(b) Massive dendritic ulcer found in a Nigerian child with measles. (Courtesy, Mr John Sandford Smith.)

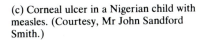

(c) Corneal ulcer in a Nigerian child with measles. (Courtesy, Mr John Sandford Smith.)

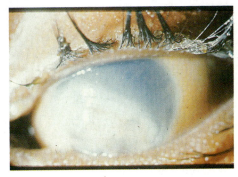

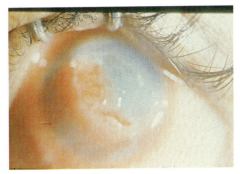

(d) Severe corneal ulcer with vascularisation associated with secondary invasive organisms. (Courtesy, Mr John Sandford Smith.)

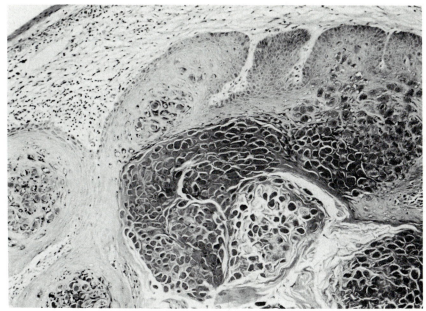

Figure 13.7.   Molluscum contagiosum, low-power view showing inclusion bodies (H and E × 100). (Courtesy, Dr. Richard Blight.)

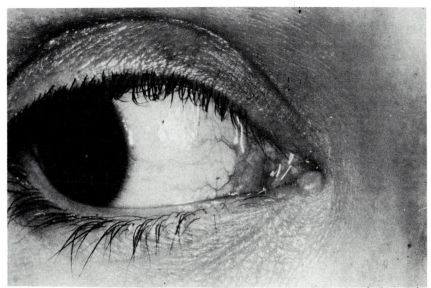

Figure 13.8.   Molluscum contagiosum at the inner angle of the right eye. A secondary conjunctivitis was present. These lesions may easily be missed.

replicate in the nucleus of vertebrate cells. In the virion their nucleic acid occurs as a cyclic double-stranded molecule. Apart from the human wart virus and the virus causing progressive multifocal leucoencephalopathy, a further interest lies in the fact that polyoma virus and simian virus 40 have been important tools for unravelling the molecular and cellular events during oncogenesis.

In man, papilloma viruses have been observed in a variety of warts and papillomas arising in skin and mucous membrane. Until recently it was considered that these tumours were caused by a single virus, the human papilloma virus. But advances have led to a reappraisal of this concept of infection with a single virus. There appears to be a genetic heterogeneity which indicates that several different types of papilloma virus infect man, each characterised by a distinct base composition and antigenic structure. It is possible that specific human papilloma virus may be preferentially associated with different types of skin warts.

The papilloma virus has a virion diameter of 45 nm and a genome of 3×10^6 daltons. The characteristic icosahedral shape of the papilloma virus is also found in the polyoma virus.

Clinical Aspects of Ocular Infection

Many clinical types of warts and papillomas can occur in the skin of the lids and conjunctiva, which are thought to be caused by papilloma viruses. The tumours are characterised histologically by proliferation of the cells of the epithelium which may be thrown into folds producing papillomatous protrusions and downward extension of the dermal papillae. The epithelium shows acanthosis and parakeratosis. Papilloma virus particles have been described in the superficial epithelial cells in ultra-thin sections of the skin tumours. Papillomata situated on the lid margin may be hidden amongst the lashes in patients with chronic catarrhal conjunctivitis. In addition a keratitis may be associated with multiple punctate epithelial erosions. Multiple papillomata may occur on the conjunctiva in the lower fornix or at the inner angle (Figure 13.9). They are usually pedunculated growths with a raspberry-like appearance with finger-like processes, and may recur after excision. Papillomata may be also found at the limbus, and may rarely spread on to the corneal surface, and also they may arise from the bulbar conjunctiva. Recurrent juvenile papillomata can sometimes be severe, producing recurrent disease in the fornices with spread on to the tarsal plates (Figure 13.10).

Treatment

In patients with chronic conjunctivitis with persistent epithelial erosions, removal of lid warts can be surprisingly beneficial. Papillomata of the conjunctiva can be removed with ease, although where the lesions are multiple (Figure 13.10) there can be considerable difficulties. Control of the lesions illustrated in this figure was achieved by means of multiple applications of cryotherapy.

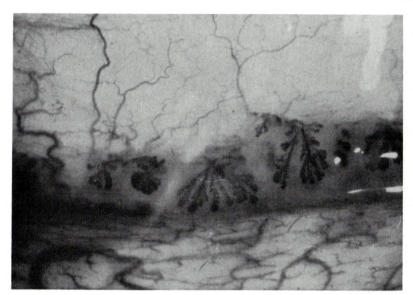

Figure 13.9.   Sessile conjunctival papillomata in the lower conjunctival fornix.

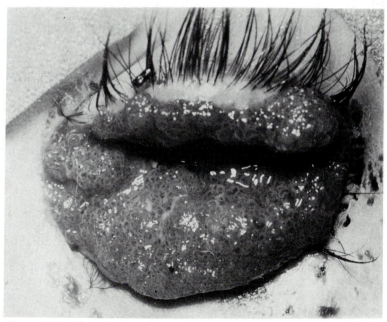

Figure 13.10.   Generalised papillomatosis of the conjunctiva in a four-year-old girl.

RIFT VALLEY FEVER

An arbovirus is, by definition, one that multiplies in a blood-sucking arthropod and is transmitted by bite to a vertebrate. Arthropod viruses comprise a convenient epidemiological grouping, but also embrace viruses from families as diverse as the togaviruses, or bunyaviruses. There are 300 known arboviruses; approximately 100 of these are capable of infecting man, and only about 40, mainly togaviruses, produce significant disease, although some of these, notably the encephalitides and the haemorrhagic fevers, rank among the most lethal of viral diseases. In their natural environment arboviruses alternate between an invertebrate vector such as the mosquito, tick, sandfly or gnat, and a vertebrate host. Mosquito-borne arboviruses are endemic in the tropics and are responsible for sporadic epidemics in temperate zones where arthropod transmission is seasonal. Man becomes involved by accident in the natural cycle of the arboviruses by intruding into the natural environment where the human is usually a foreign host.

Togaviruses consist of small, icosahedral cores 20–40 nm in diameter enclosed within a tightly fitting envelope. By virtue of a glycoprotein peplomer projecting from the envelope togaviruses haemagglutinate but only under certain conditions. The reaction is widely used in the laboratory and in epidemiological studies. Bunyaviruses are larger (90–100 nm), fragile enveloped RNA viruses of helical symmetry more closely resembling an orthomyxovirus than a togavirus.

Rift valley fever is an arthropod-borne viral disease primarily affecting domestic animals, with occasional involvement of man. A number of studies have reported ocular complications in suspect rift valley fever patients. Macular and paramacular oedema with retinal exudates and haemorrhages have been reported (Siam *et al.*, 1980). In 1977 an extensive epidemic occurred in the Nile delta area of the United Arab Republic of Egypt. Numerous cases of encephalitic, ocular and fatal haemorrhagic disease were reported. Macular and paramacular lesions were apparent which were often bilateral. Haemorrhage and oedema were frequently associated with the lesions and vasculitis, retinitis and vascular occlusion were also observed. Approximately half of the patients experienced permanent loss of vision. The visual symptoms and signs were associated with encephalitic, febrile and haemorrhage illnesses during the epidemic.

PARAMYXOVIRUSES

The paramyxoviruses are named according to the morphological resemblance to the orthomyxoviruses with which they were originally classified. It is now recognised that the two groups differ in important characteristics in relation to the nature of the viral nucleic acid and its replication. All human paramyxoviruses are important causes of respiratory infection in children. The para-influenza and respiratory syncytial viruses are responsible for most of the croup, bronchiolitis, and pneumonitis in infants today. Measles and mumps are familiar diseases to every parent.

The paramyxoviruses are larger than orthomyxoviruses, and more pleomorphic, ranging from 150–300 nm in diameter. They are enclosed in a loose lipoprotein envelope which is fragile, rendering the virion vulnerable to destruction by storage, freezing and thawing, or even preparation for EM. The particles often appear distorted on EM and may rupture to reveal the internal nucleocapsid. The RNA occurs in a single molecule. The RNA is negative in polarity and is accompanied by a transcriptase. A haemagglutinin is to be found in the envelope of all paramyxoviruses, a neuraminidase in most, and a haemolysin in some. There is no group antigen, although mumps and five of the para-influenza types are related serologically to at least one other member of the group. Measles virus shares antigenic determinants with the viruses of distemper of dogs and rinderpest of cattle. All the paramyxoviruses can be grown in embryonated eggs, sometimes after appropriate adaptations have been introduced. They are all easily handled in cultured cells. Primary cultures of human or simian kidney, diploid strains of human fetal fibroblasts and, for some serotypes, heteroploid human cell lines are all suitable. These viruses do not cause extensive cell destruction. Carrier cultures can readily arise. Syncytium formation is a regular feature with acidophilic inclusions in the cytoplasm and on occasions in the nuclei of the giant cells. Replication of the virus takes place in the cell cytoplasm.

Measles is perhaps the best known of the childhood diseases. There is a characteristic maculopapular rash, conjunctivitis, and coryza. It is not widely appreciated that it can be a dangerous disease; encephalomyelitis occurs often enough to make measles a more significant killer than poliomyelitis was in the days before vaccination against either disease. The rare and fatal subacute sclerosing panencephalitis is a late manifestation of early measles infection. The widespread use of an effective live vaccine has reduced the incidence of measles in many parts of the Western world. After an incubation period of between 9 and 12 days a prodromal syndrome of fever, upper respiratory-tract infection, coryza, cough and conjunctivitis combine to make a sick child. The diagnosis can be established by the detection of Koplik's spots, which are macules or ulcers with a bluish-white centre appearing on the mucous membrane of the inner surface of the cheek. Three days later the exanthem appears on the head and spreads progressively during the ensuing one or two days on to the chest, trunk and limbs. The flat macules fuse to form blotches. They are slow to fade and leave the skin temporarily stained. Complications include otitis media and pneumonia due to secondary invaders.

A fatal giant-cell pneumonia has been reported which may occur sometimes without the typical rash in immunodeficient children. Encephalomyelitis is a severe complication in less than 1 out of every 1000 patients, which induces a mortality of 15 per cent.

Subacute sclerosing panencephalitis can develop in children or adolescents, usually in males from rural areas, a few years after an earlier measles infection. The patient suffers a progressive loss of cerebral function ending in spasticity, death and coma after six months.

Prior to the introduction of a vaccine, slightly less than 10 per cent of infants entering a population would be expected to suffer an attack of measles. However, where careful attention is paid to the reporting of measles in some parts of the world by direct questioning of parents, the level can be in the region of 80 per cent. Serological tests indicate that at least 98 per cent of subjects at the age of 18 years have had experience of the measles antigen. It appears therefore that the true incidence of measles is essentially equal to the number of surviving children (Black 1976). Since a vaccine was introduced, the number of reported cases has fallen to below the former value (Noah, 1982). In highly populated parts of the world the measles virus causes epidemics every two to five years and an epidemic would be expected to last between three and four months. Measles occurs in most countries except those which are remote and isolated. The strains of virus from different areas are indistinguishable and antibody in sera has identical specificity. The patterns of epidemiology and the average age at infection together with mortality vary from one region of the world to another. Where epidemics have occurred in populations who have not previously experienced the disease the mortality has been high. The mortality can be reduced by appropriate medical aid. It is probable that racial differences in host response to infection by the measles virus do exist, but differences in morbidity and mortality rates are also related to population size, overcrowding, living standards, and previous history of infection within the community.

Dekkers (1981) has stressed that measles is a public health problem in many developing countries. Children suffer measles at an earlier age (8–36 months) compared to Europeans. The mortality has been calculated as ranging between 6·5 to 8·6 per cent. The morbidity is also considerable; there may be a stomatitis, laryngotracheitis, and gastro-enteritis. Bronchopneumonia, otitis media, and ocular damage may also occur. 1 per cent of measles children in such communities are said to sustain ocular damage. In the United Kingdom, fatality rates were calculated to be 1:10,000 in 1976.

Ocular Disease

Conjunctivitis and keratitis may occur in association with measles. The conjunctiva may become red and a mucopurulent discharge may be produced, these signs being associated with similar changes in the upper respiratory tract. Elevated papules can appear in the conjunctiva, particularly involving the outer half of the lower tarsal plate. Superficial punctate keratitis and epithelial erosions have been reported, giving rise to the photophobia which is a characteristic symptom of the disease. The severity ranges from small, round, punctate epithelial deficits with unilateral involvement, to multiple stellate epithelial defects with some confluence of erosions in patients with bilateral changes. The keratitis usually consists of fine superficial epithelial punctate lesions. The changes are mostly found in the centre of the cornea in the interpalpebral zone (Deckard and Bergstrom, 1981). The importance of measles keratitis relates to the severity of the disease when it occurs in the malnourished and immunodeficient. Although the keratitis may be benign, secondary infection may occur with staphylococci, streptococci, pneumococci and *H. influenzae*. Recently it has been found that a proportion of patients with severe measles keratitis have associated herpes simplex virus infection of the cornea (Plates IV *b, c, d* Sandford-Smith *et al.*, 1981). It is considered that severe disseminated virus infection is a cause of acquired immunodeficiency, and the appearance of the herpes simplex virus under these conditions is therefore not very surprising. A delayed deposition of lipid at the corneal periphery is sometimes seen in an adult patient with a history of an attack of severe measles keratitis in childhood (Figure 13.11).

Dekkers (1981) has investigated the status of ocular disease following measles in Kenya. The prodromal conjunctivitis in measles was catarrhal and was of diagnostic value. Koplik's spots were observed in the conjunctiva. The epithelial keratitis was associated with the rash. Corneal ulcers could eventually complicate measles. The ulcers appeared to have no particular characteristics which made them distinguishable from other diseases. Perforation occurred. A dense leucoma or adherent leucoma could ensue, or phthisis bulbi. Dekkers showed that at least 76 per cent of children with measles in Kenya had early

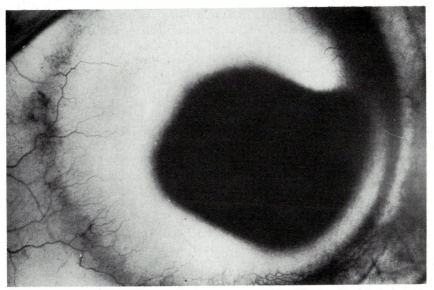

Figure 13.11. Peripheral lipid keratopathy in a patient with a history of particularly severe measles and secondary conjunctivitis in childhood. This is a rare manifestation.

keratitis. At the earliest stage, the state of nutrition appeared not to influence the severity of the keratitis. Out of 188 children, 4 per cent developed central corneal erosions. Such corneal erosions would create a high risk of the development of secondary corneal ulceration. The increased production of collagenase which has been noted in cases of vitamin-A-dependent kerato-malacia probably occurs in severe measles keratitis. Malnutrition plays an important part both in the severity of the measles, and in the onset of corneal disease, leading to post-measles blindness. The prevention of post-measles blindness should involve measles vaccination.

Where measles keratitis occurred it is mandatory that topical treatment with prophylactic antibiotics should be carried out. Education against the use of traditional medicines should be widespread. Such local remedies include various types of powders, minerals, such as copper stone and copper sulphate, foodstuffs such as honey, breast milk, orange juice, egg yolk, many varieties of plant, cows' urine and aspirin tablets. Improvement in nutritional status would also be of obvious benefit. Where evidence of associated herpetic keratitis is found, then the use of antiviral therapy can only be beneficial. It remains a possibility that a herpes simplex vaccine in subjects at risk of combined viral infections would also help to counteract the effect of the herpes simplex virus in an immunodeficient group of patients.

MUMPS

A common contagious disease of children and young adults, mumps is characterised by inflammation of the salivary glands. Occasionally the lacrimal gland can be involved (Figures 13.12 and 13.13). A simple conjunctivitis is relatively common and can be associated with subconjunctival haemorrhages. Diffuse episcleritis has been recorded. Stromal keratitis may occur with visual loss. Recovery may occur some three weeks after the onset, but occasionally permanent scarring remains.

NEWCASTLE DISEASE

The virus of Newcastle disease, which produces fatal pneumonitis in fowl, was reported to produce human disease in 1943. It may be associated with an attack of unilateral follicular conjunctivitis and punctate keratitis (Hales and Ostler, 1973). The diagnosis is made from the history of contact with infected birds, together with a rise of antibody titre and isolation of the virus.

VIRUS DISEASE ASSOCIATED WITH OPTIC NEURITIS

There is an association between optic neuritis, usually of a retrobulbar type, and demyelinating disease which is well recognised. Both optic neuritis and internuclear ophthalmoplegia are common ocular complications of multiple sclerosis. Virus infections which have been associated with optic neuritis include measles, mumps, chickenpox with or without encephalitis, post-viral and para-viral infections, infectious mononucleosis and herpes zoster.

A relationship between antibody to measles virus and multiple sclerosis, together with subacute sclerosing panencephalitis, has been suspected for some years. The titre of measles antibody in the latter is striking enough to be of diagnostic value in the individual patient, but in the case of multiple sclerosis the increased titre of circulating measles antibody cannot easily be discerned by group comparisons between patients with MS and carefully matched controls. Some surveys have indicated that multiple sclerosis patients demonstrate slight increase in mean antibody titre against measles virus but also other viruses as well. Studies have been made on genetic aspects in relation to measles antibodies in both the serum and the CSF of multiple sclerosis patients. All serological differences between MS patients and other persons are relative, not absolute. The data which has been reported has

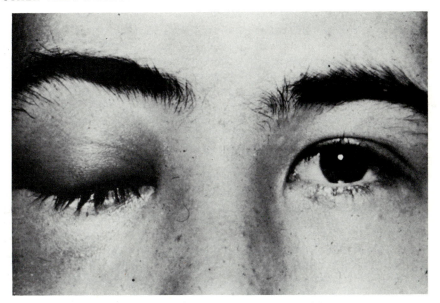

Figure 13.12.   Right dacryo-adenitis in a patient with mumps.

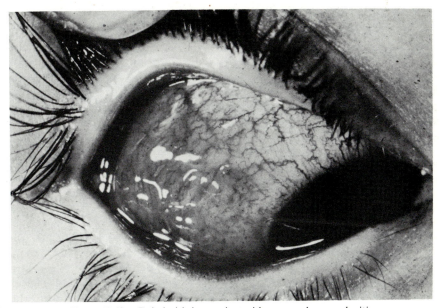

Figure 13.13.   Episcleritis in a patient with mumps dacryo-adenitis.

involved small comparative surveys in different parts of the world. An important new feature is that a specific antibody for one antigen of the virus, a haemolysin, predominates over antibody to the other structural antigens of the virus in the same way as antibody to measles virus exceeds antibody to other viruses in circulating titre and in the frequency with which it is found in the CSF. Recent studies have suggested that lymphocyte responses to measles are suppressed in MS patients (Utermohlen and Zabriskie, 1973). Measles virus has also been isolated from the brain of an MS patient on one occasion (Field *et al.*, 1972), but so have other viruses, which makes such a finding hard to evaluate. Studies on migrants from areas of high to low incidence of MS indicate that a precipitating event in MS occurs in adolescence. It is possible that the measles infection occurs late in life instead of early, as also appertains to subacute sclerosing panencephalitis. In addition to the possible role of measles virus, there are other possible predisposing factors. Thus, assessment of the HL-A antigens has revealed an unusually high proportion of HL-A 3 and 7 tissue antigens. It seems possible that there is an autoimmune mechanism in addition, because antimyelin antibodies can be demonstrated. Further investigation is required to define these associations and their possible relevance to the disease processes (Fraser, 1980).

The Role of Viruses in the Development of Ocular Tumours

The role of viruses in the development of ocular tumours has been summarised by Daniel Albert (1980). The foundation for the study of cancer viruses was laid down following the work of Ellerman and Bang (1908) and Rous (1911), where oncogenic viruses were isolated from certain avian tumours. Three groups of DNA viruses and one type of RNA virus are considered to be possible causes for human cancer. The oncogenic DNA viruses are the herpesviruses, the papovaviruses (papilloma viruses), polyoma viruses and simian virus 40 and the adenoviruses. The herpesviruses are widely considered to be the most likely candidates to produce cancer in humans. Certain parallels have been drawn between Burkitt's lymphoma and retino-blastoma which has been discussed by Zimmerman (1970).

It was noticed in the early 1960s that human adenoviruses are oncogenic in hamsters and mice, but there is relatively little evidence to support a role for them in the development of human malignancy. Oncogenic RNA viruses were originally discovered in the cancers of chicken and mice (Rouse, 1911; Gross, 1951). Genetic information is expressed in some human tumour cells which suggests that an RNA virus might be involved. Convincing evidence that such viruses are a cause of human neoplasms is at present lacking (Levy, 1977; Gross, 1976; Spiegelman *et al.*, 1974).

There has been some evidence for the presence of virus particles in human ocular tumours, although this has not been very convincing. An electron-microscopic search was made in 54 human ocular malignancy melanomas, where virus particles were identified in five specimens (Albert, 1979). Intra-ocular tumours have been induced by papovaviruses and adenoviruses (Albert, 1980). Polyoma viruses have been used to induce mixed tumours bearing some resemblance to uveal melanomas *in vitro*. Adenovirus 12 infection in hamster ocular tissues involve the neural retina, and bear some resemblance to human retinoblastoma (Albert *et al.*, 1968).

Recently an ocogenic RNA virus, the feline sarcoma virus, has been used to induce ocular melanomas in cats (Albert, 1979). The lesions occurred in the iris, and were associated with increased pigmentation. The tumours were noted to be capable of extrascleral extension. The question as to whether viruses cause neoplastic disease in the human remains unanswered. The final information that is required must lie in the study of mechanisms which play roles in pathological processes induced by persistent viruses. This may eventually throw light on factors which determine the characteristics of a defined group of neoplastic lesions (Albert, 1980).

REFERENCES

ALBERT, D. M. (1979). The association of viruses with uveal melanoma. *Trans. Amer. Ophthal. Soc.*, **77**, 365.

ALBERT, D. M. (1980). The role of viruses in the development of ocular tumours. *Ophthalmology*, **87**, 1219.

ALBERT, D. M., RABSON, A. S. and DALTON, A. J. (1968). *In vitro* neoplastic transformation of uveal and retinal tissue by oncogenic DNA viruses. *Invest. Ophthal.*, **7**, 357.

ASTLE, J. N. and ELLIS, P. P. (1974). Ocular complications in renal transplant patients. *Ann. Ophthal.*, **6**, 1269.

BERGER, B., WEINBERG, R. S., TESSLER, H. H., WYHINNY, G. G. and VYGANTAS, C. H. (1979). Bilateral cytomegalovirus panuveitis after high dose cortiosteroid therapy. *Amer. J. Ophthal.*, **88**, 1020.

BLACK, F. L. (1976). *Viral Infection of Humans: Epidemiology and Control*. Ed. A. S. Evans. Chichester: John Wiley & Sons.

BROUGHTON, W. L., CUPPLES, H. P. and POWER, L. M. (1978). Bilateral retinal detachment following cytomegalovirus retinitis. *Arch. Ophthal.*, **96**, 618.

CHUMBLEY, L. C., ROBERTSON, D. M., SMITH, T. and CAMPBELL, R. J. (1975). Adult cytomegalovirus inclusion retino-uveitis. *Amer. J. Ophthal.*, **80**, 807.

COULSON, A. S., LUCAS, Z. J., CONDY, M. and COHN, R. (1974). An epidemic of cytomegalovirus disease in a renal transplant population. *West. Med.*, **120**, 1.

DE VENECIA, G., ZU RHEIN, G. M., PRATT, M. V. and KISKEN, W. (1971). Cytomegalovirus inclusion retinitis in an adult. A clinical histopathologic and ultrastructural study. *Arch. Ophthal.*, **86**, 44.

DECKARD, P. S. and BERGSTROM, T. J. (1981). Rubella keratitis. *Ophthalmology*, **88**, 810.

DEKKERS, N. W. H. M. (1981). *The Cornea in Measles*. (Monographs in Ophthalmology, No. 3). Ed. W. Junk. The Hague: Kluwer.

EGBERT, P. R., POLLARD, R. B., GALLAGHER, J. C. and MERIGAN, T. C. (1980). Cytomegalovirus retinitis in immunosuppressed hosts. II. Ocular manifestations. *Ann. Intern. Med.*, **93**, 664.

ELLERMAN, V. and BANG, O. (1908). Experimentelle Leukämic bei Hühnern. *Zbl. Bakt., I. Abt. Orig.*, **46**, 595.

EPSTEIN, M. A., ACHONG, B. G. and BARR, Y. M. (1964). Virus particles in cultured lymphoblasts from Burkitt's lymphoma. *Lancet*, **1**, 702.

FIALA, M., CHATTERJEE, S. N., CARSON, S. C., POOLSAWAT, S., HEINER, D. C., SAXON, A. and GUZE, L. B. (1977). Cytomegalovirus retinitis secondary to chronic viraemia in phagocytic leukocytes. *Amer. J. Ophthal.*, **84**, 567.

FIALA, M., CHATTERJEE, S. N., PAYNE, J. E., STACEY, B., COSGROVE, D. and BERNE, T. V. (1976) Holoendemic cytomegalovirus infection in renal transplant recipients. *Yale J. Biol. Med.*, **49**, 67.

FIALA, M., PAYNE, J. E., BERNE, J. V., MOORE, T., HENLE, W., MONTGOMERIE, J. Z., CHATTERJEE, S. N. and GUZE, L. B. (1975). Epidemiology of cytomegalovirus infection after transplantation and immunosuppression. *J. Infect. Dis.*, **132**, 421.

FIELD, E. J., COWSHALL, S., NARANG, H. K. and BELL, T. M. (1972). Viruses in multiple sclerosis. *Lancet*, **2**, 280.

FINE, R. N., GRUSHKIN, C. M., MALEKZADEH, M. and WRIGHT, H. T. (1972). Cytomegalovirus syndrome following renal transplantation. *Arch. Surg.*, **105**, 564.

FRASER, K. B. (1980). The relationship between antibody to measles virus and multiple sclerosis. In: *Recent Advances in Clinical Virology*. Ed. A. P. Waterson. Edinburgh: Churchill Livingstone.

GISPEN, R. and BRAND-SAATHOF, B. (1972). White pox virus strains from monkeys. *Bull. Wld. Hlth. Org.*, **46**, 585.

GROSS, L. (1951). 'Spontaneous' leukaemia developing in C3H mice following inoculation, in infancy, with AK-leukaemia extracts or AK-embryos. *Proc. Soc. Exp. Biol. (N.Y.)*, **76**, 27.

GROSS, L. (1976). The role of C-type and other oncogenic virus particles in cancer and leukaemia. *New Engl. J. Med.*, **294**, 724.

HALES, R. H. and OSTLER, H. B. (1973). Newcastle disease conjunctivitis with subepithelial infiltrates. *Brit. J. Ophthal.*, **57**, 694–697.

HASWELL ELKINS, M., BALACHANDRAN, N. and HUTT-FLETCHER, L. M. (1983). Induction of immunoglobulin synthesis by cytomegalovirus. *International Herpesvirus Workshop, Oxford*, p. 105.

HO, M., SUWANSIRIKUL, S., DOWLING, J. N., YOUNGBLOOD, L. A. and ARMSTRONG, J. A. (1975). The transplanted kidneys as a source of cytomegalovirus infections. *New Engl. J. Med.*, **293**, 1109.

LEVY, J. A. (1977). Endogenous C-type viruses in normal and 'abnormal' cell development. *Cancer Res.*, **37**, 2957.

MARENNIKOVA, S. S., SELUHINA, E. M., MALCEVA, N. M., CIMISKJAN, K. L. and MACEVIC, G. R. (1972). Isolation and properties of the causal agent of a new variola-like disease (monkeypox) in man. *Bull. Wld. Hlth. Org.*, **46**, 599.

MASUYAMA, Y., FUKUZAKI, M., BABA, Y. and SAWADA, A. (1981). Histopathological study of adult cytomegalic inclusion retino-uveitis. In: *Herpetic Eye Diseases*, p. 495. Ed. R. Sundmacher. Munich: J. F. Bergman Verlag.

MEISLER, D. M., BOSWORTH, D. E. and KRACHMER, J. H. (1981). Ocular infectious mononucleosis manifested as Parineud's oculoglandular syndrome. *Amer. J. Ophthal.*, **92**, 722.

MENSER, M. A., HARLEY, J. D. and HOUSEGO, C. J. (1966). Possible chemical factors in the postnatal development of rubella cataracts. *Lancet*, **2**, 771–2.

MILLS, P. V. (1977). Ocular cytomegalic inclusion disease in the adult. *Trans. Ophthal. Soc. U.K.*, **97**, 501.

NIEDERMAN, J. C., McCULLUM, R. W., HENLE, G. and HENLE, W. (1968). Infectious mononucleosis: clinical manifestations in relation to E.B. virus antibodies. *J. Amer. Med. Ass.*, **203**, 205.

NOAH, H. D. (1982). Measles eradication policies. *Brit. Med. J.*, **284**, 997.

POLLARD, R. B., EGBERT, P. R., GALLAGHER, J. C. and MERIGAN, T. C. (1980). Cytomegalovirus retinitis in immunosuppressed hosts. I. Natural history and effects of treatment with adenine arabinoside. *Ann. Intern. Med.*, **93**, 655.

POLLARD, R. B., EGBERT, P. R., GALLAGHER, J. C. and MERIGAN, T. C. (1981). Infections with cytomegalovirus in adults and the natural history and treatment of cytomegalovirus retinitis. In: *Herpetic Eye Diseases*, p. 481. Ed. R. Sundmacher. Munich: J. F. Bergmann Verlag.

PORTER, T., CROMBIE, A. I., GARDNER, P. S. and ULDALL, R. P. (1972). Incidence of ocular complications in patients undergoing renal transplantation. *Brit. Med. J.*, **3**, 133.

ROUSE, P. (1911). Transmission of a malignant new growth by means of a cell-free filtrate. *J. Amer. Med. Ass.*, **56**, 198.

SANDFORD-SMITH, J. H. and WHITTLE, H. C. (1981). Corneal ulceration following measles in malnourished Nigerian children. *Child Care Hlth. Div.*, **7**, 91.

SHIOTA, H., YAMANE, S. and OGAWA, T. (1981). Treatment of vaccinial keratitis with various new antivirals. *6th Congress of the European Society of Ophthalmology, Brighton, 1980*. London; Academic Press.

SIAM, A. L., MEEGAN, J. M. and GHARBAWI, K. F. (1980). Rift Valley Fever ocular manifestations: Observations during the 1977 epidemic in Egypt. *Brit. J. Ophthal.*, **64**, 366.

SIMMONS, R. L., LOPEZ, C., BALFOUR, H., KALIS, J., RATTAZZI, L. C. and NAZARIAN, J. S. (1974). Cytomegalovirus: clinical virological correlations in renal transplant recipients. *Ann. Surg.*, **180**, 623.

SPIEGELMAN, S., AXEL, R. and BAYJ, W. (1974). Human cancer and animal viral oncology. *Cancer*, **34**, 1406.

TAYLOR, D., DAY, S., TIEDMANN, K., CHESSELS, J., MARSHALL, W. C. and CONSTABLE, I. J. (1981). Chorioretinal biopsy in a patient with leukaemia. *Brit. J. Ophthal.*, **65**, 489.

UTERMOHLEN, V. and ZABRISKIE, J. B. (1973). A suppression of cellular immunity in patients with multiple sclerosis. *J. Exper. Med.*, **138**, 1591.

ZIMMERMAN, L. E. (1970). Changing concepts concerning the pathogenesis of infectious diseases. *Amer. J. Ophthal.*, **69**, 947.

Index

Index